Dr E B Garrood

D1125875

An Introduction to

Clinical Anatomy by Dissection of the Human Body

R. D. LAURENSON, M.D.

Professor of Anatomy
University of Alberta
Faculty of Medicine
Edmonton, Alberta, Canada

Illustrations by
Mrs. D. M. Hutchinson, Medical Illustrator

W. B. SAUNDERS COMPANY
Philadelphia   London   Toronto

W. B. Saunders Company;   West Washington Square
                           Philadelphia, Pa. 19105

                           12 Dyott Street
                           London, WC1A   1DB

                           833 Oxford Street
                           Toronto 18, Ontario

An Introduction to Clinical Anatomy by Dissection of the Human Body
                                                ISBN 0-7216-5650-1

Print No.:   9   8   7   6   5   4   3   2

TO

PROFESSOR R. D. LOCKHART

with whom it all began

Preface

The purpose of this book is to make certain that medical students spend their time in the gross anatomy laboratory to their best advantage, not just going through the motions of dissection, but learning the facts their clinical instructors use and expect students to know. This book, therefore, is clinically oriented. Very definitely so. All the clinical material included in the book has been verified by clinicians who are active in clinical practice and interested in teaching. The candid textual criticism of the clinicians who took part in reading the manuscript was indispensable. Their contribution is acknowledged on p. vii. The contribution of clinicians who gave additional help is acknowledged later in this preface.

A second purpose of this book is to reduce the amount of homework a student of gross anatomy seems to be required to do. His studies in the laboratory, therefore, must be meaningful and relevant; he must learn, as he goes along, the very words and phrases his clinical tutors utter daily in hospital. Thus, if the student trains himself to learn by participation in the laboratory, by seeing and by doing, he can accumulate most of his fundamental knowledge of anatomy during laboratory hours. By doing so he avoids the hours of tedious reading called for when laboratory work and text are apart.

This text is the outcome of many progressive changes—call it streamlining, if you will—introduced by me into the laboratory courses in gross anatomy I have taught for 12 years now. The time had come, as I expected it would, when no present dissecting manual could fulfill my requirements. A text had to be written. Because the changes made have always been received with such favorable comment, I publish the text, confident that it will be of service to other medical schools and sure that it will make the students' gross anatomy studies more attractive, more efficient, and more to the point. My initial efforts to revise the dissection of the human body, encouraged by Professor R. D. Lockhart and Dr. J. V. Basmajian, gathered force in recent years in this department, headed by Dr. T. S. Leeson. Without his encouragement when the final radical changes were mooted, I would not have had sufficient experience to write this book. I am indebted to the editor of the Anatomical Record for permission to use techniques I have already published: A Rapid Exposure of the Facial Nerve, Anatomical Record, v. *150*, pages 317-318, 1964; A Rapid Method of Dissecting the Middle Ear, Anatomical Record, v. *151*, pages 503-506, 1965; Dissection of

v

the Orbit, Anatomical Record, v. *152*, pages 537-540, 1965; A Method of Removing the Brain, Anatomical Record, v. *156*, pages 229-234, 1966.

Several colleagues made special contributions. I owe special thanks to Dr. R. J. Bury for his personal interest in the preparation of the method of dissection and of the text on the inguinal canal; in a quiet, helpful manner he brought forth his clinical experience in this contentious area. My thanks to Dr. B. J. Greenhill is acknowledged by declaring him coauthor of the sections on the limbs; he spent many hours in the laboratory to help me grasp the clinical point of view; he read and reread the appropriate text. You will observe that Dr. T. R. Nelson is also a coauthor, of the section on the Female Pelvis; without the benefit of his careful teaching enriched by his extensive clinical experience, my knowledge of the anatomy here would have remained sterile.

In addition to these contributions, it became very obvious when the first few illustrations were delivered that Mrs. D. M. Hutchinson would make a substantial contribution to the success of the book. It is indeed a pleasure to have Mrs. Hutchinson's talents acknowledged on the title page.

Colleagues in the department were my guides as I searched for a word, a meaning, an interpretation. Dr. F. B. Cookson, Dr. E. O. Hagen, Dr. K. D. McFadden, Dr. H. Ross, and Professor W. R. Salt were always ready to rescue me in my moments of despair.

Once the manuscript had been read by my clinical colleagues and had been reviewed by me, most of it was read by three students: Mr. George Marien read the Head and Neck and the Limbs; Mr. Lawrence Jewell, the Abdomen; Mr. Ralph Edwards, the Thorax. Their helpful criticism brought us still nearer to perfection. Above all, it was most reassuring to know the text was easy to read.

Finally, I acknowledge the sustaining interest of succeeding classes of medical students, whose patience and enthusiasm allowed me to "try something else." Medical students are deeply interested in perfection and progress, and they soon lose interest in old-fashioned methods. To them, for making the age-old dissection of the human body come alive, I am forever grateful.

R. D. Laurenson

Acknowledgments

In reading the manuscript, these clinicians gave unreservedly of their knowledge and practical experience that this book might achieve its purpose.

T. A. S. Boyd — Associate Professor of Ophthalmology, Faculty of Medicine, University of Alberta.

C. M. Couves — Associate Professor of Surgery, Faculty of Medicine, University of Alberta.

J. A. L. Gilbert — Professor of Clinical Medicine, Faculty of Medicine, University of Alberta.

J. M. Hagen — Instructor in Anaesthesia, Faculty of Medicine, University of Alberta.

R. C. Harrison — Professor of Surgery, Faculty of Medicine, University of British Columbia.

S. Kling — Assistant Clinical Professor of Surgery, Faculty of Medicine, University of Alberta.

W. H. Lakey — Associate Professor of Surgery, Faculty of Medicine, University of Alberta.

W. C. MacKenzie — Dean, Faculty of Medicine, University of Alberta.

I. MacDonald — Clinical Professor of Surgery, School of Medicine, University of Southern California.

G. K. Morton — Clinical Professor in Surgery, Faculty of Medicine, University of Alberta.

H. T. G. Williams — Assistant Clinical Professor in Surgery, Faculty of Medicine, University of Alberta.

How To Use This Book

The order of dissection: thorax, abdomen, pelvis, lower limb, head and neck, and upper limb, need not be adhered to but it should be known that the order is the outcome of experience and experiment. Various methods have been tried to solve the difficulties of moving an intact, and usually heavy, corpse to reach easily all aspects of the upper and lower limbs. It was found that once the torso had been dissected, the vertebral column could be sectioned and the pelvis divided to free the lower limbs; likewise for the upper limbs.

Students dissecting the cadaver in this way have had no difficulty. Indeed, they have found it much easier and more stimulating because the parts are easier to handle. Clinicians assisting in the gross anatomy course considered the order of dissection to make good sense because to a large extent it followed systemic pathways.

At the urgent request of many students, steps in dissection have been separated from descriptive text and given item numbers; descriptive text applicable to the part just dissected is indicated by a heading in large type.

Certain sections are introductory and should definitely be read and digested before proceeding with the dissection. They are designed to be studied at home.

Wherever necessary in order to bring together a series of items or facts, summaries have been included. It is recommended that the student himself summarize the remainder of the text. In this way he will consolidate what he has learned from the introductory passages, the dissection, the descriptive passages, and from other aspects of the teaching program.

As the great John Hunter once said:

> *"A man can never know how much he knows till he*
> *arranges his knowledge, and then he can tell*
> *how defective it is . . . ."*

Contents

Part 7   THE UPPER LIMB: The Organ of Manual Activity
          by R. D. Laurenson and B. J. Greenhill

PART 1

INTRODUCTION

Chapter 1

Skin

The student of gross anatomy is encouraged to remove skin rapidly and not to waste time looking for cutaneous nerves. As he flays the body, however, he should remember a silly yet profound remark that "skin lies between the doctor and his patient," and that skin is one of the first structures inspected by a doctor in his quest for a diagnosis. The doctor knows well that the diagnosis may often be revealed or at least suggested, by changes in the skin. Therefore time spent on a study of the gross anatomy of skin and its derivatives is time well spent, even though the microscope provides a much better opportunity to study this tissue in detail. Clinically, the color of the skin is very important.

Basic Gross Anatomy

Two layers can be identified in skin, more easily in the living than in the dead. The epidermis is the white, nonvascular layer, some of which peels off after a sunburn. Deep to the epidermis is the dermis, a felt of connective tissue containing neurovascular structures, lymphatics, and a considerable amount of elastic fibers. Deep to the dermis is the superficial fascia, often loaded with fat. The epidermis is locked to the dermis; the dermis is bound by interlacing fibers to the superficial fascia (Fig. 1-1). As a result of these interconnections, all three layers are held when the skin is pinched. Furthermore, when skin is removed from a cadaver, the plane of separation is most likely to be in the superficial fascia.

In general, skin contains hair follicles, sebaceous glands, and sweat glands. Hair follicles and sweat glands lie deep to the dermis, actually in the superficial fascia; sebaceous glands lie in the dermis; nails are part of the epidermis. These structures, hairs, glands, and nails, are by some authors (Leeson and Leeson, 1966) termed derivatives in keeping with their embryology, but they are often spoken of as appendages. In addition the dermis contains arteries, veins, nerves, and lymphatics.

1

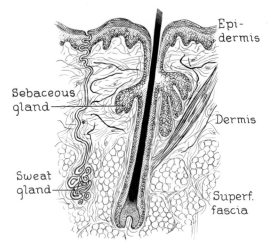

Figure 1-1. Diagram to show the two layers of skin and its appendages and their relationship to the superficial fascia.

Throughout his dissection the student should observe how skin varies from region to region, from the coarse, very thick variety on the back of the neck to the thin, freely movable variety on the anterior aspect of the forearm. He should also note the distribution of body hair and recall from his personal experience the areas of the body where sweat glands and sebaceous glands are particularly numerous.

Conservation of Body Fluid

This is a most important function of skin. If more than 20 per cent of the 2 square meters of skin covering the body (Table 1-1) is destroyed, as much as 500 ml. of plasma per hour can ooze from the surface denuded of skin. If this happens, obviously the individual will die unless the denuded area is effectively covered, and the lost plasma replaced.

Table 1-1. *Surface Area of Body Regions*

REGION	% SURFACE AREA
Head and neck	9
Right upper limb	9
Left upper limb	9
Front of trunk	18
Back and buttocks	18
Right lower limb	18
Left lower limb	18
Perineum	1
	100% total body surface

Body Temperature

Another important function of skin is the regulation of the temperature of the body. This function is under the control of the hypothalamus, linked to the blood vessels of the skin through the autonomic nervous system (see p. 338). In the skin the small blood vessels are maintained in a semicontracted state (Fig. 1-2) by vasoconstrictor fibers of the sympathetic part of the autonomic nervous system.

When the blood vessels are constricted further the skin is pale and cold, and when the vessels are dilated the skin is red and warm. Sweating, too, is under the control of the sympathetic nervous system, and when sympathetic fibers are cut the area affected becomes red, warm, and dry. Thus the hypothalamus regulates body temperature by its indirect control of both the caliber of skin vessels and the amount of sweat.

Importance of the Cutaneous Vessels

The following clinical facts may help to vivify the student's concept of the skin he will soon remove with abandon from the entire cadaver.

The arterial blood supply of skin is vital for its survival, and the quality of skin depends essentially on its metabolism, which in turn is dependent upon a sufficiency of blood. If skin is slowly deprived of arterial blood its character will change. It must be made clear, however, that aging occurs in skin and its derivatives and that there is a debate concerning the prime factors responsible for the changes seen with age. However, disease of blood vessels, with narrowing of their lumen, is sufficiently common in elderly people that most cadavers show some evidence of changes in skin associated with vascular disease. Some of the following changes may be seen on gross inspection. The surface is smooth and glossy and the skin is thinner than usual, hairs have disappeared, and the nails are thicker than usual; in life the skin would

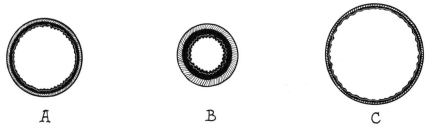

A B C

Figure 1-2. Diagram to explain what is meant by vasoconstriction and vasodilation. A is the control, showing moderate vasoconstrictor activity. B shows vasoconstriction, increased vasoconstrictor activity; the skin would be pale and cold. C shows vasodilation, decreased vasoconstrictor activity; the skin would be red and warm.

have been less elastic and sweat and sebaceous glands might have ceased to function; the skin would have felt cool. Such atrophic changes are most often seen on the skin of the toes and dorsum of the foot. Therefore, when you dissect the foot of the cadaver, take time to study the condition of the skin. Compare your findings with the appearance of your own skin, on the back of the hand for example.

Lymph Drainage from Skin

Lymph, which is a colorless fluid from the tissue spaces of the body, is collected from skin into microscopic lymph vessels draining into macroscopic superficial lymph nodes (Fig. 1-3). Ultimately, all lymph flows into the venous system. Although the lymphatic system branches throughout the body, it can never be satisfactorily demonstrated in the cadaver. Nevertheless, the student must appreciate the presence of the lymphatic system, for its functions are very significant in the spread and treatment of disease.

Cutaneous Nerves

Little attention is paid to cutaneous nerves in the removal of skin from an embalmed cadaver, for accurate dissection of those nerves involves hours of tedious and patient toil that are not now available to the undergraduate. Nevertheless, sensory innervation of the skin is important because the loss of sensation in part of the skin, spoken of clinically as an area of sensory loss, is a highly significant finding in the examination of the nervous system. Fortunately, the areas of sensory innervation are beautifully illustrated in most textbooks, to which the student should refer as his experience grows, for he can expect to have the sensory innervation of the body discussed in some detail in other parts of his teaching program.

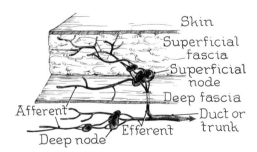

Figure 1-3. The relationship of the lymphatic system to the deep fascia. See also text on p. 8.

Referred Pain

No account of skin, however brief, is complete without reference to the problem of referred pain. Referred pain is a problem because there is a great deal to be learned about the anatomy and neurophysiology of the pathways of pain and because, clinically, the origin of a pain may be extraordinarily difficult to locate. For example, in gallbladder disease, pain is commonly experienced in the skin over the right shoulder. The explanation of referred pain is beyond the scope of this text; it is sufficient to realize that the cause of a pain may be remote from the area of skin where the pain is felt.

In conclusion, additional facts about skin will be brought to the dissector's attention as he proceeds, but while he removes the skin from each region, this much he should recall:
1. Basic gross anatomy of skin and its normal color
2. Conservation of body fluid
3. Regulation of body temperature
4. The importance of cutaneous arteries
5. Lymph drainage
6. Sensory innervation
7. The problem of referred pain

Chapter 2

Fascia

There are three forms of fascia, superficial fascia, deep fascia, and areolar tissue; the third one is also called fascia in anatomy texts. Superficial fascia was mentioned briefly as a layer deep to the dermis (p. 1). The deep fascia lies deeper still, adjacent to the musculature. These two fasciae are spread more or less over the entire surface of the body. Apart from their regional differences, however, they differ from each other in two obvious ways, namely fat content and disposition. The superficial fascia is easily recognized by the presence of fat, which is often abundant. Further, over a large extent of the body it is a distinct layer that, along with skin, can be stripped quite easily off the deep fascia (Fig. 2-1). In contrast, the deep fascia is recognized by the absence of fat, which causes its light gray color, its membranous form, and its strength, especially in each limb, where it occurs as a distinct tubular investment. Deep fascia cannot be stripped extensively because of its

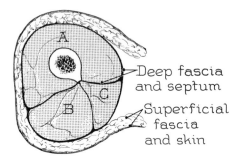

Deep fascia
and septum

Superficial
fascia
and skin

Figure 2-1. Superficial fascia and skin can be stripped off the deep fascia. Deep fascia is attached to the skeleton mainly by septa. (A, B, and C refer, respectively, to the extensor, flexor, and adductor compartments.)

attachments to bone by way of partitions known as septa, passing from its deep surface to gain attachment for example, to the length of the shaft of a long bone (Fig. 2-1); deep fascia is also attached to the extremities·of long bones in the vicinity of joints.

Areolar Tissue

What has just been said concerning superficial and deep fascia refers essentially to the surface of the body. As the student proceeds to dissect more deeply he will meet further and sometimes quite extensive sheets of areolar tissue investing structures and organs and commonly labeled fascia in atlases and textbooks. Such internal layers are named according to their site or according to the organ or structure they lie upon or invest. They are usually less robust and more translucent than the definitive deep fascia and may or may not have high fat content. Thus it may be said that by their very texture, internal layers of fascia are more deserving of the name areolar tissue. Be that as it may, the term fascia is so widely accepted and so readily used that the student can expect to find the term applied to supporting tissue anywhere within the body.

Fat

Cadaveric material gives quite the wrong impression of the true nature of superficial fascia. In life, fat is soft, not hard, and liquid, not solid; in respectable amounts it is responsible for the pleasing shape of the female form. Liquid fat occurs in microscopic amounts within the cytoplasm of each fat cell; obviously there must be a very great number of fat cells present when fat is visible. Thus the superficial fascia is a reservoir of fat with a blood supply adjusted to the metabolism of either the use or storage of fat. In abnormal conditions, however, vast amounts of fat accumulate in the superficial fascia, making the individual not just overweight, but obese. Furthermore, when there is a heavy layer of fat on the outside of the body much fat will be present inside, not only surrounding vital organs but even infiltrating their very substance. "Obesity is the most common nutritional disorder at the present time in America, Great Britain and most European countries and gives rise to more ill health than all the vitamin deficiencies put together."*

Deep Fascia in the Living

The student must not consider the deep fascia a functionless entity because he finds in the cadaver that the fascia is wrinkled and slack. Such findings are due to the shrinkage of underlying muscles, which, possibly, is due to the embalming, and certainly to the dehydration during dissection. In life the deep fascia is smooth with a degree of tension as it fits snugly over the contours of the underlying musculature. The fascial attachments to bone create fibroosseous compartments (A, B, C, Fig. 2-1) in which changes in pressure occur during muscle action. Pressure changes are of significance in assisting the return of venous blood from the limbs, especially from the lower limbs (Fig. 46-3). Furthermore, the nature of deep fascia and bone does not allow much adjustment to the increase in pressure that can occur in hemorrhage and edema. Therefore, in some instances it may be necessary to slit the deep fascia in order to restore the compartmental pressure to normal.

To conclude this account of fascia the student is offered some advice. Fascia is described at length and in detail in all standard texts. It is, however, quite unnecessary for the student to read extensive accounts of fascia, for as his experience grows, not just in the gross anatomy laboratory, but in his clinical work too, he will gain a knowledge of fascia sufficient for all practical purposes. The synopsis of fascia presented in this book is sufficient for a beginner.

Superficial Neurovascular Structures and the Deep Fascia

From the point of view of terminology, as applied particularly to veins and lymphatics, a further consideration of deep fascia is essential. The terms deep and superficial, when applied to veins and lymphatics, are used with reference to the deep fascia. It follows that superficial veins are superficial, i.e., external to the deep fascia, while deep veins are deep (internal) to it (Fig. 2-2). Eventually, superficial veins pierce the deep fascia to join deep veins streaming toward the heart. The

---

*Davidson, L. S. P.: The Principles and Practice of Medicine. 8th Ed. Edinburgh, E. & S. Livingstone Ltd., 1966.

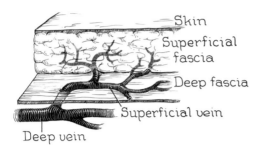

Figure 2-2. The relationship of veins to the deep fascia. See also Figure 1-3.

superficial veins of the limbs and neck are easily identified in life, particularly when they are distended; in the cadaver they are found close to the external surface of the deep fascia, at some depth from the skin surface if much superficial fat is present. The spots where superficial veins pierce deep fascia are easily found.

The superficial veins provide an extensive network, or anastomosis, or collateral circulation, that can shunt blood from one part of the circulation to another part. For example, the superior vena cava drains most of its blood from the upper half of the body while the inferior vena cava drains the lower part. When one or other of these veins is obstructed, blood may still reach the heart by alternative routes, including the superficial veins of the thoracic and abdominal wall.*

Lymphatics

Lymphatics are also classified as superficial and deep in relation to deep fascia (Fig. 1-3). Superficial lymphatic vessels eventually pierce deep fascia to join deep lymphatic vessels to form ducts or trunks emptying into the deep venous system.

Then, because all major arteries and nerve trunks lie beneath the deep fascia, it follows that arteries (with their corresponding veins) and nerves of the skin must pierce the deep fascia. Thus, as skin and superficial fascia are removed, many delicate neurovascular structures piercing deep fascia and crossing through the superficial fascia to reach skin will break. Most cutaneous nerves—and do *not* waste time searching for them—can be identified at the spots where they pierce deep fascia, and illustrations of these are to be found in any major anatomy text.

---

*Lockhart, R. D., Hamilton, G. F., and Fyfe, F. W.: Anatomy of the Human Body. London, Faber & Faber Ltd., 1959, Figure 877, p. 581.

Part 2

THORAX

Chapter 3

Introduction to the Thorax

The contents of the thorax are:
- Right and left pleural cavities
- Trachea, bronchi, and lungs
- Pericardium
- Heart, major arteries, and veins
- Esophagus
- Thoracic and mediastinal ducts
    - Lymph nodes
- Nerves (right and left)
    - Phrenic
    - Vagus
    - Recurrent laryngeal
    - Intercostal
    - Sympathetic trunk and thoracic splanchnic
- Thymus

It is possible to reach any of these structures by appropriate incisions through the chest wall.

The chest wall coverings are:
- Skin
- Subcutaneous tissue, which, in the female, contains the mammary glands
- Muscles of the upper limbs, many of which are attached to the scapulae

The chest wall itself consists of:
- Rib cage (sternum and vertebral column)
- Intercostal muscles
- Parietal pleura. This layer is not normally looked upon as part of the chest wall. Nevertheless, it adheres to the internal aspect of the wall and is an important layer in a surgical approach to the thoracic contents.

Inferiorly there is no wall as such. Instead, the thorax is separated from the abdomen by the diaphragm.

Superiorly, structures of the neck and upper limb enter or leave the thorax through the thoracic inlet. This inlet will be reviewed thoroughly when the root of the neck is dissected. Meanwhile, as an introduction, note the oblique plane of the inlet and its boundaries, namely the body of the first thoracic vertebra, the first ribs and their costal cartilages, and the manubrium sterni. The clavicles and scapulae are *not* boundaries of the thoracic inlet, although in a surgical approach to the inlet they have to be taken into account.

ITEM 3-1. Bony Landmarks (To be identified on a skeleton.) Beginning posteriorly with the thoracic vertebral column, identify:

The spinous processes of the thoracic vertebrae

The articulation of a rib, first with bodies of the column and then with a transverse process

The angle of the rib

The junction of the rib and costal cartilage, termed a costochondral junction

The costal groove on the inferior and internal aspect of the rib.

The sternum:

The suprasternal notch and the adjacent sternoclavicular articulations

The sternal angle (Fig. 6-2)

The xiphisternal junction

Surgical Approaches to Thoracic Contents

Unfortunately the rigidity of embalmed tissue prevents us from adapting surgical procedures in our anatomic dissection of the chest wall as we will do in the dissection of the anterior abdominal wall. Nevertheless, because of the keen interest of students, brief accounts of certain methods of opening the chest at operation are given here. There are two main routes; the interior can be reached laterally through the rib cage or through the midline by splitting the sternum.

When a lateral route is used the patient is placed on his side and the position of the upper limb is adjusted to get maximal exposure of the posterolateral chest wall (Fig. 3-1). The surgeon must take three layers into consideration, the skin and mammary glands, the muscles of the shoulder joint and scapula, and the rib cage and intercostal muscles. Once the rib cage is reached there are several procedures to choose from. It may be sufficient to remove a few inches of rib. On the other hand, to reach deep structures posterior to the heart almost the entire length of one or more ribs may have to be removed and the ribs above and below spread widely apart by an instrument called a rib spreader. On occasion it may be possible to gain access to the depths of the thorax not by cutting out a rib, but simply by cutting the intercostal musculature between two adjacent ribs and spreading those ribs

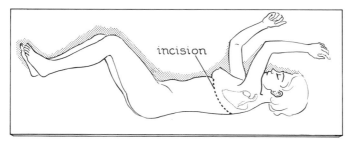

Figure 3-1. Typical position of a patient for thoracotomy. For further detail see text.

widely with the spreader. In the process the parietal pleura is incised, and, as a result, wide exposure of the pleural cavity is achieved. The level at which a surgeon makes his entry depends on the location of the structure he seeks.

The method of removing ribs may surprise you. The periosteum upon the external surface of a rib is slit lengthways, then entirely released from the rib over the required distance, but not cut. The actual bony rib is then cut in two places and the portion in between removed; the intact strip of periosteum left behind is slack enough to be displaced from the operating field. In time, bone regenerates from the periosteum and the rib is restored, but never quite to its original form. You will soon realize the extent of the difference between the strength of living and embalmed periosteum.

Splitting the sternum, either in a vertical plane or on a horizontal plane, is another route into the thorax. Spreading the parts of the chest wall widely with instruments permits extensive exposure of the heart and major blood vessels.

ITEM 3-2. Opening the Thorax of a Cadaver

To explore the thorax adequately in a cadaver, it is essential to remove the entire anterior thoracic wall, which extends from one midaxillary line to another and from the level of the first costal cartilages superiorly to the costal margins inferiorly. Before this can be done, however, it is necessary to reflect the skin, mammary glands, and pectoralis major and minor muscles. Therefore, begin by making a vertical skin incision from the suprasternal notch to the xiphisternal junction.

Then, on each side: (A) Make a skin incision parallel to the clavicle, but do not cut deeply. Identify the fibers of the pectoralis major and remain superficial to them. (B) Make a third incision parallel to the costal margin. Do not cut into the external oblique muscle. (C) Reflect the skin flap you have now created as far as the midaxillary line. (D) If you are unsure about this next and final cut to release the skin flap, ask for guidance. Make a final skin incision parallel to the anterior margin of deltoid and a short one across the axilla to release the skin flap entirely. In doing so, do not cut deeply into the region of the axilla. The pectoralis major is now fully exposed and the pectoralis minor can be seen protruding from the lateral margin of the major muscle. Retain the female mammary glands for study as described in Chapter 4.

Reflection of the Pectoralis Major. This muscle will be studied more fully in the section on the upper limb. But now is the time to observe its wide origin from the clavicle, the sternum, and the sixth and seventh costal cartilages. Superolaterally, the clavicular portion is separated from the deltoid by the deltopectoral groove, in which lies the cephalic vein.

ITEM 3-3. Identify the groove. Then incise the clavicular attachment of pectoralis major. The clavicle is narrow, so make sure the blade of the knife does not slip beyond the bone. Then, in a similar fashion, cut the sternal attachment, and finally, the costal attachments. It should now be possible to fold the pectoralis major back, off the chest wall, and thus expose pectoralis minor and subclavius.

Reflection of the Pectoralis Minor. The pectoralis minor, arising from ribs 3, 4, and 5, is inserted into the coracoid process. Deep to it lie the neurovascular structures connected to the upper limb. Between the upper border of the pectoralis minor and the subclavius extends the clavipectoral fascia, which need not be unduly disturbed at this stage of dissection.

ITEM 3-4. Cut the origin of the pectoralis minor and turn back the muscle toward the coracoid. Keep both pectoral muscles clear of the anterior chest wall with strings or clips. You are now in a position to remove a breast plate and expose thoracic contents. Chapter 5 is an essential preliminary to this exposure.

Chapter 4

The Breasts

Cancer of the female breast is common. Early diagnosis and treatment are vital. With these grave facts in mind, read an account of the surgical anatomy of the breasts, and, in doing so, take heed of the facts under these headings: hormones, elementary histology, topographical anatomy, lymph drainage, and accessory breasts.

Hormones

Throughout life the breasts, as part of the reproductive system, are influenced by hormones. At birth, the breasts of both male and female infants may, for a short time, secrete milk; maternal hormones crossing the placental barrier are responsible. At puberty the female breasts grow, with an increase of connective tissue and fat, and some increase in glandular elements. But it is not until the first pregnancy that the microscopic glandular elements responsible for the production of milk really develop. They are maintained during lactation, after which they return to their previous state. Then, at the menopause the microscopic glandular elements are largely replaced by fat and fibrous tissue. Hormones, therefore, have a far-reaching influence upon the anatomy of the breasts.

Elementary Histology

For descriptive purposes the breast may be considered in three parts, namely the nipple, glandular elements, also known as parenchyma, and supporting tissue, also known as stroma, each of which has a characteristic histologic appearance.

The Nipple

The nipple contains smooth muscle fibers, supports the terminations of the lactiferous ducts, and has a rich sensory nerve supply. It is surrounded by a circular zone of pigmented skin, the areola, which becomes darker during the first pregnancy and remains so thereafter. Sweat and sebaceous glands are found in the areola, and, in addition, areolar glands occur as minute but visible eminences upon the areola.

Glandular Tissue

Microscopic. The smallest units are, first, the alveoli, saclike dilatations whose degree of development and dilatation depend on their level of secretory activity, and second, ducts, leading from the alveoli.

In a nonpregnant, nonlactating gland (Fig. 4-1) glandular elements are inconspicuous; the characteristic appearance on microscopic examination is a preponderance of fibrous tissue and fat; ducts are much more conspicuous than alveoli.

Macroscopic. During lactation (Fig. 4-1) many alveoli together form one lobule. From each lobule a duct drains toward the parent lactiferous duct.

Many lobules make up one lobe, of which there are 15 to 20. Each lobe is drained by a lactiferous duct, so there are 15 to 20 ducts. A dilation of each duct proximal to the nipple is known as the lactiferous sinus.

The terminal orifice of each lactiferous duct upon the surface of the nipple may be seen, especially under magnification.

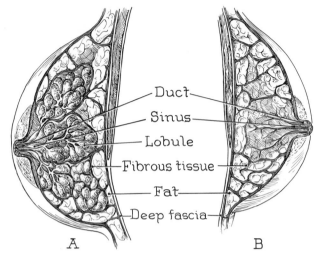

Figure 4-1.   *A.* Lactating mammary gland. *B.* Nonlactating mammary gland. See text.

The arrangement of lobes, each with its own duct, provides a segmental form to the breast tissue, which is of real importance in the diagnosis and management of discharges of a pathological nature from the "nipple," i.e., from the terminal orifice of one or more of the lactiferous ducts.

The Stroma

When all glandular elements and fat are removed the stroma, or supporting tissue of the breast, has the characteristic appearance of a coarse sponge. Bands of fibrous tissue connecting the superficial surface of the supporting stroma to the skin are known as the suspensory ligaments (ligaments of Cooper). They are notable only because a late sign of breast cancer may be an irregular dimpling of the overlying skin due to pathologic retraction of the ligaments of Cooper.

ITEM 4-1.   Read an account of the histology of the breasts (Leeson and Leeson, 1966).

Topographic Anatomy

The breasts are subcutaneous structures located in the superficial fascia. Posteriorly between the deep surface of the superficial fascia and the superficial surface of the deep fascia on pectoralis major is the retromammary space.

The extent of the glandular tissue is greater than one appreciates on viewing the female form. The tissue extends from the second to the sixth rib and from the sternum to the midaxillary line. Therefore, it is related on its deep aspect to the pectoralis major, serratus anterior, and external oblique muscles. It is estimated that two-thirds of the gland rest on pectoralis major. For descriptive purposes it is divided into quadrants. An extension of the supralateral quadrant into the axilla is termed the axillary tail.

Surgical experience dictates that the extent of mammary tissue is variable, most commonly in the degree of extension of the axillary tail and in the lateral extent of the peripheral mammary gland. Nevertheless, surgical removal of the entire breast is always an extensive surgical procedure.

The Lymph Drainage of the Breast

All aspects of the anatomy of the breast are important, but none is more important than its lymphatic drainage. The lymphatic drainage is widespread. Therefore, examination of the lymphatic fields of the breast is as important as examination of the breast itself in the diagnosis and prognosis of breast cancer.

Laterally, a very high percentage of lymph vessels from the breast drain to the ipsilateral axillary nodes. Medially, some lymph vessels drain into lymph nodes around the internal mammary artery on the deep aspect of the chest wall at the level of the second, third, and fourth intercostal spaces. Although there are not many lymph nodes located around the internal mammary artery they are nevertheless extremely important in the prognosis and treatment of cancer of the breast.

That cancer of one breast may spread to the other is presumptive evidence that there is no clear-cut division, no watershed, so to speak, of the lymphatic drainage of the anterior chest wall. Furthermore, involvement of the lymph nodes of the contralateral axilla is also known to occur. Inferiorly, some lymph drains into the lymph vessels of the anterior abdominal wall; this observation is also based on presumptive evidence from experience with the spread of breast cancer into the peritoneal cavity, the pelvis, and the liver. Superiorly, cancer cells may spread to the supraclavicular nodes, but it is not clear whether this spread is direct or indirect, via the axilla, the supraclavicular nodes being, in fact, an upward extension of the main collection of axillary nodes. With these facts in mind, it is obvious that a patient found to have breast cancer must have a complete physical examination.

Accessory Breasts

One or more small rudimentary breasts may be present somewhere along the milk line between each axilla and the groin. Apart from being an embarrassment to the individual, they too may become cancerous.

Read an account of the embryology of the breast.

DISSECTION OF THE FEMALE MAMMARY GLANDS

ITEM 4-2. Lay the deep surface of the gland on a flat surface and with a long knife (a brain knife) make an incision through the nipple, gland, and axillary tail (see *Grant's Atlas of Anatomy,* Fig. 12-1).

On one half of the gland, deep to the areola and nipple, clear away sufficient fat to expose a lactiferous duct and sinus. Usually on a cut surface of this nature one or two lactiferous ducts are exposed. Remove fat and fascia to expose one of these ducts clearly. This procedure usually exposes the dilated part of the duct, namely the lactiferous sinus. Each lactiferous duct is responsible for the drainage of one lobe, which consists of many lobules.

ITEM 4-3. Observe the stroma. You cannot fail to note the amount of fat you must remove in order to expose the stroma.

ITEM 4-4. By blunt dissection over a limited area, separate the overlying skin from stroma and identify the suspensory ligaments (ligaments of Cooper).

The brevity of this dissection is no measure of the significance of the tissues you have exposed. Brief though this dissection has been, at least it is an introduction to tissues you study in full in histology and again in pathology, and about which you will eventually make serious decisions in clinical practice.

Chapter 5

The Basic Principles of the Pleural Cavities

Each lung is almost entirely surrounded by a pleural cavity. In Figure 5-1*A* the lung is represented by a fingertip and the pleura by a balloon. In Figure 5-1*B* the fingertip has been replaced by a section of lung and the balloon by the pleura. The arrow indicates the site where structures enter or leave the lung. Those structures are known collectively as the root of the lung, and the cleft where they enter the lung is the hilus.

The one layer of pleura immediately adjacent to the lung surface is termed visceral pleura while the outermost layer, which lines all the surrounding surfaces that confine the lung, is termed parietal pleura. In Figure 5-1*B* the single asterisk indicates the true state of affairs rarely illustrated in medical texts. Thus, in life, the pleural cavity is a *potential* cavity. It becomes an actual cavity when it is occupied by fluid or air (Fig.

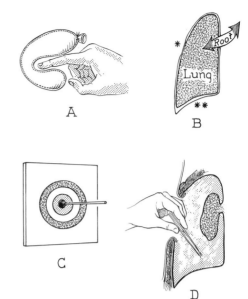

Figure 5-1. The pleural cavity, C and D illustrate a clinical principle explained in the text below. The explanation is too simple according to modern biophysical research on the pleural cavity.

5-1B double asterisk). No doubt, in the cadaver the lung is partially collapsed, transforming the potential cavity into an actual one.

In life, the parietal pleura is held to, but not fixed to, the visceral pleura by a very thin film of fluid. Observe in Figure 5-1C that the greater the pull on the sucker the more negative the pressure between the sucker and the board. In other words, the pull leads to an increase in negative pressure. Now, if the sucker is moist and the board smooth or shiny, you can demonstrate how easy it is to slide the sucker from one location to another. Imagine, then, that the sucker is the chest wall and the board a lung with the potential pleural cavity between them occupied by a thin film of moisture and possessing a negative pressure. When the chest wall moves out during inspiration there is an increase in negative pressure in the pleural cavity; the lung must expand and air must enter. In other words, the expansion of lung tissue is controlled by the movement of the chest wall, not by the intake of air. This is a concept you must grasp, for it is fundamental not only in the physiology of respiration but also in the application of that physiology in anesthesia and thoracic surgery.

The Continuity of the Pleural Surface

The dotted line inside the balloon in Figure 5-1A illustrates the continuity of the internal surface. Although in Figure 5-1B the lung is fully expanded and the pleural cavity reduced to a minimal capacity, the pleural surface is still continuous. To open the pleural cavity (Fig. 5-1*D*) the surgeon incises the parietal pleura; the lung tends to collapse because it is exposed to atmospheric pressure.* Note that hands or instruments in the cavity are separated from the lung and all adjacent structures by one layer of pleura (Fig. 5-1*D*). This will be the state of affairs in the pleural cavity of the cadaver where, in order to reveal subpleural structures, you will have to peel off pleura.

The Mediastinum

There are two pleural cavities. Between them there is a mass of structures, including the heart, and that mass is called the mediastinum. It will shortly be described in more detail. Meanwhile, note that the edges of the intact pleural cavities can be reflected to expose the mediastinum (Fig. 5-2). Thus it is not always necessary to open one or the other pleural cavity in order to reach mediastinal structures.

Naming the Pleura

Stress has been laid upon the continuity of the pleural surface. For descriptive purposes, however, the parietal pleura is named according to sites. For example, the parietal pleura lining the rib cage only is called costal pleura. Then there are the diaphragmatic and mediastinal pleura. Where do they lie? And finally there is the apical pleura, also known as the cervical pleura or the cupola, which protrudes through the thoracic inlet to the level of the neck of the first rib.

Pleural Recesses

At certain regions the pleural surface is sharply angled (Fig. 5-2) when seen on section. The line along which this occurs is called a line of pleural reflection, and the pleural cavity at the reflection is termed a pleural recess. Two recesses are noteworthy, the costomediastinal recess referred to previously (Fig. 5-2) and the costodiaphragmatic recess. In many ways, perhaps, the latter is more important because a minimal quantity of abnormal fluid may gravitate into its depths and remain undetected by the dull observer. You will have the opportunity to explore the depths of the recesses once you are in the pleural cavity.

---

*In surgical operations, the degree of collapse of the lung is under the control of the anesthetist.

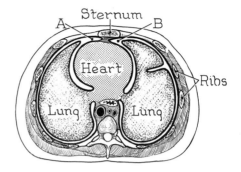

Figure 5-2. Cross section of thorax. *A* and *B* indicate the costomediastinal recesses. Both *A* and *B* may be peeled laterally to expose the pericardium surrounding the heart. See also Figure 6-3.

Hollow Organs or Structures Related to the Pleural Cavities

The significance of this relationship is thus: if a hollow organ related to the pleural cavity ruptures through the pleural surface, then inevitably the contents of that hollow organ spill or even pour into the pleural cavity. By the end of your dissection of this region you will have learned that the following hollow organs or structures are related to pleura: thoracic duct, esophagus, aortic arch and thoracic aorta, intercostal vessels, trachea, and bronchi.

The amount of chyle entering one or other pleural cavities from a ruptured thoracic duct depends on the stage of digestion; if digestion is of limited extent it may be several days before a chylothorax becomes obvious. The amount of fluid from the esophagus depends on the quantity swallowed and the amount regurgitated from the stomach. Rupture of the aorta usually causes an immediate disaster. In a less urgent but equally mortal circumstance, several pints of blood from ruptured intercostal vessels may accumulate in the pleural cavity after ribs have been fractured. Do not, therefore, underestimate the capacity of a pleural cavity.

Rupture of the trachea and lung surface may be considered together. If air enters the pleural cavity, the negative pressure essential for normal respiration is destroyed. Respiration, however, can proceed as long as the amount of air leaving the cavity is equal to the amount of air entering. Sometimes a "flap valve" forms, especially when the surface of the lung ruptures; then air accumulates in the pleural cavity (tension pneumothorax); death is inevitable if steps are not taken to reduce the tension.

The Pleural Cavities and the Mediastinum

In the cadaver the mediastinum is an immovable mass, whereas in life it possesses a considerable range of movement in all directions, but particularly from side to side. To prove this sometime, lie on your left side and observe your heartbeat; then observe it again while lying on your right side. The normal central position of the mediastinum in life depends on several factors. In the present context, one factor is the balance of pressures in the pleural cavities. If this balance is altered, as, for example, by the entry of air into one pleural cavity, mediastinal structures are shifted out of their normal position to the opposite side. They may shift to a degree sufficient to embarrass the heart's action. Therefore, after thoracic surgery steps are taken to equilibrate the pleural cavity pressures in order to center the mediastinum.

You will get the opportunity to pursue these topics more fully in your clinical years. They are introduced to you now to draw attention to the pleural cavities, empty spaces readily ignored by the eager dissector, but of great clinical importance to the competent physician.

Chapter 6

The Pleural Cavities

Removal of the Breast Plate

ITEM 6-1. On each side, identify the digitations of the serratus anterior. Using an electric autopsy saw, section the second to the sixth ribs just anterior to the tips of those digitations. Do not thrust the saw deeply. Try to cut bone only, leaving parietal pleura intact.

ITEM 6-2. Inferior to the sternoclavicular articulations, section the sternum. Just inferior to level of the sixth costal cartilages, cut across the sternum.

A breast plate is now free to be removed, and you should remove it in such a way as to preserve the costomediastinal recesses. This means you must elevate the breast plate alone, leaving parietal pleura undisturbed. It is difficult to begin this procedure, but, once begun, it is easy to peel off the breast plate, leaving behind, to some extent at least, the costomediastinal recesses as in Figure 5-2.

ITEM 6-3. In the process, each internal thoracic (mammary) artery must be severed superiorly at the level of the first intercostal space and inferiorly at the level of the sixth costal cartilage.

Intercostal Space

Examination of an intercostal space (Fig. 6-1). On each side of the chest wall there are now several sections of an intercostal space for you to examine. In clinical practice, when it is necessary to aspirate fluid from

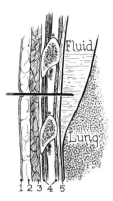

Figure 6-1. Number 5 indicates the pleural cavity. What layers are represented by numbers 1, 2, 3, and 4?* The needle has passed through those layers to enter the pleural cavity. The student will know from his specimen that all these layers are normally in contact. The spaces are shown here to make it easier for the student to distinguish the layers.

the pleural cavity a needle is passed through an intercostal space. In doing so a scrupulous technique is required, but for the time being it is the anatomy of the space that deserves your attention.

The skin, subcutaneous tissue, and overlying muscles can be ignored while you explore the intrinsic anatomy of the space. Three thin layers of muscle may be identified, namely the external, internal, and innermost intercostal muscles. Between the internal and innermost muscles, and sheltered to some extent by the subcostal groove, lie the intercostal neurovascular structures. The parietal pleura is immediately internal to the innermost intercostal muscle.

ITEM 6-4.   Observe the directions of the intercostal muscle fibers and identify the neurovascular structures.

Variation in the Anatomy of a Typical Intercostal Space. Posteriorly, between the vertebral column and the angles of the ribs, the internal intercostal muscle is replaced by a thin membrane. In the same location, the intercostal neurovascular structures have not yet reached the shelter of the subcostal groove, so they are exposed, so to speak. The site chosen for aspiration of the pleural cavity clearly depends on where the abnormal fluid is located. Commonly, however, the needle is passed through the space at a point just beyond the angles of the ribs. Then the exact location of the neurovascular structures is known.

Anteriorly the external intercostal muscle is replaced by a membrane. Anteriorly, also, the subcostal groove disappears and the intercostal space narrows, so the intercostal neurovascular structures are again without the shelter of the rib above. Finally, the innermost intercostal muscles do not form a complete sheet. They are most highly developed in the area between the angles of the ribs and the costochondral junctions. This means that a needle entering the intercostal space between the vertebral column and the angle of the rib transfixes one sheet of muscle, the external intercostal muscle; the internal intercostal muscle has been replaced by a membrane and the innermost intercostal muscle is absent.

---

*1 is the skin, 2 is fat, 3 is overlying muscle, and 4 is intercostal muscle.

ITEM 6-5.   Review the anatomy of an intercostal space with the aid of a skeleton, and, using a dissector's probe, practice passing the tip of the probe through an intercostal space of a cadaver into the pleural cavity (Fig. 6-1).

THE MEDIASTINUM

It is appropriate to consider now the various parts that the mediastinum is divided into for descriptive purposes (Fig. 6-2).

A transverse section through the mediastinum at the level of the second costal cartilages divides it into superior and inferior regions. The second costal cartilages join the sternum at the sternal angle (the angle of Louis) and lie at the level of the fourth thoracic vertebra.

There are no further divisions of the superior mediastinum, but the inferior mediastinum is divided into anterior, middle, and posterior parts, termed the anterior mediastinum, middle mediastinum, and posterior mediastinum. It must be stressed here and now that those three parts are subdivisions of the inferior mediastinum and that the superior mediastinum has no subdivisions.

The middle mediastinum is considered first because it is central to the other mediastinal regions. It contains the heart enclosed in pericardium, parts of the great vessels, and the lung roots. Observe (Fig. 6-2) that the ascending aorta, a, is intrapericardial and lies deeply in the middle mediastinum.

The anterior mediastinum is the space between the middle mediastinum and the posterior surface of the sternum. In other words, it is anterior to the pericardium, and is the space you have just exposed in removing the breast plate. The costomediastinal recesses of pleura protrude into the anterior mediastinum. In fact, the right and left pleural cavities may overlap to an extent that a strong needle thrust through the middle of the sternum would transfix both cavities and, possibly, the anterior edges of the lungs.

The Anterior Mediastinum

Thymus

The notable structure in the anterior mediastinum is the lower end of the thymus gland extending downward from the superior mediastinum. View this gland with keen interest under a microscope as well as in its gross form in a cadaver, for today it is under intensive investigation in the field of immunity. In the cadaver the remnants of the thymus gland lie mainly in the superior mediastinum and are barely distinguishable from surrounding fat. The thymus is removed at surgical operation through a midline split in the sternum.

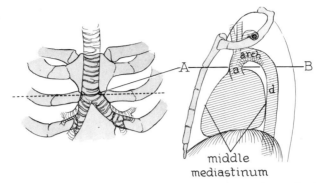

Figure 6-2. The plane *AB* divides the thorax into the superior mediastinum, above the plane *AB*, and the inferior mediastinum. The latter is subdivided into anterior, middle, and posterior parts (see text). In the cadaver the bifurcation of the trachea is found to be level with *AB*. The ascending and descending parts of the aorta are represented by the letters a and d. The position of the former alters with the heart beat.

The Posterior Mediastinum

The posterior mediastinum lies posterior to the middle mediastinum and anterior to the vertebral column, and contains the esophagus, the thoracic descending aorta and other longitudinal structures to be exposed in the course of dissection (d, Fig. 6-2).

The superior mediastinum, superior to all the other mediastinal regions, contains the esophagus, the trachea, the arch of the aorta and the roots of its branches, and major veins returning toward the heart. The trachea, subcutaneous in the root of the neck, enters the superior mediastinum directly posterior to the suprasternal notch. Palpation of the trachea in this site helps a doctor to localize the position of the entire mediastinum (Fig. 6-2).

Points to Note Concerning the Mediastinum

In life, the structures found in the mediastinum are not held rigidly in place. Accordingly, the plane of division between the superior and inferior mediastinum is not a rigid boundary, but it is useful in an initial review of the topographic anatomy of the mediastinum.

The fibrous pericardium lies entirely within the boundaries of the middle mediastinum and blends with the outer coat of the major vessels at the level of the sternal angle. The ascending aorta situated in the middle mediastinum lies entirely within fibrous pericardium. The arch of the aorta lies entirely in the superior mediastinum, and the descending thoracic aorta lies entirely in the posterior mediastinum.

ITEM 6-6. To expose the pericardium, reflect the pleurae to each side as in Figure 6-3. The pleural cavities behind the sternum overlap, so

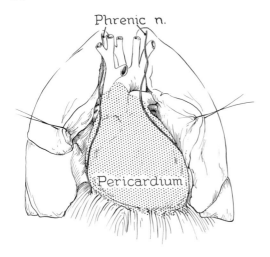

Phrenic n.

Pericardium

Figure 6-3. The costome-diastinal recesses peeled off the pericardium to expose the phrenic nerves. Each nerve is sandwiched between peri-cardium and pleura.

you will have to gently peel one cavity away from the other. To make sure you identify correctly each cavity, slip the fingers of the left hand into the right costomediastinal recess and the fingers of the right hand into the left recess. With some manipulation you should be able to peel the pleurae far enough to the right or left to expose the pericardium.

Exposure of the Pericardium

The pericardium is a loosely fitting sac enclosing the heart and the adjoining vessels. Three layers are present; the first two are inseparably fused. The layers are: (1) a solitary fibrous layer, (2) a parietal serous layer that lines the internal aspect of the fibrous layer, and (3) a visceral layer upon the surface of the heart and the adjoining vessels. On the surface of the heart this layer is frequently named the epicardium.

Continuity of parietal and visceral serous layers exists here, as well as in the pleural cavities, the peritoneal cavity, and around each testis. However, the principle of invagination that applies to these other regions does not quite apply to the heart; the development of the transverse sinus of the serous pericardium does not conform. Otherwise, the principle of invagination would be applicable.

The pericardial cavity is close to being an actual cavity in that the pericardium does not fit snugly around the heart, for an obvious reason. Be that as it may, it can enlarge to become an obvious cavity filled with fluid, which may be blood from a rupture of the heart wall. On inspection of a chest radiograph revealing enlargement of the cardiac shadow, it is necessary to decide if the enlargement is due to an increase in cardiac muscle, to an increase in the size of the heart chambers, or to an accumulation of fluid in the pericardial sac.

The pericardium is not essential for survival and is often removed when it is diseased.

ITEM 6-7. Opening the Pericardium

Upon the anterior surface of the heart towards the diaphragm make a horizontal incision between the left and right phrenic nerves and vessels (Fig. 6-4). At each end of this incision make a vertical incision superiorly, to the limit of the pericardium. These incisions create a flap of pericardium that you can turn back.

ITEM 6-8. Observe the external coarse solitary layer of fibrous pericardium and the two smooth shiny layers of serous pericardium. One layer of serous pericardium is adherent to the surface of the heart and the other to the internal surface of the fibrous pericardium.

ITEM 6-9. Attachment of Fibrous Pericardium to the Great Vessels

Slide a finger superiorly posterior to the flap you have just created. Push gently superiorly while you pull the flap anteroinferiorly and you will demonstrate the blending of the fibrous pericardium with the three main vessels superior to the heart.

ITEM 6-10. Reflection of Serous Pericardium

Turn the flap as far back as you can to see how serous pericardium from the posterior surface of the flap merges without any interruption with the serous pericardium upon the vessels and the heart itself. Be sure of this point — it is quite simple — before you cut and remove the flap.

ITEM 6-11. Attachment of Pericardium to the Diaphragm

The firm attachment of the pericardium to the central tendon of the diaphragm is of significance in the physiology of the thorax. Confirm that they are attached to each other.

ITEM 6-12. Further Exploration of the Pericardial Cavity

Slip a hand under the apex of the heart. Lift the heart superiorly and anteriorly. In doing so you will demonstrate that the heart has considerable mobility, even in a cadaver. In the process you can identify

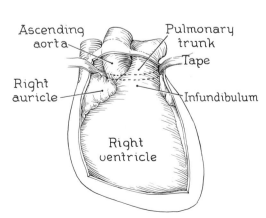

Figure 6-4. The pericardium is opened. A tape passes through the transverse sinus.

the intrapericardial part of the inferior vena cava, and at a more superior level, the intrapericardial part of the pulmonary veins.

Two fingers can usually slide up posterior to the heart into a recess bounded on each side by pulmonary veins. This recess, the oblique sinus, is posterior to the left atrium. Thus the pericardial cavity is the immediate relationship of the left atrium as it is of the other three chambers.

ITEM 6-13.   Transverse Sinus of the Pericardial Cavity

This is an important landmark in heart surgery. To see why, slip the tip of the index finger of your left hand in between the superior vena cava and the ascending aorta. This is a little difficult in a cadaver because of the rigidity of the vessels, but persevere. Now curl the finger slightly so that the tip slides posterior to the ascending aorta. Push the finger to the left and the tip should appear on the left side of the pulmonary trunk. In Figure 6-4 a tape has been slipped through the transverse sinus, a maneuver common enough in cardiac surgery because, assisted by the tape, the surgeon has control over the blood flow in either the aorta or the pulmonary trunk.

ITEM 6-14.   Review

Identify the fibrous pericardium and its attachment superiorly to the superior vena cava, ascending aorta, and pulmonary trunk, and inferiorly to the diaphragm. Identify the other major vessels, the pulmonary veins, and the inferior vena cava. Identify the transverse sinus. Last, if you are unsure of the location of the four chambers of the heart in situ, give this your attention now because the next stage of dissection is the removal of the heart by cutting the major vessels.

Chapter 7

Basic Plan of the Heart

The dotted line on Figure 8-1 shows the plane of section upon which this description is based. Figure 7-1*A* is a superior view of a transverse section of the heart just below the entry of the pulmonary veins. In such a section the only orifice of a major vessel to be seen is the orifice of the inferior vena cava. Observe, however, that all four chambers of the heart are seen; the left atrium is posterior; the right atrium is on the right; the right ventricle is anterior; the left ventricle is posterior and to the left.

B, in Figure 7-1, is a superior view of a heart; the location of each chamber is indicated. A dotted circle shows where the ascending aorta

A

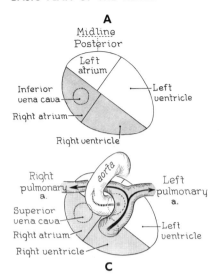

B

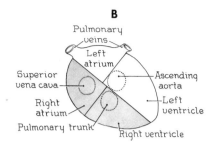

Figure 7-1. Sections of the heart. For explanation see text. Figure 8-1 indicates the plane of the section.

leaves the left ventricle; another where the pulmonary trunk leaves the right ventricle; another where the superior vena cava enters the right atrium (note that this is vertically superior to the inferior vena cava). The pulmonary veins entering the left atrium are shown.

In Figure 7-1C the interrupted arrow indicates the direction taken by the ascending aorta, whereas the double headed arrow indicates the course of the pulmonary trunk dividing into right and left pulmonary arteries. Observe that the ascending aorta first lies inferior to the pulmonary trunk, second, is seen to the right of the trunk, and, third, lies adjacent to the left aspect of the superior vena cava and superior to the right atrium. Observe also that the right pulmonary artery first lies posterior to the ascending aorta, then lies posterior to the superior vena cava, and all the while is superior to the left atrium.

ITEM 7-1. With these facts in mind, reexamine the heart in your cadaver.

Identify the right atrium and auricle.

Identify the superior and inferior vena cava, rather, the termination of these veins within the pericardium, for they are both extra- and intrapericardial.

Identify the right ventricle. Observe how it narrows to an infundibulum, or funnel, where the pulmonary trunk begins.

Identify what you can see of the ascending aorta. Remember the very root of the aorta is posteroinferior to the infundibulum and pulmonary trunk.

Identify the apex of the heart and the left ventricle.

Identify left atrium and auricle.

ITEM 7-2. Removal of the Heart

Insert a piece of stout string into the transverse sinus (Fig. 6-4), and leave it there as a guide to the depth of the cut you will now make. Be careful where you direct the point of the knife when you cut now the ascending aorta, *before* it leaves the pericardium. Within the lumen of the aorta you will find a mixture of blood, latex, and calcified debris, sometimes as solid as brick and really difficult to cut. This material usually crumbles easily, so, with patience, you can completely sever this major vessel.

ITEM 7-3. Identify the bifurcation of pulmonary trunk and, proximal to the bifurcation, cut the trunk.

ITEM 7-4. Inside the pericardial cavity, cut the superior vena cava. In mobilizing this vessel you will have to make a small incision in the serous pericardium reflected on the posterior surface of this vessel. Usually, however, the serous pericardium in a cadaver tears all too easily.

ITEM 7-5. In a similar manner, cut the inferior vena cava.

ITEM 7-6. To cut the right pulmonary vein or veins, twist the heart to the left, not too much or you will distort the veins. Then identify the veins entering the left atrium. Sometimes the pulmonary veins, usually two in number, conjoin just before they enter the left atrium. Cut the veins half a centimeter from the left atrial wall. Use a similar procedure to cut the left pulmonary veins.

ITEM 7-7. To finally remove the heart it will be necessary to cut or tear remaining reflections of serous pericardium in the vicinity of the vessels. The heart is now free. Reidentify the four chambers and their related blood vessels.

Chapter 8

Dissection of the Chambers of the Heart

The presence of embalmed blood and latex or starch sometimes makes dissection of the heart really difficult, especially when the mixture of blood and latex is solid. Because of this possible difficulty, first let the instructors examine the heart. If the contents of the heart are really solid, make a transverse section of the heart as in Figure 8-1. In this way it is fairly easy to soften the heart by soaking it and then to extract the caked material lodged tightly in the heart chambers and orifices. Sectioning the heart in this way is not a disadvantage. In fact, it is an excellent way to gain a sound knowledge of the layout of the heart and its

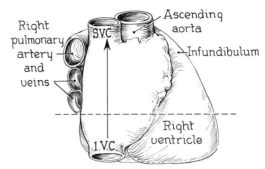

Figure 8-1. View of the heart from the right. The arrow indicates the cut to open the right atrium. The dotted line indicates the plane of the transverse section which is fundamental to Figure 7-1 *A*, *B*, and *C*.

adjoining vessels (Fig. 8-1). Indeed, it is recommended that there be one transversely sectioned heart for every 20 students.

Exploring the Chambers of the Heart

Exploring the chambers of the heart is a fascinating venture into the realm of cardiac surgery. To understand some of the concepts that guide the cardiac surgeon you should concentrate on the following:

1. Precise orientation and position of each chamber in the living heart, including its relationship to the septal wall (Fig. 7-1)
2. The vessels and how they enter or leave each chamber
3. The atrioventricular orifices
4. The valves in operation
5. The capacity of each chamber
6. The blood flow tracts, which, with the first five points established, are of ultimate importance

The six preceding points are basic to an understanding of the effect upon the entire heart of stenosis (i.e., narrowing of an orifice) and valvular incompetence (i.e., a valve cannot perform its normal function). Stenosis and incompetence are really pathological conditions and are dealt with in review after you have considered the normal anatomy of the heart.

Auricle and Atrium

Before you open the heart, the distinction between atrium and auricle must be emphasized. Each auricle is an appendage of an atrium; the cavity of each auricle is an extension of an atrial cavity. Until recent years it was common practice to call the entire chamber *auricle*; some still do. But in an age of precise operative procedures upon the heart this practice is no longer permissible. You will misconceive the meaning of reports upon cardiac surgery if you do not have the distinction between auricle and atrium clearly in mind. The following extract is an example. "The left atrium was explored by a finger passed through an incision in the left auricle."

The Right Side of the Heart

This description includes the right atrium and ventricle, but now that you have reviewed the external anatomy of the heart it is clear that the description is misleading, for the right ventricle is anterior, and the furthest right side of the heart is formed mainly by the right atrium. Another term commonly used is the venous side of the heart; the right atrium receives all venous blood and the right ventricle pumps that blood through the pulmonary circulation.

ITEM 8-1. The Right Atrium

Identify both the superior and the inferior vena cava. Make a vertical incision (Fig. 8-1) to open the superior vena cava, the right atrium, and the inferior vena cava. Turn the flaps back and flush out all debris in a sink, not a washbasin. This incision exposes the internal wall of the atrium. There are two parts to be examined, one smooth the other rough.

ITEM 8-2. Examination of the Rough Wall

Identify the crista terminalis, a vertical ridge extending between the vena caval orifices. From the crista terminalis the musculi pectinati, which are bands of muscle formed like a comb (pecten means comb in Latin), extend into the auricle.

ITEM 8-3. Examination of the Smooth Wall

Identify the interatrial wall. It may be patent, i.e., may possess an abnormal orifice, the reason for which will be explained shortly. At the anterior aspect of the wall a normal orifice, the orifice of the coronary sinus, can be found. Adjoining this orifice there is a very small, sometimes inconspicuous flap, so placed as to seem to direct blood flowing out of the coronary sinus toward the tricuspid orifice. The opening of the coronary sinus is mentioned again when the conducting system is described.

The Interatrial Wall

On inspection of the interatrial wall, evidence of its embryonic development is frequently observed. The wall is thin but, even so, a shallow circular depression known as the fossa ovalis may exist and possess an incomplete overlapping margin known as the limbus fossae ovalis. Superiorly between the limbus and the floor of the fossa, and overlapped to a degree by the limbus, an abnormal orifice, the foramen ovale, may be present connecting the right and left atrial cavities. In embryonic development this orifice is a normal occurrence that allows oxygenated blood to reach the left side of the heart without going through the pulmonary circulation. After birth, when the pulmonary circulation becomes fully established and a foramen ovale is no longer necessary, the foramen closes but, often, not entirely. A small, insignificant orifice may be left.

The size of the orifice, however, does become significant when it allows a sufficient volume of recently oxygenated blood from the lungs to be shunted from the left atrium into the right atrium thence into the right ventricle to reenter and overload the pulmonary circulation. The size of the orifice is also significant in cardiac catheterization, when the tip of the catheter may proceed through the foramen ovale into the left atrium and beyond, instead of through the tricuspid orifice into the right ventricle and from there into the pulmonary trunk.

ITEM 8-4. Examine the right atrioventricular orifice, also known as the tricuspid orifice.

Observe the three major cusps of the tricuspid valve, and check by Figure 8-2 that they are named septal, anterior, and inferior (sometimes called posterior), according to their anatomic position. Look for additional smaller cusps. You can examine these cusps more thoroughly after you have opened the right ventricle.

ITEM 8-5. Pulmonary Valve

Look into the pulmonary trunk and identify its cusps, usually three in number. Your point of view will be greatly improved if you trim carefully with scissors to remove the "excess" of the trunk down to the level of the cusps. Each cusp possesses a nodule at the center of its free margin. The pocket formed by each cusp is called a sinus. Where adjacent cusps meet is called a commissure.

ITEM 8-6. Opening the Pulmonary Trunk, Its Orifice, and the Infundibulum (Fig. 8-3).

Always look before you cut with scissors. Look into the pulmonary

Figure 8-2. Transverse section of the heart. 1. Aortic cusp, mitral valve. The asterisk indicates the location of the vestibule of the ascending aorta. 2. Septal cusp, tricuspid valve. 3. Anterior papillary muscle connected to the septum by the moderator band.

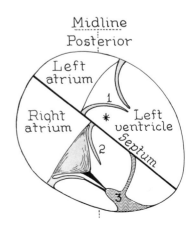

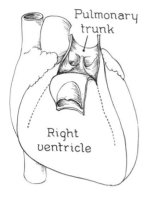
Pulmonary
trunk

Right
ventricle

Figure 8-3. Dotted lines indicate incisions to open right ventricle. See text.

trunk and identify the three cusps of the pulmonary valve. With straight scissors make two cuts into the trunk, one cut on each side of the right cusp; i.e., make it into a commissure. Continue the cut nearer the right atrium along a line parallel to the right coronary artery lying in the atrioventricular groove. Continue the other cut parallel to the interventricular groove. Check frequently that you are not cutting tissue other than the wall of the right ventricle. A large flap somewhat triangular in shape with one cusp of the pulmonary valve near the apex can now be turned down to reveal the internal architecture of the right ventricle. Gently but steadfastly probe and wash out all debris from the ventricular cavity.

ITEM 8-7. The Infundibulum

By opening and closing the flap, you can explore the external shape, the wall, and the internal appearance of the infundibulum, the narrowing portion of the right ventricle preceding the actual pulmonary trunk. Note that the muscular ridges, so characteristic of the internal ventricular wall, are absent from the infundibulum.

ITEM 8-8. Interior of the Right Ventricle

Identify the anterior, posterior (also called inferior), and septal walls. Observe the muscular ridges called trabeculae carnae cordis (translated literally, "ridges fleshy of the heart") and note the papillary muscles. The anterior papillary muscle is attached to the flap you prepared in Item 8-6. The posterior papillary muscle springs from the posterior wall (there may be a group of smaller papillae instead of one large solitary papilla). There is little or no evidence of papillary muscle formation on the septal wall, although chordae tendineae do attach thereon.

Reidentify the cusps of the tricuspid valve (you have already examined these from their atrial aspect), noting particularly the line of attachment of the septal cusp, to be mentioned again under conducting system.

Study the distribution of the chordae tendinae connecting the papillary muscles to the margins and mural (*murus*—wall, Latin) surfaces of the cusps. Chordae from at least one papillary muscle are attached to two cusps (Fig. 8-2) this arrangement is very obvious in the vicinity of a commissure where two cusps meet.

Test the patency of the tricuspid orifice by seeing how many fingertips fit into the orifice from its atrial aspect. In a normal heart — and one not unduly affected by embalming — the size is three fingertips.

Two ridges within the interior of the right ventricle are named. The moderator band, (Fig. 8-2) also known as the septomarginal trabecula, bridges the interval between the septal wall and the anterior papillary muscle. It is not always present as a conspicuous bridge. The second named ridge, the supraventricular crest, is invariably present. As its name implies, it arches over the cavity of the ventricle. It lies posterior to the infundibulum. To identify the crest, slide the tip of a finger from the infundibulum toward the atrioventricular orifice. In doing so the fingertip slides under the crest.

ITEM 8-9. Right Flow Tract

Consider now the direction of blood flow. Blood descends through the superior vena cava and ascends through the inferior vena cava into the right atrium. Coronary sinus blood comes into the atrium through the coronary sinus orifice.

From the atrium through the tricuspid orifice into the right ventricle, blood flow is horizontal and in a left anterior direction. This direction is spoken of as the inflow tract, in contrast to the outflow tract. The outflow tract is at an angle, thus:

$$\underline{60° \diagdown \text{outflow}}$$
$$\text{inflow}$$

It includes the infundibulum and pulmonary trunk. Confirm that the supraventricular crest is superior to the inflow tract and posterior to the outflow.

The Left Side of the Heart

This description includes the left atrium and ventricle, but now that you have reviewed the external anatomy of the heart it is clear that the description is misleading, for the left ventricle faces posteriorly as well as to the left, and the left atrium is definitely posterior in its location. The apex of the heart is that small, but not unimportant, part of the left ventricle occupying the left side of the anterior surface of the heart. In other words the apex, part of the left ventricle, can be seen on inspection of the anterior aspect of the heart.

This side of the heart is also called the arterial side; oxygenated blood is received into the left atrium from the lungs; the left ventricle pumps that blood into the systemic circulation.

ITEM 8-10. The Left Atrium

The best exposure of the internal anatomy of this atrium is obtained by making a horizontal cut between the orifices of a pair of right and left pulmonary veins. Usually there are two pulmonary veins on each side, but sometimes they are conjoined as one. The horizontal cut creates two flaps, which can be reflected, one up and the other down, sufficiently to explore the atrial cavity.

Observe that almost the entire internal wall of the atrium possesses a smooth surface. The internal aspect of the auricle is different and displays musculi pectinati.

ITEM 8-11. The Interatrial Wall

Now that both right and left atria are open for inspection, reconsider the anatomy of the interatrial wall. Observe the fossa ovalis, the limbus, and, possibly, the foramen ovale. Check the translucency of the wall.

ITEM 8-12. Examine the left atrioventricular orifice, also known as the mitral, and as the bicuspid orifice.

While identifying the valve cusps, note that the description implied in *bicuspid* is erroneous. See for yourself. There are additional smaller cusps. There may be a total of four cusps, not just two, so the term *bi*cuspid is inaccurate. Postpone consideration of the nomenclature of the two major cusps until you have opened the left ventricle. Then it will be easier to understand the several names given to each cusp.

ITEM 8-13. The Aortic Valve

To improve your viewing of this valve, trim carefully the wall of the aorta, to within a centimeter of the orifice of the coronary arteries. Each coronary orifice is frequently referred to as an ostium, which means opening.

The nomenclature of the cusps presents difficulty to the beginner. To avoid confusing you at this stage, it is recommended that you name the cusps and sinuses according to the coronary arteries. Thus there is a right coronary cusp, sinus, and ostium and a left coronary cusp, sinus, and ostium. The third cusp and sinus are then described as noncoronary.

The Coronary Circulation

A study of the coronary circulation may be made when three chambers of the heart are open to the extent that you can relate the position of the vessels to the chambers. If you wish, however, you may postpone consideration of the coronary circulation until you have opened and explored the left ventricle. In opening the left ventricle it is necessary to sever either the circumflex or the interventricular branch of the left coronary artery and the beginning of the coronary sinus. Experience has shown that such procedures cause no real difficulty in the study of the coronary circulation.

ITEM 8-14.   Opening the Ascending Aorta, Its Orifice, the Aortic Vestibule, and Left Ventricle

In the process of the dissection, if the interior of the left ventricle is not being exposed with ease do not cut further until you have consulted an instructor. Figure 8-5. demonstrates what the final dissection should look like.

Hold the heart in your left hand with the apex toward the tips of your fingers (Fig. 8-4). Look carefully into the ascending aorta and observe whether the cusps are placed as in Figure 8-4*A* or *B*. Explore with the fingers of your right hand the precise location of the coronary and noncoronary sinuses. Identify the commissure nearest the apex. That commissure may be the one between the left coronary sinus and the right coronary sinus, i.e., between 1 and 2 in Figure 8-4*A* or between the left coronary sinus and the noncoronary sinus, i.e., between 1 and 3 in Figure 8-4*B*. With straight scissors, cut longitudinally through that commissure, toward the left ventricle. The cut separates two cusps. Continue to cut gradually toward the apex to open the left ventricle. In doing so you will inevitably cut either the interventricular branch of the left coronary artery (Fig. 8-4*A*) or the circumflex branch *(B)*. The termination of the great cardiac vein and the beginning of the coronary sinus are also cut.

Continue the cut toward the apex of the heart, opening the cavity of the left ventricle as you proceed. You will at first encounter fibrous tissue, not muscle. The fibrous tissue you encounter is the wall of the aortic vestibule, which is nonmuscular.

Observing carefully before making any cuts, continue the incision through muscle as far as the apex of the heart. You are now in a position

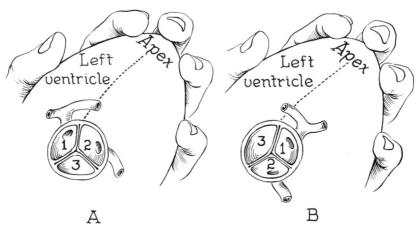

A   B

Figure 8-4.   Two different hearts. *A.* The aorta is rotated to the left. *B.* The aorta is rotated to the right. 1. Left coronary aortic sinus. 2. Right coronary aortic sinus. 3. Noncoronary aortic sinus. The dotted lines indicate the incision to open the left ventricle. In *A* the line intersects the interventricular branch, and in *B* the circumflex branch of the left coronary artery.

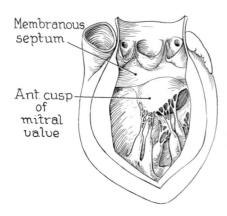

Membranous septum

Ant. cusp of mitral valve

Figure 8-5. The left ventricle opened. The exposed surface of the anterior (aortic) cusp of the mitral valve of your specimen should be examined with care. Refer to the practical demonstration of the left flow tracts on p. 37.

to open the ventricle and explore its interior. Because of the length of the incision and the rigidity of the embalmed tissue, you may have difficulty seeing the interior to best advantage. To meet this difficulty obtain a short plastic or wood rod, 4 or 5 cm. long, and insert it in order to keep the ventricular walls apart (Fig. 8-5).

Gently wash out and probe out all debris until the atrioventricular cusps, the chordae tendineae, and the papillary muscles are clearly seen.

ITEM 8-15. The Left Atrioventricular Orifice

Consider the nomenclature of the two major cusps. The cusp adjacent to the aortic vestibule is anterior, according to its anatomical position (Fig. 8-2), but it is frequently referred to as the aortic cusp because of its proximity to the aorta. This is one instance when a descriptive term, aortic, is more helpful than a positional term, anterior. There can be no doubt which cusp is under consideration if the term aortic is used. The other major cusp is called posterior, posterolateral, sometimes mural, and even ventricular.

ITEM 8-16. Lesser Cusps

Operative procedures upon the left atrioventricular valves has drawn attention to the presence of lesser cusps. Examine the regions of the commissures of the two major cusps, and in all probability you will find lesser cusps.

ITEM 8-17. Further exploration of the Interior of the Left Ventricle

Identify the papillary muscles and chordae tendineae. The aortic cusp is unusual in this respect. Chordae tendineae are attached to its free margin and not to the surface facing towards the ventricle. The reason for this is explained next.

ITEM 8-18. Left Flow Tracts

Blood from each lung enters the left atrium through the horizontally disposed pulmonary veins. Blood from the left atrium streams anteriorly and to the left in a nearly horizontal plane. The aortic cusp of the left atrioventricular orifice is on the right of this stream.

From the ventricular cavity, the blood streams superiorly and to the right, into the aortic vestibule, and on into the ascending aorta. The aortic cusp is to the left of this stream. Thus blood flows freely over both surfaces of the aortic cusp and this is the accepted reason why the chordae tendineae are attached only to the free margin of the aortic cusp.

ITEM 8-19. Practical Demonstration of the Left Flow Tracts

Students who have difficulty visualizing the left flow tract can resolve their difficulty in this way: Rest the apex of the heart on the palm of the left hand. Thrust the thumb of the right hand into the left atrium and onward through the atrioventricular orifice into the left ventricle. Keep the thumb there while you insert the index finger of the same hand into the ascending aorta and beyond into the left ventricle. The tip of the thumb and index finger meet and represent the left flow tract, the thumb representing the inflow tract and the index finger the outflow tract. Gradually slide the thumb and index finger out of the heart. If all is well, the thumb will slide over the atrial surface of the aortic cusp while the finger slides over its ventricular surface. This is really a simple demonstration. Seek help if the technique is not clear.

At the same time test the patency of the left atrioventricular orifice, which under normal conditions admits the tips of two fingers from the atrial aspect.

Chapter 9

The Skeleton of the Heart, the Heart Muscle, the Conducting System, and the Septal Wall

The four chambers of the heart work together as a unit. True, there is variation in the function of each chamber, but there is not gross evidence of this variation under normal circumstances, when the heart maintains a steady flow of blood through both the systemic and the pulmonary circulation. Basic to an understanding of the integrative action of the chambers of the heart is a knowledge of the so-called skeleton of the heart, the gross arrangement of cardiac musculature, and the layout of the conducting system.

SKELETON OF THE HEART

The skeleton of the human heart is fibrous tissue, not bone, although in some animals bone is present. Special techniques are necessary to reveal the heart's entire skeleton, but the membranous part of the interventricular septum is a visible projection of the fibrous skeleton and forms a key part of the interventricular wall; it is the only visible evidence of the existence of a fibrous skeleton. It is discussed further below.

The rest of the skeleton, which can be seen under a microscope (Fig. 9-1), consists of four rings of fibrous tissue. Each ring bounds an orifice, namely the right atrioventricular orifice, the pulmonary orifice, the left atrioventricular orifice, and the orifice of the ascending aorta. The rings are known as the tricuspid, pulmonary, mitral, and aortic rings; their proximity to each other should be noted.

ITEM 9-1.   Place the heart so that the apex is pointing away from you. By pushing the *left* index finger through the already opened left atrium, place the tip of that finger within the mitral ring (i.e., within the left atrioventricular orifice). Through the right atrium place the tip of the *left* thumb in the tricuspid ring. Then push the *right* thumb into a sinus of the aortic valve and the *right* index finger into a sinus of the pulmonary valve. Observe how close the tips of your fingers and thumbs are to each other.

Orientation of the tricuspid and mitral rings in particular aids the student to correctly orient the heart. Both rings are nearly vertical, and the right atrioventricular ring (tricuspid) is anterior to the left atrioventricular ring (mitral).

The dimensions of the atrioventricular rings are also of some importance. Normally the tricuspid ring is nearly 12 cm. in length, while the mitral ring is smaller, and, normally, not more than 10 cm. At autopsy, when the width of each ring is measured, a measurement without question greater than the normal figure is presumptive evidence that the ring is dilated, and, therefore, that the valve mechanism has been incompetent. Obviously there is an element of human judgment in any decision of this kind.

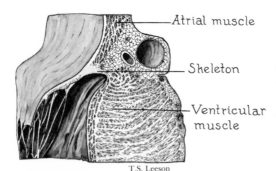

Atrial muscle

Skeleton

Ventricular muscle

T.S. Leeson

Figure 9-1. Section of the heart wall at the junction of atrium and ventricle. Observe that atrial and ventricular muscle fibers have separate attachments to the skeleton of the heart.

ITEM 9-2.   Examination of the Membranous Part of the Interventricular Septum (Abbreviated Here to Membranous Septum)

A cross section of the heart shows clearly the site and connections of the membranous septum. Observe on a cross section that: (1) The septum connects the thin interatrial wall to the thick muscular part of the interventricular wall. (2) The septum separates not just ventricle from ventricle, but also the left ventricle from the right atrium. (3) The septal cusp of the tricuspid orifice is attached to the "middle" of the membranous septum and divides it into an atrial part and a ventricular part.

ITEM 9-3.   Examination of an Intact Membranous Septum

Using the heart whose chambers you have opened and explored, review the position and relationships of the membranous septum. With a probe or other instrument, elevate the septal cusp of the tricuspid valve and examine the ventricular part of the membranous septum obscured from view by the cusp. Then on the left side, observe the proximity of the aortic valve and the aortic cusp of the mitral valve to the membranous septum.

DEFECTS IN THE MEMBRANOUS SEPTUM

Most congenital septal defects occur in the region of the membranous septum. A defect means that the septum is incomplete and, therefore, in its simplest form, it means that there is a communication between left and right ventricles. If, however, the defect is on the atrial side of the attachment of the septal cusp of the tricuspid orifice, then the left ventricle and right atrium are in communication.

An operative procedure to close a septal defect is often complicated by the fact that the orifices of the ascending aorta and the pulmonary trunk are not exactly in their normal position. The orifice of the ascending aorta, for example, may override the incomplete interventricular septum so that the lumen of the aorta and the cavity of the right ventricle are in communication. A further complication in the repair of septal defects is the proximity of the conducting system, to be discussed further on, after a necessary comment about the gross arrangement of cardiac muscle.

MUSCULATURE OF THE HEART

The arrangement of muscle bundles throughout the heart wall is more complex than one appreciates on casual observation. Special dissections are necessary to demonstrate how the muscle bundles are arranged in spirals. The swirling arrangement of straps of muscle entering and leaving the vortex of the apex of the heart explains to some extent the uniform "punch" of each heartbeat.

Perhaps of more importance to the clinical student is that the atrial musculature is independent of the ventricular musculature. The line of separation is at the atrioventricular junction, or, more precisely, at the atrioventricular fibrous rings, at the skeleton of the heart (Fig. 9-1). Accordingly, under certain circumstances, atria and ventricles may beat independently. Synchronization of atrial and ventricular contractions depends entirely upon the efficiency of the conducting system.

Until 1893 there was no clear concept of how impulses pass from atria to ventricles. Then Wilhelm His, Jr., a clinician and the son of a professor of anatomy, announced: "I have succeeded in finding a muscle bundle which unites the auricular and ventricular walls . . ." (Hudson 1966). This was the atrioventricular bundle, known thereafter as the bundle of His.

CONDUCTING SYSTEM

Shortly, you will read that the atrioventricular bundle passes through the membranous septum. In the event of a membranous septal defect, the bundle usually lies in the margin of the defect, and the surgeon is acutely aware of its presence. The bundle is the only physiologic link between the atrial and ventricular musculature, a fact of supreme importance in the synchronization and regulation of the heart's action. Therefore operative procedures to close a septal defect must not damage such a vital link. In looking for the conducting system in your specimen you face the same dilemma as the cardiac surgeon, for the conducting system is not visible except microscopically when special stains are used to distinguish it from cardiac muscle. Furthermore, it is so small that is is measured in millimeters. There are four main parts to be named, and the position of each part can be roughly indicated:

1. The sinoatrial node, measuring only a few millimeters, is located on the external surface of the heart at the junction of the anteromedial aspect of the superior vena cava and the right auricle, at the upper end of the sulcus terminalis, a vertical linear depression on the external surface of the heart at the base of the auricle.

2. The atrioventricular node, also measured in millimeters, lies deep inside the heart in the interatrial wall, on the ventricular side of the orifice of the coronary sinus.

3. The atrioventricular bundle proceeds from the atrioventricular node through the membranous septum towards the "apex" of the muscular part of the interventricular septum, where it spreads into right and left parts, commonly called right and left bundles. Each bundle proceeds from the ventricular wall into a ventricle and spreads into a fine network.

4. This microscopic fine network is composed of fibers called *Purkinje fibers*, located upon the surface of the papillary muscles and the trabeculae carneae.

ITEM 9-4. Locate the sites of the conducting system. In doing so, reidentify the moderator band. When present, the band transmits some of the conducting system from the interventricular wall to the anterior wall of the right ventricle.

THE PACEMAKER, THE SINOATRIAL NODE

Written upon the pages of the history of medicine are many discoveries that spring from a combination of chance and meticulous research. A fascinating example is the discovery in 1906 of the sinoatrial node by Flack, a medical student who was left one summer afternoon to cut serial sections of a mole's heart while his mentor, Arthur Keith, went for a bicycle ride. When Keith returned, a greatly excited Flack bade him examine a strange structure under the microscope (Hudson, 1966). It was the sinoatrial node, and, later, brilliant research by Lewis and the Oppenheimers (1910) confirmed the node as pacemaker of the heart. Thus a clever observation by a medical student opened up a new line of research into the physiology of the conducting system, a subject of even greater interest today because of the artificial pacemaker. The outlook of patients crippled by disorders of the conducting system has been completely changed by the development of the artificial pacemaker. Clearly, you must study carefully the anatomy and physiology of the entire conducting system.

THE SEPTAL WALL

Finally, your attention is drawn especially to the septal wall, not only because it contains most of the conducting system, but also because of the thickness of the muscular part of the interventricular septum. Both require an adequate blood supply because of their highly specialized metabolism. For some curious reason medical students forget this important region in describing the blood supply of the heart.

ITEM 9-5. Review the anatomy of the septal wall.

Chapter 10

The Coronary Circulation

The Importance of the Coronary Arteries

Listen to a patient with occlusive coronary artery disease tell how he must halt until the pain across his chest (angina pectoris) passes off, and then you will know how much we depend upon the adequate oxygenation of heart muscle in our daily lives. According to Hudson (1965), the heart muscle extracts more oxygen than any other organ. Clearly, the vessels bringing blood to heart muscle must be in good condition, but so must the blood itself; the blood must also be adequate in volume. Thus, anoxia, anemia, and hemorrhage can all contribute to ischemia of heart muscle.

Accordingly in the practice of medicine the coronary circulation cannot be isolated from the rest of the body, although in learning names of vessels and their pattern isolation is permissible, indeed essential.

ITEM 10-1. On an isolated heart, with the aid of *Grant's Atlas of Anatomy* Figure 437, identify the recognized parts of each coronary artery, namely the ostium and the definitive artery and its branches. At autopsy and during subsequent investigations each part is scrutinized by the pathologist seeking evidence of arterial disease.

The Nomenclature of the Left Coronary Artery

Textbooks differ in describing the left coronary artery. In most recent textbooks, the left coronary artery is described as being short, quickly dividing into a circumflex branch and an anterior interventricular branch (Fig. 8-4). By some authors, however, the circumflex branch is regarded as the continuation of the left coronary artery; the artery, then, is long and has only one named branch, the anterior interventricular. Students must be familiar with both descriptions, although the first description given is the one to be preferred, and is the one used hereafter.

ITEM 10-2. Look for anomalies such as coronary arteries arising from a pulmonary trunk. Now answer this question. If a coronary artery does arise from the pulmonary trunk, in what direction will blood flow in the artery? To or from the pulmonary trunk?* This is one example of

---

*Answer: *to* the pulmonary trunk.

blood being diverted from one side of the heart to the other; clinically it is called a "left to right shunt."

ITEM 10-3. Try to identify the artery to the sinoatrial node and to the atrioventricular node. Neither is easy to find on the heart of a cadaver, so do not delay. They may arise from either the right or left coronary arterial system.

ITEM 10-4. On a cross section of the heart, reexamine the muscular interventricular septum and identify one or two of the septal branches of the interventricular arteries. These arteries have been cut across and can be identified by the presence of latex.

The Function of the Coronary Arteries

A 336-page monograph, *The Coronary Arteries*, by William Fulton, published in 1965, is a measure of the attention recently paid to these arteries and their diseases. Therefore, an aspiring clinical student must have a basic knowledge of the coronary arteries, but he must not be doctrinaire in applying this knowledge to patients because of the individual variations known to occur in the area supplied by each coronary artery. The accepted basic pattern is as follows:

The left coronary artery supplies most of the left ventricle, and that part of the wall of the right ventricle adjacent to the anterior interventricular groove and the two-thirds of the interventricular septum adjacent to that groove. The right coronary artery supplies the remainder of the right ventricle, the small portion of the left ventricle adjacent to the posterior intraventricular groove, *and* the remaining one-third of the septum.

In 55 per cent of hearts, the right coronary artery supplies the sinoatrial node with blood (therefore in 45 per cent of hearts the supply is from the left coronary system) (Hudson, 1965). Commonly, the right coronary system supplies the region of the atrioventricular node.

Anastomoses

In 1965 Fulton showed that there are anastomoses between the branches of the left and right coronary arteries. He showed also that the right coronary artery, for example, can supply all of the heart if the left artery is occluded. Some contemporary debate centers upon how rapidly and effectively one or the other artery can take over in event of acute arterial occlusion. In an acute occlusion, it is inevitable that some heart muscle will perish (by infarction) before the supply of blood via an anastomosis becomes effective. But prompt diagnosis and correct long term management can do much to prevent a person suffering a cardiac infarction from becoming a cardiac cripple as a result of extensive infarction of cardiac muscle.

Read an account of the coronary arteries.

Veins

In dealing with the coronary circulation it is common practice for the undergraduate to dwell almost exclusively upon the anatomy of the coronary arteries and to ignore the venous system except for the coronary sinus. This is permissible; the student may review the venous system from *Grant's Atlas of Anatomy*, Figure 438.

Lymph Vessels

The heart, like all muscle, has a lymphatic drainage whose vessels cannot be seen unless special techniques are employed. Unlike the coronary arteries and veins, which are confined to the heart itself, the lymph vessels from the heart penetrate the pericardium and drain into mediastinal lymph nodes. It is said that heart muscle has an abundant lymphatic drainage, which is presumably in continuous flow, unlike the lymph flow from limb muscles, which is only obvious during physical exercise.

Nerve Supply

Ramifying upon the surface of the heart, especially near the sinoatrial and atrioventricular nodes and upon the surfaces of the coronary arteries, are fibers of the autonomic nervous system. Sympathetic, parasympathetic, and afferent (afferent to the central nervous system, and also described as sensory) fibers are all included, and their functional responsibilities are of great interest indeed to the physiologist and pharmacologist. Unfortunately the fibers cannot be displayed in the gross anatomy laboratory.

These fibers, or their parent fibers, arise from the cardiac plexus and must inevitably penetrate pericardium in order to reach their goal.

The cardiac plexus is exposed in the next stages of dissection.

Review

The internal anatomy of the heart is not easy; it may challenge the most experienced cardiac surgeon, to whom the internal anatomy of the heart seems different when the heart is beating, open, and on the pump. Furthermore, from both an academic and a practical point of view, a clear concept of the basic embryology of the heart and an understanding of how anomalies of the heart occur help one to grapple with the anatomy of the normal heart. But stick to embryology texts that are simple and concise! Of the different ways to review the anatomy, perhaps for a student who will soon embark upon basic training in the diagnosis of heart disorders, the following review will be most useful.

The main purpose of the heart is to pump blood into both the systemic and the pulmonary circulations. To assist in this purpose, the valves in the flow tract are so designed that they maintain the flow in one direction. Accordingly, valvular disease has a profound effect upon the efficiency of the heart in performing its purpose. Let us suppose the aortic valve is diseased. It may be narrower than usual because of stenosis or wider than usual (incompetence). Without the benefit of the valve in either allowing or maintaining the onward flow of blood into the aorta, the left ventricle must make an additional effort. In time this effort will fail (left ventricular failure). Thereafter an increased strain will fall upon the left atrioventricular (mitral) ring until, eventually, the mitral valve ceases to function effectively. Then left atrial failure occurs, the lungs become congested with blood (pulmonary congestion), and the blood pressure in the pulmonary circulation rises. And so, relentlessly, deterioration of cardiac and pulmonary function goes on.

This is not the time or place to delve deeply into the clinical aspects mentioned briefly in the previous paragraph. This is the time, however, for you to consider thoughtfully the following sequence of anatomic structures. It is a sequence cardiac physicians and surgeons have imprinted clearly in their minds, and one they use daily in establishing the diagnosis of a disordered heart. In following the sequence, it will become clear to you that the anatomic structures are in reverse order in relation to blood flow.

Peripheral (arterial) circulation, including the entire aorta
Aortic valve
Left ventricle
Left atrioventricular (mitral) valve
Left atrium
Pulmonary circulation in the lungs and including the pulmonary
    arteries and trunk
Pulmonary valve
Infundibulum
Right ventricle
Right atrioventricular (tricuspid) valve
Right atrium
Venous system, draining blood from the head and neck, liver,
    kidneys, and lower limbs

ITEM 10-5.   When the pulmonary valve is stenosed (i.e., narrowed) does this normally affect the left ventricle?

ITEM 10-6.   The left atrioventricular valve (the mitral valve) is stenosed. Does this affect the pulmonary valve? Why?

L'ENVOI

In writing this section it has been a real temptation to refer extensively and vividly to all the exciting, wonderful, and worthwhile technical advances in the diagnosis and treatment of heart disease. Instead, a somewhat sober account has been given, with reference to highly specialized techniques carefully avoided, because it is still held by those who know that:*

Diagnosis in heart disease can usually be made from a carefully taken history and a detailed physical examination, but in some cases accessory methods of examination, such as radiology and electrocardiography, are required, and occasionally it is necessary to make use of highly specialized techniques such as cardiac catheterization and angiocardiography.

Chapter 11

Relationships of the Left Atrium

At least one experienced anatomist holds that if a student can describe the major relationships of the left atrium then he must have a clear idea of the anatomy of the thorax. So far, in dissecting the heart you have exposed relationships of the left atrium within pericardium, and by now you should be able to list these relationships and state their anatomical direction. Now you must expose relationships of the left atrium external to pericardium. Let us begin with the posterior ones first, by venturing into part of the posterior mediastinum, well aware that the entire posterior mediastinum will be reviewed later.

ITEM 11-1. Confirm that the immediate posterior relationship of the left atrium is pericardial sac. After pericardium was cut open and the pulmonary veins cut to release the heart a portion of pericardium remained in situ. It can be identified extending between the orifices of the right and left pulmonary veins (*Grant's Atlas of Anatomy*, Fig. 441). Posterior to this portion of pericardium lies the esophagus.

ITEM 11-2. Look before you cut. Make a vertical incision through the pericardium, midway between the right and left pulmonary veins. Peel each edge of the incision laterally to expose the esophagus. (*Grant's Atlas of Anatomy*, Fig. 442). Cut away "surplus" pericardium to leave the esophagus in full view.

---

*L. S. P. Davidson: *The Principles and Practice of Medicine.* 8th Ed. E. & S. Livingstone Ltd., Edinburgh and London, 1966.

Left Atrium and Esophagus

It is commonly said that the esophagus is a posterior relation of the left atrium, but it is implicit that the pericardium lies between them, as you have just demonstrated. The relationship of the esophagus to the left atrium is significant in radiology. A radiograph of the chest taken in an oblique direction (this is called a right anterior oblique projection, or simply R.A.O.), while there is barium sulphate in the esophagus, will reveal indentations in the esophagus. One of the indentations may be an enlarged left atrium pressing the posterior pericardium into the esophagus; as you may have surmised, however, the indentation could be caused by excess fluid in the pericardial sac. Other indentations of the esophagus seen on R.A.O. projections are caused by the arch of the aorta and the left bronchus. Today, angiocardiography and other equally specialized techniques have largely replaced barium sulphate studies for assessing the size of the left atrium. Nevertheless the relationship of esophagus to atrium remains not just interesting but important.

The Pulmonary Trunk and Arteries

The pulmonary artery to each lung conveys deoxygenated blood (low in oxygen, but not entirely without it) while the pulmonary veins return blood in which the normal level of oxygen has been restored (oxygenated) to the heart. Observe that deoxygenated does not mean that the blood is lacking completely in oxygen. The terms venous and arterial are often used in place of deoxygenated and oxygenated. Here, you will note, the pulmonary artery conveys venous blood.

ITEM 11-3. Identify the pulmonary trunk. If you made a nice clean cut across the trunk when you removed the heart you can easily identify the remainder of the pulmonary trunk proximal to its bifurcation. Cut through the bifurcation to disconnect the right pulmonary artery from the left. "Peel" each artery as far toward the lung root as you can. Observe how each artery leaves the pericardium. Beyond the pericardium, on the left side, you will be hampered somewhat by a band of fibrous tissue between the left pulmonary artery and the aorta. This band is the ligamentum arteriosum, the remnant of the ductus arteriosus, which was part of the fetal circulation to be discussed on p. 53. On the right you must displace the superior vena cava.

Replace the heart and confirm that the bifurcation of the pulmonary trunk and the pulmonary arteries, especially the right pulmonary artery, lie superior to the left atrium.

ITEM 11-4. Pulmonary Veins
On each side, reidentify the pulmonary veins and "peel" them as far

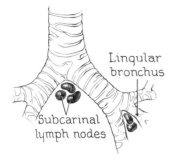

Lingular
bronchus

Subcarinal
lymph nodes

Figure 11-1. Two significant clusters of lymph nodes. Similar groups of lymph nodes are present at other similar sites.

as the root of the lung. Observe how they too are intra- and extrapericardial. Confirm the relationship of the veins to the left atrium.

ITEM 11-5.   The Bifurcation of the Trachea

Posterosuperior to the right pulmonary artery, the lower end of the trachea bifurcates into the right and left main bronchus. In the angle between the bronchi (Fig. 11-1) lies a cluster of lymph nodes. Why these nodes are sometimes called subcarinal nodes will be explained later. The nodes in a cadaver are black and granular, crumbling easily, so it is not easy to remove them intact. Even though the pulmonary arteries are displaced from the dissecting field, the bifurcation of the trachea will not be readily found until you have got rid of the pretracheal fascia passing from the anterior aspect of the trachea inferiorly to join the pericardium. Dissect until you can see the bifurcation of the trachea clearly.

Also, in this region between the pulmonary arteries and the bifurcation of the trachea lies the cardiac plexus. Do not lose time seeking the plexus even though it is important. It is not always easy to display in a cadaver.

Cardiac Plexus (Part of the Autonomic Nervous System)

Although this plexus is often described as having superficial and deep parts relative to an approach to the arch of the aorta from the left side, it is adequate to refer simply to *a* cardiac plexus. On each side the cardiac plexus merges imperceptibly with a pulmonary plexus.

From the cardiac plexus, autonomic fibers penetrate the pericardium to reach the nodal areas of the heart and the coronary vessels.

ITEM 11-6.   For Review

By restoring the heart to its original position, observe how the anatomy here fits together. The left atrium, the most posterior chamber of the heart, and also central in position, is on a level with the right and left pulmonary veins; superior to the left atrium is the bifurcation of the pulmonary trunk; posterosuperior to the pulmonary bifurcation lies the bifurcation of the trachea; posterior to the left atrium is found the esophagus after removal of pericardium.

The juxtaposition of the left main bronchus to the upper left atrium is utilized clinically in the measurement of left atrial pressure. With a bronchoscope the clinician views the "floor" of the left main bronchus, then thrusts a needle designed for this purpose through the floor into the left atrium. It would be out of place here to describe the apparatus and the precise technique. Suffice it to say that once the anatomic facts are recognized and their significance realized, it is as if a bright light had been cast upon an otherwise dark and exclusive region of the thorax.

ITEM 11-7. The Lung Root

In addition to the lymph nodes and vessels and the pulmonary nerve plexus, at each lung root there are a bronchus, pulmonary artery, and two veins. You have already taken the artery and veins as far as you can toward the lung. Now, by slipping your curved scissors posterior to the bronchus, free the bronchus and trace it to the lung root.

ITEM 11-8. Removal of the Lung

The pulmonary artery and veins are already disconnected. Now— about one inch from the tracheal bifurcation—sever each bronchus. Some pleura around the lung root will still be in situ. Remove the lung from the thorax cage, incising the remaining pleura at the lung root as you proceed. Throughout you will be tearing the pulmonary plexus; the plexus is important, but do not delay, for it is rarely seen easily or adequately in a cadaver.

Lymph Nodes

While the regional drainage of the lymph nodes you are exposing is simple to understand, the names applied to the various groups of nodes can at times be very confusing. Essentially, the nodes receive lymph from the lungs and heart.

From each lung the sequence of nodes is as follows: pulmonary (isolated nodes inside the lung), bronchopulmonary (clusters of nodes at the hilum of lung where lung tissue and bronchus meet), tracheobronchial (present in the angles between trachea and bronchus—hence divided into a superior and inferior group for descriptive purposes); and tracheal (the name is self-explanatory).

Tracheal nodes belong to a larger group called mediastinal nodes, located throughout the superior mediastinum. Two lymph trunks, the right and left bronchomediastinal trunks, drain this large group of nodes by joining the subclavian vein of their own side. Thus lymph from each lung soon returns to the venous system, and, mark you, to the venous system close to the heart and thus to the beginning of the pulmonary circulation.

Recent work, however, demonstrates that this is not the whole story and that lymph from the lower lobe of the left lung reaches nodes on the right side of the root of the neck. Hence, in looking for evidence of spread of cancer from that lung, both sides of the neck must be examined.

Clinically, the bronchopulmonary nodes are generally referred to as the hilar nodes, a term which more than likely includes some tracheobronchial nodes as well. The hilar nodes are radiopaque. Therefore they are visible as a gray "shadow" on a radiograph, especially when they are enlarged.

Pulmonary Plexus (Part of the Autonomic Nervous System)

The primary purpose of each pulmonary plexus seems to be to control the caliber of the bronchi and the secretions from the myriads of mucus-secreting glands throughout the bronchial mucosa. Drugs that mimic the activity of the sympathetic nervous system, sympathomimetic drugs, cause the bronchi to dilate, so easing respiration. Then again, drugs that are parasympatholytic block the activity of the parasympathetic system and so reduce the amount of mucus secretion that the bronchial mucosa is dry. There are other examples, but enough has been said to show that the control of the caliber of the bronchi and their secretions through the administration of drugs is an important part of clinical medicine. And these important effects are mediated through the pulmonary plexus, which a student rarely sees properly in the gross anatomy laboratory.

ITEM 11-9. Review

By inspecting the heart, lungs, and mediastinum, confirm your ability to identify the major structures you have cut or exposed.

Establish in your mind the anatomy of the pulmonary circulation, which includes the right ventricle, pulmonary trunk, right and left pulmonary arteries, the capillary vessels in each lung, the right and left pulmonary veins, and the left atrium.

Before you dissect each lung and study the distribution of bronchi, arteries, and veins, it is suggested that you now journey into the superior mediastinum to view the trachea from which the right and left bronchi stem.

Chapter 12

The Superior Mediastinum

Pleura must be removed to expose most of the mediastinal structures. Specific instructions for its removal will not be given. Therefore verify, always, a structure's relationship to pleura.

Largely as a result of advances in thoracic and vascular surgery, our understanding and awareness of diagnostic problems in the superior mediastinum has increased to a remarkable degree. Include the root of the neck and the cervical spine and it can be said that the increase is truly dramatic. This entire region absolutely commands the function of both upper limbs, the head and neck, and, to a great extent, also the function of the lower part of the body. It has been likened to a vast cloverleaf, with arterial, venous, and nerve highways and with respiratory and alimentary throughways, a distributing center, if you like, a key region. Combine your knowledge of the anatomy of the superior mediastinum with that of the neck and you are well established to diagnose peripheral problems, especially in the upper limbs and head, and, to some extent, in the lower part of the body as well. From now on, therefore, you must not divorce the anatomy of the superior mediastinum from that of the neck even if, for practical reasons, they are not dissected together in the anatomy laboratory.

The structures to be sought are: (1) The innominate veins and the superior vena cava, (2) The arch of the aorta and branches, (3) the trachea, (4) the esophagus, (5) the vagus nerves and the left recurrent laryngeal nerve, (6) lymph nodes, (7) fascia, (8) intercostal nerves and sympathetic trunk (9) anomalous structures. The thymus gland has already been identified.

Between the trachea and the manubrium there are two vascular planes, a superficial venous plane and an arterial plane close to the trachea. Behind the trachea lies the esophagus, then the vertebral column. (*Plane* is used here to mean a specified level or depth.)

ITEM 12-1. The Venous Plane

Identify the right and left innominate veins joining to form the superior vena cava. Each innominate vein arises from the junction of a subclavian and internal jugular vein, usually at the level of the sternoclavicular joint. Realize that the superior vena cava is at the end of the venous line from the upper limbs and the head and neck. Acute occlusion of this major vein may produce venous congestion of those regions, with a characteristic appearance. What would you expect the appearance to be?

Take heed of the azygos vein, the last tributary of the superior vena cava and an important collateral connection with the field of drainage of the inferior vena cava.

ITEM 12-2.   The Arterial Plane

This plane consists of the arch of the aorta and its branches. Identify and study the arch first.

The Arch of the Aorta

Because this part of the aorta may be somewhat sinuous in your cadaver and because it is usually incorrectly illustrated, let us deal with its normal orientation first. The normal aortic arch is directed backward. Thus the posterior "pillar" of the arch is essentially directly posterior to the anterior "pillar." Illustrations from an anterior view are erroneous if they show clearly the posterior pillar. This fact is applied in the interpretation of chest radiographs wherein, in perfect anteroposterior projections, the arch of the aorta appears as a hump, spoken of as the aortic knuckle. When the radiologist sees more of the aortic arch than this he speaks of unfolding of the aorta, meaning that the arch is wider and more sinuous than normal; probably in your cadaver the arch of the aorta is unfolded and somewhat dilated because such features are characteristic of old age.

The ligamentum arteriosum connects the arch of the aorta to the left pulmonary artery; the significance of this anatomy is dealt with further on, after the study of the arterial plane is complete.

On the left side of the aorta lies the vagus nerve, and underneath the arch, posterior to the ligamentum arteriosum, curves the left recurrent laryngeal nerve. The right and left recurrent laryngeal nerves are considered together after further dissection.

Medial to the aorta (i.e., on its right side) are the trachea and esophagus. In advanced degrees of arterial disease associated with aneurysm, the aneurysm compresses and may even erode into those tubular structures. When erosion is of such a degree to produce a vast and sudden hemorrhage, death is inevitable. Proximally the arch is a continuation of the ascending aorta while distally it continues on as the descending thoracic aorta.

ITEM 12-3.   Branches from the Aorta

Identify, from anterior to posterior, the brachiocephalic (still often called innominate), the left common carotid, and the left subclavian arteries. The brachiocephalic artery bifurcates posterior to the right sternoclavicular joint into right subclavian and right common carotid arteries. Be on the alert for anomalies; occasionally, for example, the left vertebral artery springs from the arch and the right subclavian artery arises independently and passes posterior to the esophagus. Occasionally an artery to the thyroid gland is found arising from the arch (arteria thyroidia ima — *ima* means lowest).

The Fetal Circulation. On p. 94 you are told that freshly oxygenated blood from the placenta enters the fetus via the umbilical vein, traverses the liver via the ductus venosus, and reaches the right atrium via the inferior vena cava. Eventually the blood leaves the fetus through the two umbilical arteries to return to the placenta.

From the right atrium most of the blood bypasses the pulmonary circulation through the foramen ovale, which opens, as you recall, into the left atrium. Some blood does pass through the right atrioventricular orifice into the right ventricle, thence into the pulmonary trunk. Little or none of this blood, however, reaches the lungs, for it is shunted into the aorta via the ductus arteriosus connecting the left pulmonary artery to the aorta just distal to the origin of the left subclavian artery. The ductus arteriosus should close after birth, and normally does, so that only a band of fibrous tissue, the ligamentum arteriosum, remains. Patent ductus arteriosus, however, is quite common and, in brief, the surgical treatment is ligation.

ITEM 12-4. Review the fetal circulation. What is the difference between ductus arteriosus and ductus venosus?

The Trachea in the Thorax. The trachea is located partly in the neck and partly in the thorax.

ITEM 12-5. Identify the trachea in the thorax and observe its close relationship to adjacent structures, the arch of the aorta and what else? Did you include mediastinal lymph nodes? You should have, because enlargement of any of the tissues or structures in the superior mediastinum causes pressure upon the trachea. Did you include pleura?

ITEM 12-6. Press firmly on the trachea in your neck and you will experience an irrepressible desire to cough. In like fashion, a persistent dry cough may be due to pressure upon the trachea from enlarged or abnormal mediastinal structures.

Trachea: Anomalies. The trachea, as an airway to the lungs, normally does not support any branches before the bifurcation. Occasionally a bronchus to the right upper lobe arises before the bifurcation. Clinically, the possibility of an anomaly is to be kept in mind and the embryology of a region reviewed when a disease pattern seems unusual.

ITEM 12-7. Trachea: Carina

Slip the tip of each little finger into the proximal stump of the right and left bronchus. If the stumps are short enough the tips of the fingers will meet. Internally, the obvious edge where the bronchi part company is called the carina, meaning keel (of a boat), but here the keel is uppermost (like an upturned boat when the season is done). The subcarinal lymph nodes (another name for inferior tracheobronchial nodes) lie in the angle between the bronchi inferior to the carina.

The Carina

This is an important landmark in bronchoscopy (the examination of the trachea and bronchi with an instrument, a bronchoscope). Normally the carina is nearly sagittal in direction, i.e., anteroposterior, and has a fairly definite edge. Displacement and distortion of the carina lead the examining clinician to suspect disease in the vicinity of the tracheal bifurcation; when the subcarinal nodes (Fig. 11-1) for example, are enlarged with tumors the carina becomes widened posteriorly and immobile. Certainly other information is essential for a final accurate diagnosis.

From a therapeutic point of view, the mucous membrane at the carina and near it is said to be one of the several more sensitive areas of the airway that are concerned with the cough reflex. It is probable, therefore, that the region of the carina is the last line of defense against a foreign body such as a peanut. Once a foreign body is past the carina and beyond this sensitive area, then the foreign body may remain "silent," but with serious consequences, somewhere in the bronchial tree, more than likely in the right tree because of the direction of the right bronchus. Furthermore, in postural drainage of the lungs (see later) secretions gravitating to the carina usually precipitate a pronounced cough and, as a result, are expectorated.

ITEM 12-8.   Right Lung to Left Lung and Vice Versa

Reexamine the carinal region and the direction of the main bronchi. Realize how easily fluid from one bronchial tree can reach the other tree by swilling over the carina as water swills over the freeboard of a boat. This is a point of great practical importance, not only in the spread of infection from one lung to the other but also in the management of patients with excessive amounts of fluid in one or the other bronchial tree.

ITEM 12-9.   Lymph Nodes and Fascia

While lymph nodes are plentiful in the superior mediastinum, and some can be found in a cadaver, fascia is not plentiful. But, for reasons not clearly understood, there are diseases that prompt the proliferation of fibrous tissue to a degree that the thin-walled veins of the superior mediastinum, the superior vena cava, for example, are compressed. Accordingly, the absence of conspicuous fascia, or fibrous tissue, from the superior mediastinum of a cadaver, should not lead you to dismiss such tissue from your mind.

ITEM 12-10.   The Esophagus in the Thorax

Check the relationship of esophagus to the pleural cavities. From your observations, which pleural route would you use to reach the esophagus above the arch of the aorta? And below the arch?

ITEM 12-11.   Esophagus and Left Bronchus

Observe how the esophagus tends toward the left, emerging, as it does, from posterior to the trachea, to lie posterior to the left bronchus.

Esophageal Anomalies

Anomalous connections between esophagus and trachea or left bronchus are highly unlikely in an elderly cadaver. In newborn infants, however, they do occur; the lower end of the esophagus fails to develop a lumen (atresia: *a*—negative; *tresis*—hole) and a false passage (fistula) between trachea and esophagus may be present. It is a deadly disorder, for fluid can easily enter the airway and lead to serious pulmonary infection, which is usually fatal in the newborn infant. Expert diagnosis and treatment have changed the prognosis of these anomalies from hopeless to hopeful. Thus every newborn infant must have a complete physical examination and be carefully observed until feeding is established.

The right and left recurrent laryngeal nerves are identical in distribution to nearly all the muscles and to some of the mucous membrane of their respective sides of the larynx, but their course to the larynx differs. The right nerve recurs beneath the right subclavian artery while the left recurs beneath the arch of the aorta. Either nerve may be involved in an adjacent disease process with an identical effect upon the voice. Accordingly, when disorders of vocalization are being investigated, both nerves must be considered and the variation in their respective pathways kept in mind.

ITEM 12-12. The Left Recurrent Laryngeal Nerve

Identify the vagus nerve upon the arch of the aorta. Pull it to the left, i.e., toward you if you are at the left side of the cadaver.

Disappearing inferior to the arch and posterior to the ligamentum arteriosum, the left recurrent laryngeal nerve should be recognized.

Now, while retaining hold of the recurrent nerve, pull the arch of the aorta to the left, away from the trachea (if need be, trim off the aorta to the level of the ligamentum arteriosum). Now you should see the recurrent nerve ascending to the cleft between the trachea and the esophagus. There will be bronchopulmonary and tracheal lymph nodes in this vicinity. Also, the recurrent nerve feeds some branches into the cardiac plexus as well as branches to the trachea and esophagus. Do not confuse one of these for the recurrent nerve.

Expose the nerve as far as you can superiorly towards the neck, on its way to the larynx. Observe again the close relationship of the nerve to the aortic arch, the left bronchus, and the bronchopulmonary nodes.

ITEM 12-13. The Right Recurrent Laryngeal Nerve

The vagus nerve on the right lies adjacent to the lateral aspect of the trachea. It is oblique and looks like a narrow strap. Identify it first. Now trace the vagus nerve superiorly to the point where it appears posterior to the subclavian vein and anterior to the subclavian artery.

Here, pull the vagus nerve inferiorly and scrutinize the inferior aspect of the artery. You should see the right recurrent laryngeal nerve curving inferior to the artery and then proceeding medially. The nerve soon disappears from view. At this stage of dissection only a short length of the nerve can be exposed. Nevertheless, it is quite important to see that this nerve is directly related to the cervical pleura and is separated from the apex of the right lung only by the pleural cavity.

ITEM 12-14. An Exercise in Applied Anatomy

A patient with a noticeable change in the modulation and "explosive" quality of his voice has his chest x-rayed. The radiologist suspecting that one or the other laryngeal nerve is involved in some disease would scan particularly carefully two regions of the chest. What are they?

ITEM 12-15. Proceed now to explore the hilum of each lung—yes, each lung, because there is a difference in their anatomy. Then explore the rest of the pleural cavity and the mediastinum.

Chapter 13

Lungs

Do not be misled by the shrunken, solid, waterlogged cadaveric lungs. In life each lung fills its side of the thorax, is radiolucent (i.e., allows through sufficient x-rays to darken a radiograph), and is buoyant.

ITEM 13-1. On each side, confirm the extent of the lung in the following manner. Superiorly, slip the fingers of one hand posterior to the first rib, push the fingers superiorly toward the summit of the pleural cavity. Press the finger anteriorly and demonstrate that this part of the pleural cavity, named the cupola, and apex of lung, rise above the clavicle.

ITEM 13-2. Inferiorly and posteriorly, slip the fingers of one hand into the costodiaphragmatic recess. Estimate the level of your finger tips with reference to the vertebral column. Next slide the fingers anteriorly over diaphragmatic pleura towards the anterior costal margin. Then, keeping the fingers close to the costal margin, slide them along the costodiaphragmatic recess to return to your point of departure posteriorly. The base of the lung is related to the diaphragmatic surface you have just outlined.

Although a breast plate has been cut out and also the heart removed you can still assess the area of lung surface related to the vertebral column and mediastinum and to the rib cage.

ITEM 13-3. Now identify the apex, base, and mediastinal and costal surfaces of the lungs of the cadaver.

THE FISSURES OF THE LUNG

ITEM 13-4. The Oblique Fissure

Observe on a right lung how the oblique fissure separates the upper and middle lobes from the lower lobe and, on the left lung, the upper lobe and its lingula (lingula means tongue) from the lower lobe.

ITEM 13-5. The Horizontal Fissure

When it is present a horizontal fissure separates middle lobe from upper lobe. The fissure is a solitary structure, a feature of the right lung, and has no replica in the left lung.

ITEM 13-6. Grasp how fluid may be loculated (i.e., isolated in a pocket) in any part of these fissures.

SURFACE ANATOMY OF THE LUNGS

Medical textbooks deal adequately with this topic, which is fundamental to successful physical examination of the chest. In dealing with this topic, however, the preclinical student rarely detects five indispensable facts to be considered now:

First, the upper lobe of the lung is related to more of the chest wall than meets the eye. On inspection, the scapula and clavicle overlay so much of the upper chest wall that the inexperienced student confines his examination to an anterior area between clavicle and nipple. The experienced clinician, however, realizing that much of the upper lobe is also related to the lateral chest wall, will examine the upper lobe through this aspect of the wall as well; to do so he asks the patient to raise his arm. Confirm for yourself that raising your arm exposes a considerable area of chest wall.

Second, the middle lobe is an anterior part of the right lung. The lobe is wedge-shaped, with the apex posterior, in a cleft between upper and lower lobes; the anterior base is related to the fourth to sixth costal cartilages. Therefore this lobe has no direct relationship to the posterior chest wall. However, as has been stated, the middle lobe does have a relationship to the anterior chest wall between the fourth and sixth costal cartilages. It is precisely in this region that the clinician would examine the middle lobe.

Third, the "base" of the lung refers clinically, not to the anatomical base, which is related to the diaphragm and, therefore, is inferior, but to the lower limits of the posterior surface of the lower lobe. To listen to the base of the lung the clinician applies his stethoscope to the posterior chest wall approximately at a level with the tenth thoracic vertebra.

Fourth, because of the dome shaped form of the diaphragm, certain well-recognized abdominal organs lie within the shelter of the rib cage and are overlapped peripherally by the lungs in the pleural cavities. In physical examination of the chest, the presence of the liver, which is solid, and of the stomach, which is hollow, must always be kept in mind. At times, also, enlargement of the spleen, and, rarely, enlargement of a kidney may affect the findings upon physical examination of the chest.

Fifth, consider the bulk of a lung, its breadth in particular — examine a cross section of lung if one is available — and you must agree that it is unlikely, if not impossible, that a small but serious lesion in the center of the lung can be detected by physical examination alone. For this reason, chest radiography is absolutely essential in detecting diseases of the lung; mass radiography, therefore, is an integral part of modern medicine. Nevertheless, giving a good physical examination of the chest is still important, as you will learn, and you will be successful at it only if your knowledge of the surface anatomy of the lungs and pleural cavities is sound.

Into each lobe proceeds a bronchus with a nerve plexus and an artery, and from each lobe emerges a vein and lymphatic vessels.

ITEM 13-7.   In each lung, now explore the divisions of the main bronchus and accompanying structures. In doing so, do not become embroiled in details. Clearly a chest surgeon must know precisely where the bronchus artery and vein lie in relationship to each other when he removes a lung (pneumonectomy), a lobe (lobectomy), or a segment of lung (segmental resection). At your present stage of training, it is sufficient for you to identify the bronchi and realize that they have companion vascular structures.

ITEM 13-8.   Right and left upper lobe bronchi

At the hilum of each lung, tear away lung tissue, displacing artery and vein, until you have the upper lobe bronchus in clear view. Meanwhile, look out for lymph nodes. Compare the distance of each upper lobe bronchus from the carina.

The right upper lobe bronchus was frequently called eparterial (*epi*

Table 13-1. *Bronchopulmonary Segments*

RIGHT LUNG	LEFT LUNG
Superior lobe	Superior lobe
1. Apical	1 and 2. Apicoposterior
2. Posterior	3. Anterior
3. Anterior	4. Superior lingular
Middle lobe	5. Inferior lingular
4. Lateral	Inferior lobe
5. Medial	6. Apical (superior)
Inferior lobe	7. Medial basal (cardiac)
6. Apical (superior)	8. Anterior basal
7. Medial basal (cardiac)	9. Lateral basal
8. Anterior basal	10. Posterior basal
9. Lateral basal	
10. Posterior basal	

is Greek for upon) because it lay superior to the right pulmonary artery; although this nomenclature has been abandoned in favor of, simply, right upper lobe bronchus, *eparterial* still appears in some texts.

   ITEM 13-9. On the left side expose the bronchus to the lingula. It is the first branch of the left upper lobe bronchus. Confirm that the lingular bronchus is proceeding into the lingula.

   ITEM 13-10. On the right side, expose the bronchus to the middle lobe. Usually, inferior to the point of origin of this bronchus, in the angle between it and the remainder of the bronchial tree, lies a conspicuous cluster of lymph nodes. Observe how enlargement of these nodes could compress the middle lobe bronchus and obstruct the free passage of air into the middle lobe. Similar groups of nodes occur at other similar sites (Fig. 11-1); strictly speaking, they are pulmonary, because they are located well inside the lung, but they are often referred to as bronchopulmonary in order to emphasize their close relationship to the bronchus nearby.

   ITEM 13-11. That each lobe can be divided into two or more segments was a discovery of great surgical significance; it did, in fact, revolutionize lung surgery. The segments and their bronchi are extremely well illustrated in most texts. Guided by colorful illustrations (*Grant's Atlas of Anatomy*, Figs. 424-427), a Huber lung model if one is available, and the line drawing and table (Fig. 13-1), remove lung tissue in order to expose the origins of the segmental bronchi in each lung.

Postural Drainage

   There are many times in the practice of medicine when the assistance of gravity is sought. In the care of the chest, for example, when it is

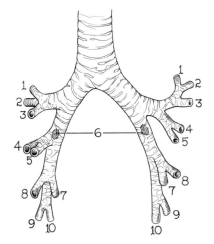

Figure 13-1. Lobar and segmental bronchi. The bronchi are named in Table 13-1. Observe that, on the left, 1 and 2 have a common origin and so do 7 and 8. Thus the former segment is named apical-posterior and the latter anteromedial basal.

necessary to promote drainage from all or part of the bronchial tree, the posture of the patient is adjusted to bring the maximal influence of gravity to bear on the bronchus to be drained. It must be clearly understood, however, that the aim is to bring gravity's influence to bear on an affected bronchus, not necessarily on the trachea, as you will now see.

ITEM 13-12. Using the right lung, in which you have just recently exposed the middle lobar bronchus and the apical bronchus of the lower lobe, position the lung so that the middle lobar bronchus is vertical. In life this would be so when the shoulders are slightly lower than the rest of the body and the left side of the body is slightly lower than the right. In this way, secretions are guided towards the carina, a sensitive area where the cough reflex springs to life. Keep the middle lobe bronchus vertical and note that the position of the trachea is far from vertical. Thus it is not always necessary to put a patient into a jackknife position, a position in which the trachea is vertical, in order to achieve postural drainage.

ITEM 13-13. What posture achieves drainage of the upper lobes, the lingula, and the lower lobes?

The previous section dealt with an aspect of the application of gravity in therapeutic medicine. Consider now a preventive aspect.

ITEM 13-14. While reviewing the apical segmental bronchus you dissected, position the lung as if it were in a recumbent patient (i.e., one *on* his back). Observe that fluid in the bronchial tree can readily gravitate into this bronchus, small though it is. To drain this small bronchus, what position must the patient adopt?

Awareness that gravitation of foreign matter into a segmental bronchus so often has serious consequences is one reason why the posture of an unconscious patient is changed regularly. Maximal drainage and maximal aeration of all parts of the lungs is achieved by changing the position of the patient.

With these basic facts in mind, reconsider the anatomy of the bronchial tree.

Sputum

The matter coughed up and spat from the mouth, for example in the course of a "cold in the chest," is the sputum. The sputum is to be distinguished from the spittle, or spit, which is another name for the saliva secreted into the mouth. Patients rarely distinguish between sputum and spit. To the patient the terms are synonymous, but a clinican must distinguish between them. Sure that the matter expectorated has come from the patient's chest and not from his mouth, the clinician can deduce a great deal about the state of the heart and lungs from the quantity, color, presence of red or brown streaks of fresh or altered blood, and microscopic examination of the sputum.

Sputum is not an anatomic term. It is introduced here to alert you to the importance of the secretions present, in life, on the surfaces of the bronchial tree, which is arid in the embalmed cadaver.

Chapter 14

Posterior Mediastinum and Vertebral Column Region

Pleura must be removed in order to expose most of these structures. Specific instructions for its removal will not be given. Therefore verify, always, a structure's relationship to pleura.

By definition, you recall, the posterior mediastinum is a subsection of the inferior mediastinum and, therefore, strictly speaking, lies below the level of the fourth thoracic vertebra (Fig. 6-2). However, you should also recall that this level is arbitrary, based as it is on the findings in a cadaver. Furthermore, all the structures located in the posterior mediastinum continue beyond the boundaries of the mediastinum. Thus it would be foolish to think of the posterior mediastinum as an isolated compartment. It is much better to think of it as a definable region where intermediate parts of longitudinal structures are found.

ITEM 14-1. Identify the thoracic descending aorta and trace it to where it passes behind the diaphragm to leave the thoracic cage. The arbitrary level is the twelfth thoracic vertebra.

ITEM 14-2. Identify some of the important branches of the descending thoracic aorta; the bronchial arteries have been seen already. Trace out at least one typical intercostal artery, and realize that esophageal branches do occur, difficult though it is to find them in the cadaver.

ITEM 14-3. Read an account of radicular arteries (p. 143).

The significance of the entire aorta will become clear to you when you have displayed the abdominal aorta and read its account (p. 142). Meantime, grasp that the thoracic aorta may be considered part of a conduit for blood from the heart to the periphery, but it is not inert. In life, powerful pulses urge onward a torrent of blood.

ITEM 14-4. Identify the entire thoracic esophagus. Observe how at first it lies posterior to the trachea, then passes anterior to the aorta, and then veers to the left to leave the thorax through the diaphragm. Veering to the left, the esophagus lies posterior to the left bronchus. Recall how it lies posterior to pericardium and the left atrium.

See if you can find a fairly substantial artery from the aorta to the esophagus. In a cadaver it lies about level with the dome of the diaphragm. Such a branch is typical of the many smaller branches that stem from adjacent definitive vessels. These many small arteries nourish the esophagus and must be preserved as far as possible in surgical procedures. A surgeon, operating upon and mobilizing the esophagus, is greatly concerned lest he diminish its blood supply. Why? Because he knows that incisions into the esophagus will not heal without a sufficient supply of arterial blood.

Revise the relationship of esophagus to the pleural cavities.

ITEM 14-5.   Identify the Thoracic Duct

This slender duct lies posterior to the esophagus and may not be easily identified, unless digestion was in an active phase before death, which is unlikely. During digestion the thoracic duct is distended with chyle, a product of the small bowel consisting of lymph and emulsified fat. The duct lies adjacent to the right side of the aorta (it enters the thorax through the aortic opening). Be alert. The unwary dissector sometimes confuses the duct with the larger, more readily identifiable azygos vein, which lies nearby.

Trace the thoracic duct superiorly to where it crosses posterior to the esophagus before continuing superiorly to the root of the neck, where it joins the venous system.

Take into consideration the relationship of the duct to the pleural cavity. While you have been exposing the duct you have been destroying mediastinal pleura.

ITEM 14-6.   Sympathetic Trunk

Strip off pleura to expose the sympathetic trunk. It is a series of strands of nerve fibers linking small masses of tissue called ganglia (singular ganglion). Usually there are twelve ganglia on each side, but do not attempt to count them, for they are often fused, and it is quite unnecessary to identify them all.

THORACIC SYMPATHETIC SYSTEM

Four parts of the sympathetic system in the thorax deserve careful consideration apart from the sympathetic trunk itself, (1) the splanchnic nerves, (2) the cardiac nerves, (3) the rami communicantes (to one intercostal nerve, for example), and (4) the stellate ganglion (this name is applied to the solitary ganglion present when the inferior cervical sympathetic ganglion and the first thoracic ganglion are fused. Fusion is common).

ITEM 14-7.   Splanchnic Nerves

The splanchnic nerves proceed anteriorly from the sympathetic chain on to the lateral aspect of the bodies of the thoracic vertebrae.

Thence they descend to penetrate the diaphragm to join the celiac ganglion, a major ganglion that lies on the anterolateral aspect of the abdominal aorta, in the vicinity of the celiac artery.

ITEM 14-8. Cardiac Nerves

You may not find these easily but you must know of their existence because, within them, afferent (going *toward* the central nervous system) fibers exist. Thus they convey impulses from painful stimuli in the heart muscle back to the central nervous system. See if you can identify branches from the sympathetic trunk to the region of the tracheal bifurcation where the cardiac plexus lay. But do not delay.

ITEM 14-9. To identify rami communicantes select an easily identifiable ganglion adjacent to an intercostal space. Pull the ganglion medially, and in other directions if need be; then clear away fat and fascia with a blunt instrument to expose the very very short rami strung between the intercostal nerve and the sympathetic ganglion. One expects to find two rami, but there may be only one.

ITEM 14-10. Stellate Ganglion

The relationship of this ganglion to the pleural cavity and the apex of the lung is important because cancer of the apex of the lung may obliterate the pleural cavity and infiltrate the sympathetic ganglia at the superior part of the thorax. The outcome of this disaster should become clear to you after reading review of the autonomic nervous system.

A word of encouragement to the student:

No doubt the autonomic nervous system, at the present stage of dissection, is a nightmare of words and a jungle of nerves. This is because the autonomic nervous system is widespread throughout the body, and rarely is there a region of the body to be dissected in which there is no evidence of the autonomic nervous system. Therefore, be patient — when you have completed dissection of the body is the time for you to study the autonomic nervous system more comprehensively. Then you will realize that the autonomic nervous system is, in fact, a very well organized system, and one that is easy to understand.

ITEM 14-11. Intercostal neurovascular structures

Select a conveniently located intercostal space to demonstrate how an intercostal vein, artery, and nerve assemble at the vertebral end of the space.

Consider the relationship to pleura and note how they lie horizontal in the space which is sloping inferiorly and laterally. Accordingly the neurovascular structures soon reach the "shelter" of the rib above; this point you can soon verify by removing innermost intercostal muscle as far laterally as the angle of the rib.

In practice, these findings mean that in paracentesis thoracis (tapping or needling the pleural cavity) the clinician inserts his needle at the angle or beyond the angle of the rib where he knows the precise location of intervening neurovascular structures. It must be clear to you, however, that the choice of site for a paracentesis depends, without question, on the site of the abnormal fluid. Relate your findings to what was said on p. 21.

REFERENCES

Davidson, L. S. P.: The Principles and Practice of Medicine. 8th Ed. Edinburgh, E. & S. Livingstone Ltd., 1966.

Fulton, W. F. M.: The Coronary Arteries. Springfield, Ill., Charles C Thomas, 1965.

Grant, J. C. B.: An Atlas of Anatomy. Baltimore, Williams & Wilkins Co., 1962.

Hudson, R. E. B.: Cardiovascular Pathology. London, Edward Arnold Publishers Ltd., 1965.

Leeson, C. R., and Leeson, T. S.: Histology. Philadelphia, W. B. Saunders Co., 1966.

Lockhart, R. D., Hamilton, G. F., and Fyfe, F. W.: Anatomy of the Human Body. London, Faber & Faber Ltd., 1959.

PART 3

ABDOMEN

Chapter 15

Introduction to the Abdomen

The Contents of the Abdomen

The peritoneal cavity

The gastrointestinal tract, which includes the abdominal part of the esophagus, the stomach, duodenum, small bowel, large bowel, and vermiform appendix

The liver

The biliary system

The spleen

The pancreas

The suprarenal glands

The kidneys

The ureters

The major blood vessels, including the lymphatics

The sympathetic chain

The pelvic organs, female and male, that lie in the pelvis and are seen from the abdomen

It is possible to reach any of these structures by appropriate incisions through the abdominal wall.

The Layers of the Abdominal Wall

Skin

Superficial fascia, which may be abundant

Muscles and aponeuroses

Transversalis fascia

The parietal layer of peritoneum. This layer is not regarded by everyone as a layer of the abdominal wall. Nevertheless it adheres to the deep surface of the abdominal wall and is taken into consideration in every surgical incision through the abdominal wall.

The Extent of the Abdominal Wall

When the beginner is asked to demonstrate what he believes to be the extent of the abdominal wall, he usually indicates an area no greater than a handbreadth across the front of his belly. Therefore, one of the first lessons to be learned in this very important area is how extensive the abdominal wall really is, because, in clinical practice, the clue to a difficult diagnosis may not be found until the entire abdominal wall has been carefully examined. As a first step toward appreciating the entire abdominal wall, the description of the following subdivisions of the wall should be read with a skeleton in view. Next, the subdivisions should be identified as far as possible on the cadaver, and on yourself at some convenient time.

The Subdivisions of the Abdominal Wall

The anterior abdominal wall
The right and left loins, also known as flanks
The posterior abdominal wall
The diaphragm, superiorly
The pelvic inlet and the right and left iliac bones, inferiorly

It must be emphasized that these walls are continuous with each other. There are no rigid boundaries between them, except for descriptive purposes.

Exercise

On a skeleton, identify the boundaries of the various subdivisions. The anterior abdominal wall is bounded on each side by a vertical line through the anterior superior iliac spine, superiorly by the right and left costal margins, and inferiorly by a line connecting each anterior superior iliac spine to the symphysis pubis. A line joining the xiphisternum to the symphysis pubis indicates the position of the linea alba, a fibrous white line that divides the anterior abdominal wall into right and left sides.

The posterior abdominal wall (See Figs. 17-3 and 17-5) is bounded on each side by a vertical line through the tip of the twelfth rib, superiorly by both twelfth ribs, and inferiorly by the crests of the pelvis. In the midline, observe the position of the bodies of the twelfth thoracic and the five lumbar vertebrae. That they jut so far forward (they are almost midway between the skin of the back and front) may escape you, yet this protrusion must be noted in order to understand the true position of the viscera on the posterior abdominal wall. In the more detailed description of the posterior abdominal wall (p. 140), the vertebrae are likened to a steep mountain range between two broad valleys.

On each side the flank (or loin) extends from the anterior boundary of the posterior abdominal wall to the posterior boundary of the anterior abdominal wall. Superiorly the flank is bounded by the costal margin, inferiorly by the iliac crest. Usually the distance between the costal margin above and the iliac crest below is very short. On the other hand, the anteroposterior distance of the flank is considerable, even in a person of slender build.

Superiorly, the abdomen is limited by the diaphragm (Fig. 15-1), an extensive dome-shaped sheet of muscle extending anteroposteriorly from the sternum to the vertebral column and from one side of the rib cage to the other. The dome of the diaphragm is level with the xiphisternal junction.

Inferiorly, the boundary is the pelvic inlet. The margin of the inlet, from the symphysis pubis to the sacral promontory, is on an oblique plane, posteroinferior to which is the true pelvic cavity, and through which the abdominal and pelvic cavities are in continuity (Fig. 15-1). On each side of the inlet the fan-shaped iliac bones complete the inferior boundaries.

Before proceeding to investigate the anterior abdominal wall and the right and left loins, the student must become familiar with the bony landmarks mentioned in this introductory section.

SKIN

Read the general account of skin and fascia (Chapters 1 and 2). The lymphatic drainage of the abdominal wall (this includes the skin of the flanks, the posterior abdominal wall, and the anterior abdominal wall) is toward the superficial nodes in each axilla and groin. Venous blood drains into tributaries of either the superior or inferior vena cava. The arterial supply of the skin of the abdominal wall comes from widely dispersed sources put arbitrarily into three groups, proximal, central,

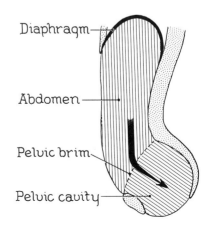

Figure 15-1. Lateral view. The arrow above the change in direction from the abdomen to the pelvis.

Diaphragm

Abdomen

Pelvic brim

Pelvic cavity

and distal, relative to the main arterial stem or system. The proximal group of vessels arises essentially from each of the subclavian and axillary arteries; the central group, namely the paired intercostal and lumbar arteries, arises in a segmental fashion from the thoracic and abdominal descending aorta; the distal group, namely the inferior epigastric and superficial circumflex iliac arteries, arises from the junction of the external iliac and femoral arteries on each side. The nerve supply of the skin has a segmental pattern that will be understood by the student if he reads an account of a typical spinal nerve and its branches.

UMBILICUS

The umbilicus is small but it is not unimportant. To be seen later are several fibrous connections between the posterior surface of the umbilicus and each internal iliac artery, the liver, the bladder, and sometimes the small bowel. These fibrous structures were, in their embryologic development, hollow tubular structures; the connections to bladder and to bowel may remain hollow and patent throughout their length after birth. Sometimes at birth the parietal peritoneum protrudes into the umbilicus to become the sac of an umbilical hernia.

Clinicians have found that the so-called obliterated umbilical vein, between the umbilicus and the liver, is usually patent but, although it is patent, it does not contain blood. It can be dilated to admit a 6 or 7 mm. probe, and, after pushing to overcome a narrowing or a valve mechanism in the liver substance, a catheter the size of a pencil can be passed through into the portal vein. This procedure may be used as a simple method of measuring the portal venous pressure and a means of introducing dyes for venography. Blood does not leak out once the tube is removed.

SUPERFICIAL FASCIA

This fascia is often loaded with fat to a depth of several inches. Fortunately for the dissector, the presence of some excess fat makes easier the demonstration of a membranous layer that reinforces its deep surface. Accordingly, two layers, a fatty layer, and a membranous layer can be identified but rarely, if ever, separated. At this point, to avoid confusion, the student is reminded that these two layers are in the superficial fascia.

Between the membranous layer and the deep fascia, in the experience of the practicing surgeon, thin people have a little loose areolar tissue and fat people larger and more loosely held lobules of fat. The membranous layer is better defined in certain areas where it can be approximated accurately with sutures, but it is demonstrable all over the abdominal wall.

Certain limits or boundaries to the membranous layer are described. Superiorly and laterally on the abdominal wall its limits are indefinite, while inferiorly, well-defined limits can be identified and are shown in Figure 15-2. The fascia is adherent to the deep fascia of the thigh along the line XC and horizontally across the perineum at CC. The same layer of fascia invests the scrotum and penis, hence the orifices shown in Figure 15-2*A*. If the student has difficulty in understanding this layout, it may be of some help to liken the fascia to the front of a swimsuit (Fig. 15-2*B*). Of course, the front of the swimsuit, representing fascia, must be fashioned to invest the penis and scrotum.

It may be many years before the student sees why it is important to know the arrangement of the superficial fascia of the anterior abdominal wall. Nevertheless, he should satisfy himself now that deep to the membranous layer of fascia is a potential space in which fluid can accumulate. That fluid is usually urine, which passes through a rupture of the membranous urethra (p. 172). This state of affairs is spoken of clinically as extravasation of urine.

DEEP FASCIA

Little need be said of the deep fascia on the abdominal wall because it is practically nonexistent. One point, however, will be discussed later, and that is how the deep fascia forms one of the coverings for the spermatic cord.

ITEM 15-1.   Dissection of Skin and Fascia (Fig. 15-3)

Examine the skin of the abdominal wall for scars from surgery or from injury. If any are present, the dissectors can expect abnormal findings within the abdomen or pelvis.

Even though the cadaver may be extremely old, examine the pubic hair and its distribution. In endocrine disorders involving the repro-

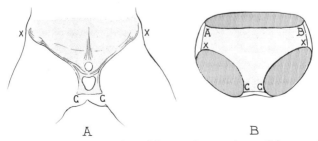

A   B

Figure 15-2. *A* is a representation of the membranous layer of the superficial fascia. *B* is a swimsuit. The front piece, AxccxB, is a visualization of the membranous layer which is fashioned to invest the penis and scrotum.

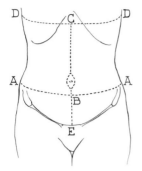

Figure 15-3. Skin incisions. For further explanation see text.

ductive system the presence or absence of pubic (and axillary) hair, and its quality and amount, must be noted and recorded.

Incise skin and superficial fascia at point A (Fig. 15-3) until the muscle fibers of the external oblique are exposed. Extend the incision medially to B. Check carefully that the incision has not penetrated either the muscle fibers or the aponeurosis of the external oblique. Continue the incision to C and then to D. Flap ABCD can now be reflected back as far as the vertebral column, *but* only at a depth that will safeguard the latissimus dorsi, serratus anterior, and trapezius muscles, which will be displayed more extensively later.

From A to A, demonstrate the potential space between the membranous layer of the superficial fascia and the external oblique muscles.

Reflect flap A B A as far as possible. It will be necessary to make a cut B E so that A B E may be reflected far enough to expose the external spermatic fascia surrounding the spermatic cord (or the round ligament in the female). Do not disturb the spermatic fascia.

Slide a finger gently downward along the cord and fascia, toward the scrotum, and demonstrate the superficial inguinal pouch. When the testis retracts, especially in infants exposed to cold, the testis comes to lie in this pouch deep to the membranous layer of fascia and external to the superficial inguinal ring. To demonstrate the adhesion of the membranous layer of fascia to the deep fascia of the thigh (XC in Fig. 15-2), slide the finger laterally from the superficial inguinal pouch.

Remove as much skin and accompanying fascia as possible.

THE MUSCLES AND APONEUROSIS OF THE ANTERIOR ABDOMINAL WALL, EXCLUDING THE INGUINAL REGION

The combination of muscle and aponeurosis forming the anterior abdominal wall (Fig. 15-4) affords considerable protection to the abdominal viscera, especially when the muscles are in trim. In addition to being a natural barrier, however, the muscles and aponeurosis may also

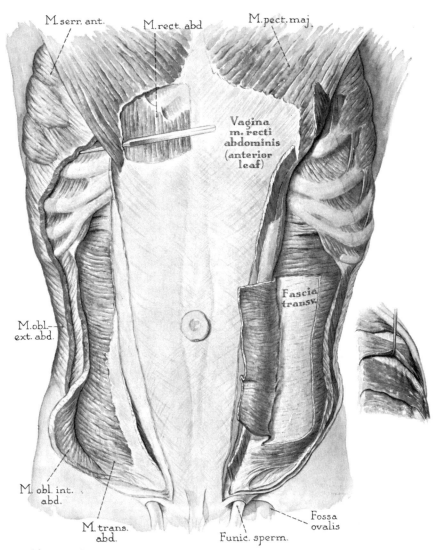

Figure 15-4. Third layer of lateral abdominal musculature. On reader's right the transverse abdominal muscle has been reflected to expose internal investing (transversalis) fascia. On left, anterior leaf of rectus sheath on one side has been partially removed (From B. J. Anson: Atlas of Human Anatomy. 2nd Ed. W. B. Saunders Co., 1963.)

be described as an extensive surgical barrier. Accordingly, numerous incisions through the wall have been described; a few of those incisions are employed here. But it is much more important to stress to the beginner that increased tone or spasm of the abdominal muscles is significant in certain acute abdominal conditions, and that this change can be detected by unhurried methodical inspection and gentle palpation of the anterior abdominal wall. Indeed, one measure of clinical perfection is the evidence that the practitioner can obtain on inspection and palpation of the abdominal muscles in a patient who has acute abdominal pain, a condition known clinically as acute abdomen. Later in your career, clinical tutors will instruct you in the precise technique of examining an acute abdomen, but, even at this stage, it is helpful to know that the abdominal muscles contract in certain acute abdominal conditions. However, they also contract when the upper and lower parts of the body are under the influence of gravity; that topic is dealt with next.

Action of the Abdominal Muscles, Gravity, and Rigidity

Normal muscle tone of the abdominal muscles plays an important part in the movements of the vertebral column as well as of the pelvis. The muscles are concerned with three basic movements, flexion forward, flexion to the side, and rotation of the trunk, all to be discussed more fully in the section on the vertebral column.

There is a tendency to underestimate the influence of gravity upon the action of the abdominal muscles. Gravity is particularly influential when the body is supine and the head or the legs are raised from the horizontal. Then the abdominal muscles contract and the abdominal wall presents a boardlike rigidity to the examining hand. In a normal person, such rigidity will diminish or disappear entirely when the head and the lower limbs are set at rest in a slightly flexed position and the upper limbs are at ease beside the body.

But, even when these requirements are fulfilled and the patient is relaxed, the abdominal muscles may remain rigid. If the rigidity is indeed involuntary, then the patient's condition must be considered abnormal until proven otherwise, for such rigidity usually signifies an underlying acute pathological intraabdominal disorder.

Movement of the Abdominal Wall

In life, quiet rhythmic movements of the abdominal wall, accompanying the respirations, are readily seen. When the diaphragm contracts to increase the dimensions of the thoracic cage, the diaphragm moves down ("down" is, indeed, an oversimplification of a complex movement). To accommodate the viscera, the abdominal wall moves out. This "down and out" movement is frequently inspected in clinical medicine, for example, in anesthesia in which the degree of diaphragmatic respiratory movement is particularly important.

THE ANTERIOR ABDOMINAL WALL AS A WHOLE

On inspection of the anterior abdominal wall, the central feature is often the pair of vertically disposed rectus abdominis muscles (Fig. 15-5). Their strength and visibility varies from person to person, but when they are strong they are conspicuous, their outline creating an aura of manliness even when they are at rest. Thus, a powerful pair of rectus abdominis muscles has long been a symbol of strength, exploited to the utmost extent by the weight lifter and recognized long since by the sculptor. Michelangelo, in his statue of David, carved in bold relief the linea semilunaris, which is the lateral margin of the rectus abdominis muscle as seen through the skin, and he gouged across the upper half of each muscle the tendinous intersections that are particularly well seen in a lean male (Fig. 15-5).

Each rectus abdominis muscle is enclosed in an aponeurotic sheath, and each sheath is incorporated into an extensive aponeurosis that occupies the central area of the anterior abdominal wall (Fig. 15-6). The anatomy of the rectus sheath is easily studied by dissection and need not be described further.

The extensive central aponeurosis is really composed of three pairs of aponeuroses (Fig. 15-6) more or less adherent to each other, and the strength of the entire central aponeurosis is due in large measure to this arrangement. An aponeurosis is a fairly tough sheet of tissue; it splits easily one way only because its fibers run parallel to each other. In the anterior abdominal wall, the direction of the fibers of each aponeurosis

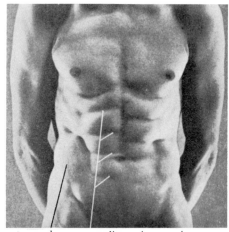

Figure 15-5. Muscles of abdominal wall 'set'. Note the fullness of external oblique bulging over the groove of the groin. (From R. D. Lockhart: Living Anatomy. London, Faber & Faber Ltd., 1963.)

external
oblique

tendinous intersections
of rectus abdominis

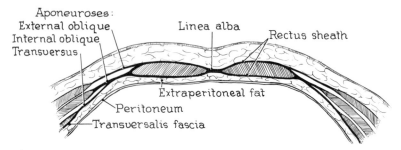

Figure 15-6. Schematic cross section of the anterior abdominal wall. For further description see text.

is different. Thus, the criss-cross of fibers that occurs when the three aponeuroses are in their anatomic position gives strength to the entire aponeurosis.

The criss-cross of fibers is particularly obvious in the midline, where the aponeuroses from the right and left sides meet and fuse to form the linea alba (Fig. 15-6). When the student cuts the linea alba he will appreciate that it is indeed an interlacement of aponeurotic fibers approaching the midline from different directions. The linea alba is a solitary central slender zone between the medial borders of the rectus sheaths and extending from the xiphoid process to the symphysis pubis. Above the umbilicus the linea alba is about 2 cm. wide, while below the umbilicus it is so narrow that the two rectus muscles are adjacent.

It has already been said that each of the three aponeuroses that contribute to the formation of the central aponeurosis is a bilateral structure. When each aponeurosis is traced laterally, it is found to be continuous with one of the three bilateral flat abdominal muscles, the external oblique, the internal oblique, or the transversus abdominis. Accordingly, the three aponeuroses have been named the external oblique aponeurosis, the internal oblique aponeurosis, and the transversus abdominis aponeurosis (Fig. 15-6).

The three flat abdominal muscles occupy the flank and span the interval between the posterior abdominal wall, the rib cage, and the pelvis. Their names indicate the direction of their fibers, but the student will soon see that the direction of the fibers in each muscle is not constant, for the direction changes at certain levels, so that, for example, some of the fibers of the internal oblique muscle become horizontal in direction.

In summary, the anterior abdominal wall consists of muscle and aponeurosis. The linea alba is a solitary central aponeurotic strip flanked by the broad rectus sheaths enclosing the vertically disposed rectus abdominis muscles, which extend from the pubic bones to the rib cage. On the lateral side of each rectus sheath is the fringe of the central aponeurotic area, and beyond that fringe lie the three flat abdominal muscles extending into the flank.

In this introduction a deliberate effort has been made to make the student view the anterior abdominal wall as a complete structure because it is believed that this will aid him considerably in examining the anterior abdominal wall of his patients. It must be pointed out, however, that it is much easier to describe an abdominal muscle and its aponeurosis or sheath in the singular, not the plural, and that is how it is done in all standard texts. The textbooks of surgery the student will use in his clinical years dwell briefly on the origins and the insertions of each of the abdominal muscles.

Transversalis Fascia

Although the transversalis fascia is not taken into consideration in routine abdominal incisions, it is quite a definite layer found laterally and posteriorly deep to the muscular part of transversus abdominis. The transversalis fascia is of great importance in the inguinal region, which is dealt with on p. 98.

ABDOMINAL INCISIONS

There are many incisions used to penetrate the abdominal wall; the location of each incision depends on the organ to be reached and the extent of the operation to be performed. In choosing an incision, the following are taken into account: the direction of muscle fibers (it is often possible to separate muscle fibers rather than cut across them), the locality of aponeurotic fibers (Fig. 15-7), and the position of nerves (cutting a nerve will paralyze the muscle fibers supplied by that nerve and so weaken the abdominal wall). The relationship of the organ to peritoneum also influences the decision, as does the personal choice of the surgeon, influenced by his range of experience. Many surgeons believe that transverse incisions anywhere in the abdomen surpass vertical incisions because transverse incisions can be made in the upper, mid, or lower abdomen, or laterally, and still lie more or less parallel to the fibers of the aponeuroses. Cutting across the rectus muscle transversely merely creates another tendinous intersection and does not weaken the muscle; such an incision can be closed more securely because there is less tendency for the sutures to cut out.

Posterior abdominal wall structures, the kidney, for example, are usually approached through an oblique incision across the loin. When you explore the peritoneal cavity, you will see how it is possible to reach the kidney and other posterior abdominal wall structures through the loin without opening the peritoneum. Unfortunately, this important in-

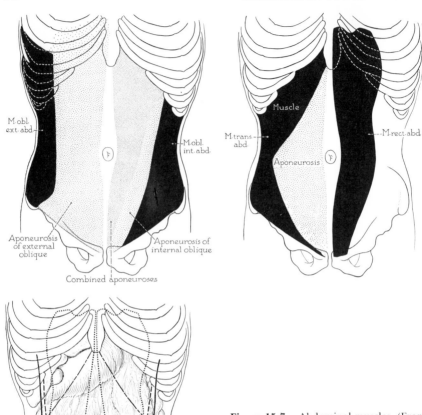

Figure 15-7. Abdominal muscles. (From B. J. Anson: Atlas of Human Anatomy. 2nd ed. W. B. Saunders Co., 1963.)

cision in its exact form does not fit in with our total plan, but the student can still glean its basic form when he comes to Item 15-7.

Commonly, incisions through the anterior abdominal wall are made through the linea alba, through the rectus sheath, and along the costal margin. These incisions are now to be made on the cadaver and, in addition, the student will have the opportunity to practice a gridiron incision, probably the most frequently used incision of all.

ITEM 15-2. Median Incision

First of all, deep to the linea alba lies parietal peritoneum, except in grossly obese specimens, in whom extraperitoneal fat and fascia are plentiful. Therefore, incise the linea alba with care.

A median incision may be made above the umbilicus or below. When the incision is made below the umbilicus, the narrowness of the linea alba must be kept in mind. In the present dissection, in order to safeguard the median umbilical ligament (p. 93), incise the linea alba from the umbilicus to the xiphoid process. In doing so, note the rasping sound indicative of the stringy nature of the linea alba, which is in fact an interlacement of tough aponeurotic fibers lacking both nerve and vessel. The lack of these structures is one reason for the use of this midline incision. Look out for extraperitoneal fat and even a sac of parietal peritoneum, which may penetrate the linea alba between its interlacing fibers, especially in the region of the umbilicus.

In the cadaver it is nearly certain that the parietal peritoneum will be incised when the linea alba is incised. If this mishap has not occurred, incise parietal peritoneum to open the peritoneal cavity (see p. 83). The full extent of the cavity will be explored later, when the entire anterior abdominal wall has been reflected. Meanwhile, review the incision and identify the cut edges of parietal peritoneum. They must be sewn together after a surgical procedure in order to close the peritoneal cavity (p. 83).

ITEM 15-3. Paramedian Incision

On each side, identify the anterior lamina of the rectus sheath. To open the sheath, make an incision parallel to and 1 inch from the midline between rib cage and pelvis. Identify the intersections of the rectus abdominis, and then retract the muscle fibers laterally, toward the lateral border of the rectus sheath where neurovascular structures are entering. Having retracted the muscle laterally and exposed the posterior lamina of the rectus sheath, or having at least grasped the method for doing so, cut across and reflect the rectus muscle in order to gain a more extensive exposure of the posterior lamina.

Note the relationship of the lateral edge of the rectus muscle to a vertical line through the pubic tubercle, especially near the tubercle. Observe the density of the posterior layer of the rectus sheath. It is usually most marked in its intermediate part. Superiorly, the rectus muscle fibers are directly related to the rib cage and to muscle fibers of the transversus abdominis. Inferiorly, the posterior lamina is also deficient below the arcuate line. The line will vary from cadaver to cadaver, not only in its height above the symphysis pubis but also in its perceptibility. Below the line the transversalis fascia completes the posterior lamina of the rectus sheath.

ITEM 15-4. Identify the superior and inferior epigastric vessels. The former is a branch from the proximal part of the arterial tree, and the latter is from the distal part; they form a significant anastomosis.

Make a small cut through the posterior layer of the rectus sheath. Open the peritoneal cavity. How would you close the cavity?

ITEM 15-5. Right Iliac Gridiron Incision

On the right side split the external oblique aponeurosis in the line of its fibers. Separate the edges enough to see the fibers of the internal oblique. Do not be surprised to find that they are transverse at this level. Thrust scissors into the fibers, open the scissors wide enough to separate the fibers. A thin layer of fascia may be identified deep to the internal oblique and superficial to the transversus. Proceed beyond this fascia by thrusting deeper still before opening the scissors, until the transversalis fascia and extraperitoneal fat appear. Then open the peritoneal cavity. In a cadaver there will be difficulty because the tissues are so stiff, but the student should persevere in order to learn the principle of one of the commonest incisions in abdominal surgery.

ITEM 15-6. Paracostal Incisions

At AB and AC (Fig. 15-8), incise along the costal margins. In cutting towards the right, the falciform ligament of the liver will be encountered and must be cut. Identify muscle and aponeurotic layers and observe that neurovascular bundles are sacrificed. Deliberately cut the parietal peritoneum.

ITEM 15-7. Removal of Abdominal Musculature and Underlying Parietal Peritoneum

Extend incisions AB and AC along the costal margin as far posteriorly as the midaxillary line. Do not cut beyond the ascending and descending colon, in order to preserve the paracolic gutters to be studied later. Continue each incision down to the crest of the ilium; the subcostal, iliohypogastric, and ilioinguinal nerves will be cut. Continue the incision anteriorly toward the tubercle on the iliac crest. A large flap has now been made. Turn the flap down and identify the structures attached to the umbilicus.

An extensive view of the peritoneal cavity is now available. Before the cavity is explored, the following account of peritoneum must be thoroughly absorbed.

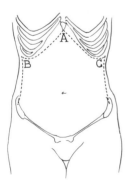

Figure 15-8.   Right and left paracostal muscle incisions and their extensions inferiorly to open widely the peritoneal cavity of a cadaver.

Chapter 16

The Peritoneal Cavity

Now that the student has a clear view of the peritoneum, he can appreciate that it is a thin membrane providing a lining to the interior of the abdominal wall as well as a covering to viscera. But he may not appreciate that the peritoneum he sees lining the abdominal wall and on the viscera are parts of the same continuous sheet. How that comes about will be explained in a simplified manner that nonetheless conveys a true basic concept of peritoneum. Then the student must take time to explore the intact peritoneal cavity thoroughly or as best he can in an embalmed cadaver.

Embalming hardens structures that are normally soft and that adapt to pressure. The fresh sheep's liver, for example, lies flat upon the slab. After embalming, the hardened liver becomes a major obstacle to exploration of the superior regions of the peritoneal cavity in the cadaver. Thus it will not be easy to reach into deeper parts of the peritoneal cavity, but it can be done. Furthermore, the nature of peritoneum changes with death and with embalming so that it tears more easily. Indeed, for a proper concept of the peritoneum, the student ought to see the viscera of the body at operation or at autopsy. If neither of these opportunities is available, the entrails of an animal can be seen in an experimental laboratory.

Two Basic Principles

In Figure 16-1, the fundamental principles of the peritoneal cavity are illustrated. In Figure 16-1*A*, a finger has invaginated a balloon without breaking the continuity of its internal surface. Note that the internal surface remains unbroken, but note particularly that this is also true in Figure 16-1*B*, although several fingers have invaginated the balloon, one of them quite deeply. The dotted lines in *A* and *B* reemphasize the continuous nature of the internal surface of the balloon and illustrate the first fundamental principle of the peritoneal cavity as follows: No matter how complex the form of the peritoneal cavity may seem, *its surface is continuous.* Thus one may trace a path from a certain point inside the balloon in Figure 16-1*A* or *B*, travel in any direction over the internal surface, and return to the point of departure, without losing contact with the surface. In the course of your dissection of the peritoneal cavity, try it and prove it.

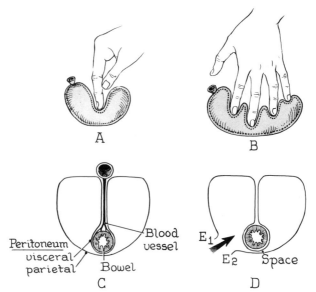

Figure 16-1.   The basic principle of the peritoneal cavity. (See text.)

Some organs invaginate the peritoneal cavity to such a degree that they are almost wholly but never totally surrounded by peritoneum (Fig. 16-1C). There must be a channel through which neurovascular and lymphatic structures can reach or leave the organ (Fig. 16-1C). To reach their destination, these structures must skirt the cavity until they find a place of entry. *Nothing passes through the peritoneal cavity.* This second fundamental principle, just stated, must also be borne in mind constantly, because the peritoneal cavity is in fact much more complex than has been demonstrated so far in simple diagrams. Nevertheless, the principles outlined so far are constant, and this the student will soon demonstrate to his own conviction.

Total Area

Infection of the peritoneum (peritonitis) is very serious and can be fatal. Aware of this possibility, doctors regard peritoneum with great respect, if not with awe. Even so, one must not underestimate the great powers of the peritoneum to resist infection and overcome gross contamination with bacteria, provided the contamination is not continuous.

The total area of peritoneum, 2 square meters, the area of one side of a door, provides sufficient surface for the absorption of certain drugs, and, alas, of lethal toxins. Warm, moist, and virtually anaerobic, the 2 square meters of peritoneum may become a vast medium for the culture of bacteria if a hollow organ perforates and its contents escape onto the peritoneum. In studying the peritoneum, make a list of all the hollow organs related to the peritoneal cavity and the nature of their contents. Proceeding from the esophagus, and including the biliary system, the urinary system, and such embryologic structure as Meckel's diverticulum, and finally the rectum, the student will make an impressive list. Perforation of a hollow organ through its peritoneal surface can be deadly.

Capacity

Furthermore, the peritoneal cavity can hold large quantities of fluid or air. Often, in disease, liters of fluid fill the cavity. But more urgently, a vascular structure may rupture through its peritoneal surface and spill several pints of blood into the cavity. Not a drop of this blood lost from the circulation is seen by the eye; without medical aid death will probably follow. Table 16-1, showing several vascular structures with their minute volume of blood, demonstrates how profuse the loss of blood might be.

In addition, rupture of an ectopic pregnancy in a uterine tube may cause a hemorrhage and, rarely, the uterus itself may rupture in pregnancy. As you identify these vascular structures in their embalmed state, remember that their solidity is unlike their state in life. In addition to these large vascular structures the student will find many major arteries and veins partially or wholly covered by peritoneum. They too may bleed into the peritoneal cavity with disastrous results.

Pancreas

It is not readily appreciated by the uninitiated that the pancreas has an extensive relationship to the peritoneal cavity. But it does, and abnormal leakage of its digestive enzymes through peritoneum into the cavity may cause serious harm.

Table 16-1. *Blood Circulation/Minute to the Liver, Spleen, and Kidneys*

STRUCTURE	WEIGHT	CIRCULATION/MINUTE
Liver	1500	1500
Spleen	170	200
Kidneys	330	1300
	2000 g.	3000 ml.

SUMMARY

In the present context, it is apparent that the abdominal organs related to the peritoneal cavity have been put into three groups, namely:

(1) Hollow organs — prone to perforate.

(2) Blood-filled structures — born to bleed.

(3) Solid organs — likely to leak.

How to deal with the wide range of clinical conditions arbitrarily put into one of the three groups will be dealt with in clinical surgery. They are introduced here simply to draw attention to the peritoneal cavity, a vast and sinister void, so easily overlooked by the beginner in his eagerness to tear through peritoneum to get at some structure or other.

Relationship of Organ to Organ

When an organ is covered partly or wholly by peritoneum it is related primarily to the peritoneal cavity. Across the cavity it will be related to other organs covered by peritoneum. In other words, the peritoneal cavity intervenes. It is common practice, however, to take the peritoneal cavity for granted and to say, for example, that the gallbladder is related to the transverse colon. Indeed, they are adjacent, but the peritoneal cavity lies between them. There are many such examples. In the end, it is permissible to adopt the common practice of omitting peritoneum, provided the student knows that the presence of the peritoneal cavity is implicit in a statement such as "the small bowel is related to the urinary bladder."

Pouches

Figure 16-1B shows also how pouches can occur. No matter how inaccessible a pouch seems to be, the student can demonstrate that there is no break in the continuity of the peritoneal surface and that a pouch is merely an extension of the peritoneal cavity. A pouch acts as a sump for fluid and as a trap for the unwary, who might leave behind instruments, sometimes large instruments, concealed in the depth of a pouch. Thus at a surgical operation, while the peritoneum cavity is open, everything brought into the operating field is accounted for before the cavity is closed, and often rubber drains are brought from the depths of a pouch to the skin surface.

Visceral and Parietal Peritoneum

The peritoneum on the surface of an organ is termed visceral peritoneum, whereas parietal peritoneum describes peritoneum lining the body wall. However, the student should not seek to define these terms too precisely because when he is in practice he will say simply "peritoneum." Peritoneum on the surface of an organ is closely applied to the organ; indeed, it is almost impossible to distinguish the thin layer of peritoneum except by its shine. The space between that layer of peritoneum and the layer on the body wall is minimal (Fig. 16-1*D*), and contains a thin film of fluid to allow mobile organs to slide easily upon each other.

Opening and Closing of the Peritoneum

The student may already know the meaning of the terms opening and closing the peritoneum. They are defined here because they are used every day in operating rooms, and the medical student must become familiar with them. *To open* the peritoneum, the parietal peritoneum lining the muscular wall has to be incised (Fig. 16-1*D*). It must surely be apparent that in the cavity the surgeon's hands are separated from an organ by a layer of peritoneum (see the arrow in Fig. 16-1*D*). *To close* the peritoneum, edges E_1 and E_2 are brought together and sutured.

Peritoneal Cavity in the Female

Most of the female reproductive viscera are covered by peritoneum. The peritoneal surface of the ovary differs histologically from the rest of the peritoneum. As a result of this difference, one may debate at length whether or not the ovary is in the peritoneal cavity. Suffice it to say that when the ovum is shed it enters the peritoneal cavity. Probable mechanical and chemotactic influences bring the ovum to the opening of the uterine tube, through which it leaves the peritoneal cavity. Thus, on each side of the female pelvis there is a small opening in the peritoneal cavity not only serving to transmit an ovum, but also sometimes allowing infection from the outside to reach the peritoneal cavity via the reproductive tract.

Nerve Supply of the Peritoneum

Consult reference books for more detailed accounts of this nerve supply. Essentially, visceral peritoneum is poorly innervated by the autonomic nervous system. Accordingly, when visceral peritoneum is stimulated, the pain experienced is vague and hard to define, but real to the patient. Personal experience testifies how real this pain can be. On the other hand, parietal peritoneum is supplied by the somatic nerves, and when it is stimulated the pain can often, but not always, be located to a precise part of the body wall (*soma*—Greek for *body*).

Examination of the Peritoneum

In an acute abdominal illness, the peritoneum is examined by gentle manual pressure on the abdominal wall. But, in addition, pressure can be exerted on peritoneum through the wall of the rectum or vagina (per rectum or per vaginam). Often, pelvic examination may clinch the decision in a difficult diagnosis and cannot be omitted from the examination of an acute abdomen. The student will have the opportunity to perform rectal and vaginal examinations when he dissects the pelvis.

Parts of the peritoneum have names not mentioned so far. Terms such as greater sac, lesser sac, mesentery, omentum, gutter, ligament, space, and retroperitoneal will be explained by demonstration in the course of dissection.

Chapter 17

Exploration of the Peritoneum

ITEM 17-1. Identify the greater omentum. It is a vascular structure, often fat-laden, suspended from the stomach and transverse colon. Its normal shape is like an apron (see anatomic illustrations) draped in front of the small intestine. Its free (unattached) margin, with right, lower, and left edges, should suggest to you that it is a mobile structure. Indeed it is. At operation it is found bunched around a source of infection, perhaps an inflamed gallbladder or appendix; it is usually the first and most conspicuous structure met upon opening the peritoneum, but in the cadaver it may well be shriveled and dry, and sometimes seems to be absent.

ITEM 17-2. Identify the stomach, which will be considered more carefully later, and observe the lesser omentum, a loose lacelike sheet of peritoneum between the stomach and the liver.

ITEM 17-3. To reveal the transverse colon, cast the greater omentum over the costal margin. Figure 17-1 shows why this maneuver is necessary. The greater omentum, attached to the anterior aspect of the transverse colon, hides the colon and its mesentery. The maneuver described here exposes the inferior surface of this mesentery. Figure 17-1 shows why its superior surface cannot be exposed without dissection.

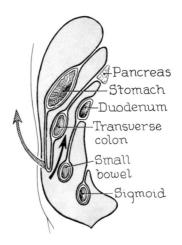

Figure 17-1. Schematic sagittal section of the peritoneal cavity. The black arrow indicates the relationship of the infracolic compartments to the greater omentum and transverse colon and the mesocolon. The compartments are exposed only when the greater omentum is pulled upward over the costal margins.

THE SUPRA- AND INFRACOLIC COMPARTMENTS

The mesentery of the transverse colon (*mesocolon* is the abbreviated term) droops across the abdomen and, for descriptive purposes, is used to divide the peritoneal cavity into supracolic and infracolic compartments (Fig. 17-2). The infracolic compartment is divided into right and left parts by the mesentery of the small bowel (Fig. 17-2). Before studying these compartments, study the mesentery of the small bowel.

ITEM 17-4. Identify the root of the mesentery of the small bowel attached obliquely across the posterior abdominal wall. The length of this attachment is only 15 cm. (Fig. 17-2), whereas the small bowel itself is 700 cm. long. Thus the mesentery narrows dramatically from a length of 700 cm. to one of 15 cm., and this explains its fluted appearance. Between its root and the bowel the mesentery measures 15 to 25 cm. The area of the mesentery, on the basis of these measurements, must be at least 1 square meter. Because of its shape and attachment, the mesentery is more mobile from side to side (i.e., right superior to left inferior and vice versa) than from superior to inferior (i.e., left superior to right inferior and vice versa). Confirm this statement. Take heed of the mesentery. Within the cadaver it is readily seen; within the patient it is often forgotten, yet the astute clinician can tell that an obscure lump he is palpating is in fact in the mesentery.

ITEM 17-5. The Peritoneal Cavity

The student now has the opportunity to confirm the three fundamental facts concerning the peritoneal cavity.

First, to confirm the continuity of the peritoneal surface, place a finger on one or the other surface of the mesentery. Keeping contact with that surface, slide the finger laterally in a horizontal direction. The finger will slide across the posterior abdominal wall, then across the peri-

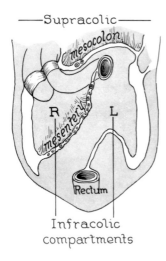

——Supracolic——

Infracolic
compartments

Figure 17-2. The mesocolon divides the peritoneal cavity into a supracolic compartment and an infracolic compartment. The mesentery divides the infracolic compartment into right and left infracolic compartments.

toneum lining the flank, on to the peritoneum, first of the anterior abdominal wall, then of the other flank, until, reaching the other side of the mesentery, the finger surmounts the small bowel to return to the point of departure.

Second, to confirm that in a mesentery neurovascular and lymphatic structures lie between two sheets of peritoneum, proceed as follows: Place an index finger on each side of the mesentery at its attachment. Slide the fingers toward the bowel. Between the fingers are two sheets of peritoneum, and between the layers of peritoneum are the structures going to and from the bowel. Thus a mesentery consists of two sheets of peritoneum suspending an organ from the posterior abdominal wall (Fig. 17-2). Note that the mesocolon has a similar plan. To confirm the presence of the neurovascular and lymphatic structures in the mesentery tear away some of the peritoneum from both aspects of the mesentery.

Third, to confirm the existence of two openings into the cavity, examine the right and left uterine tubes and the fimbriae of a female cadaver. When the fimbriae are pulled gently apart it should be possible to see and to probe a tiny opening (the abdominal ostium) connecting the peritoneal cavity and the infundibulum of the uterine tube. Female cadavers are uncommon in the dissecting laboratory, so do this at a time convenient to your colleagues. In elderly specimens the tissues may be shrunken and far from their normal state.

ITEM 17-6. Examination of the Infracolic Compartments

These compartments are exposed when the greater omentum, taking with it the transverse colon, is pulled well up over the costal margin.

Outline the triangular shape of the right compartment (Fig. 17-2), bounded on the left by the mesentery, on the right by the ascending colon, and superiorly by the transverse mesocolon. To expose the compartment, the small bowel is displaced to the left. Therefore, small bowel may be described as a content of the compartment. Note how at the inferior angle of the triangle the termination of small bowel (the terminal ileum) joins the large bowel (cecum). In theory, this arrangement means there is no direct passage between the compartment and the pelvic peritoneal cavity. The left side is different.

   ITEM 17-7. "Retroperitoneal"

   Gently strip off some peritoneum from the posterior wall of the right infracolic compartment. If the location chosen is appropriate, the anterior surface of the right kidney will be exposed. It is embedded in fat, to be considered more thoroughly later. In the meantime, recognize that the kidney is lying behind the peritoneal cavity and warrants the description retroperitoneal. Other retroperitoneal structures in this area which will be seen as the dissection advances, are the inferior part of the second part of the duodenum, the third part also, some of the head and neck of the pancreas, the right ureter and the blood vessels that cross anterior to the ureter and proceed to the right to reach the ascending colon, and other vessels that proceed inferiorly to reach the gonads. Thus, "retroperitoneal" describes structures covered by peritoneum on their anterior surface only.

   To study the left infracolic compartment (Fig. 17-2), move the small bowel to the right. The compartment is bounded to the right by the root of the mesentery, to the left by the descending colon, and superiorly by the transverse mesocolon.

   Note that the inferior angle of the compartment opens into the pelvis because of the way sigmoid colon enters the pelvis to join the rectum. Retroperitoneal structures here are the left kidney, the inferior surface of the body of the pancreas, the termination of the duodenum, the left ureter, the gonadal vessels, and the inferior mesenteric vessels and branches. Scratch away sufficient peritoneum to expose the left kidney.

THE RETROPERITONEAL SPACE

   The retroperitoneal space is a potential space located between the peritoneum and subjacent organs. It extends from as high as the diaphragm to well down into the pelvis, as well as from flank to flank. It may be transformed into an actual space by blood, a condition termed retroperitoneal hemorrhage, which may be profuse and critical.

   ITEM 17-8. Paracolic Gutters

   Identify, on the right side, the ascending colon and, on the left, the descending colon. Lateral to each there is a shallow gutter where peritoneum leaves the surface of the colon to line the abdominal wall. Each gutter extends superiorly and inferiorly. Examine the right paracolic gutter. Superiorly it is continuous with a recess posterior to the liver and anterior to the right kidney, the hepatorenal recess or pouch, also known as the right subhepatic space (p. 89). Inferiorly, a hand can slide from the gutter over the brim of the pelvis into another recess behind either the male bladder or the vagina. Stick the fingers of one hand into the hepatorenal recess (Fig. 17-6), and then slide them down the right paracolic gutter over the pelvic brim into the depths of the pelvis.

Examine the left paracolic gutter. Superiorly it is limited by a small fold of peritoneum connecting the diaphragmatic peritoneum and colonic peritoneum. In the cadaver this small structure, the phrenicocolic ligament, is not always apparent. Inferiorly, the gutter continues into the pelvis.

Caution—do not proceed further until you are certain of the paracolic gutters. They are not difficult to understand, but they are important channels in the spread of infected material from one region of the peritoneal cavity to another. Curiously, the spread is not always downward from the upper regions to the pelvis. Spread in the reverse direction happens too.

ITEM 17-9. The Supracolic Compartment

Restore the greater omentum to its normal position for an examination of the supracolic compartment. It is anterosuperior to the greater omentum and the transverse mesocolon. The arrangement of the viscera in the supracolic compartment may at first baffle the beginner, but a knowledge of the basic embryology of the region can clarify how each organ comes to its definitive position. Therefore, until he has studied thoroughly the embryology of the gut, the student must simply accept what he sees. When he considers the contents of this compartment for the first time he may divide them into two simple groups, easily seen structures and structures that are not so easily seen. The liver, gallbladder, stomach, and the proximal inches of the duodenum are easily seen, whereas the kidneys, and suprarenal glands, and spleen lie really deep.

Furthermore, in addition to actual structures within it, the supracolic compartment has numerous extensions of the peritoneal cavity dealt with under the heading Subphrenic Spaces.

ITEM 17-10. Duodenum—Its Relationship to the Supracolic and Infracolic Compartments

Identify the first part of the duodenum and the proximal part of the second part. In radiology these are commonly referred to as the duodenal cap. Keep the duodenal cap marked with a finger and remember that you are in the supracolic compartment. Now flip the greater omentum, transverse colon, and mesocolon over the costal margin to expose the fourth part of the duodenum in the infracolic

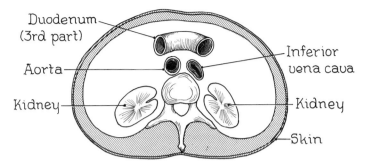

Figure 17-3.   Diagrammatic cross section of the abdomen to show how the third part of the duodenum is anterior to the vertebral column.

compartment. Mark this part of the duodenum and the adjacent duodenojejunal flexure with the fingers of the other hand. Note how near the beginning and end of the duodenum are to each other, but note particularly that the former is supracolic while the latter is infracolic. The third part of the duodenum crossing the vertebral column from right to left is well hidden. At this point the duodenum is liable to injury from blunt trauma (Fig. 17-3). The diagnosis is nearly always late and the damage hard to find at operation. When the transverse colon and mesocolon are removed, the relationships of the duodenum will be more apparent and can be considered more effectively at that time.

SUBPHRENIC SPACES

The anatomy of these spaces is really very straightforward, but their terminology may confuse not just the beginner but someone with more experience. Here the spaces are named according to the *Surgical Practices of the Lahey Clinic.* The spaces lying below (*sub*) the diaphragm (*phrene*) and below the liver are named accordingly right and left subphrenic and subhepatic spaces. You will have observed, no doubt, that the general heading subphrenic spaces includes spaces which are in fact subhepatic.

ITEM 17-11.   Right Subphrenic Spaces

Identify the falciform ligament. Place a hand to the right of the ligament between liver and diaphragm. The hand is now in the right subphrenic space. Next, slide a hand underneath the liver to lie in the right subhepatic space (hepatorenal recess or pouch) (Fig. 17-4).

If the solid form of the liver allows you to do so, slide the *left* hand into the right subhepatic space. Keep it here and slide the other hand into the right subphrenic space. Gently direct the fingers of each hand toward each other. They will become separated from each other by the coronary ligament, consisting of peritoneum extending from liver to

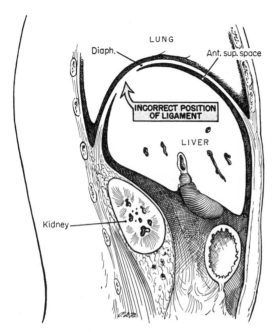

Figure 17-4. The very large areas occupied by the subhepatic and subphrenic spaces on the right side are shown. Normally the ligament indicated is closer to the kidney. Courtesy of the Lahey Clinic. Surgical Practice of the Lahey Clinic. Philadelphia. W. B. Saunders Co., 1962.

diaphragm. Such peritoneal ligaments of the liver will be seen more easily when the liver is removed.

ITEM 17-12. The Left Subphrenic Spaces

Place a hand on the liver to the left of the falciform ligament. You are now in the left subphrenic space. Observe how the left lobe tapers rapidly, and is best described as projecting into the left subphrenic space.

The real left subhepatic space is posterior to the lesser omentum and the stomach. To demonstrate its position, return to the greater omentum. About 2 inches from the edge of the stomach, cut (with restraint) into the anterior surface of the omentum. In all probability, you will open a space. If not, ask for assistance, or proceed to explore cautiously closer to the stomach—cautiously, because blood vessels to the stomach lie in this region. Once the space has been identified, gently increase the size of the opening until the fingers, if not the hand, can slide in behind the stomach. The fingers are now in the lesser sac (to be described) and may be maneuvered to touch the posteroinferior surface of the liver. This space in which the fingers now lie is the last of the subphrenic spaces to be considered, namely the left subhepatic space, which is the lesser sac.

These are detailed instructions for what are in fact very simple anatomic demonstrations. Do not waste time, therefore, but ask for a demonstration if you are in difficulty.

REVIEW

Quickly review the location of the spaces. The spaces are extensions of the peritoneal cavity, and can contain pockets of infected material (subphrenic abscess). What hollow organs prone to perforate are in the vicinity of these spaces? Furthermore, the subphrenic spaces are related through the diaphragm to each pleural cavity and lung, especially on the right side.

It is not expected that the undergraduate will become at once completely familiar with the detailed anatomy of these spaces, but he must know of their existence if he is to understand subphrenic abscess, one of the most serious complications that may arise after upper abdominal surgery, or, more rarely, as a complication of pulmonary disease.

ITEM 17-13. Greater Sac and Lesser Sac

It is appropriate now to consider these divisions of the peritoneal cavity. Identify the gallbladder. Its peritoneal surface is protruding into the greater sac. In other words, the part of the peritoneal cavity the student has examined so far is the greater sac.

Now, standing on the left side of the cadaver, and using the *left* index finger, proceed along the surface of the gallbladder to its neck and, at the same time, with the *right* hand pull the duodenum gently downward and to the left. The left index finger will arrive at a ridge, the lateral edge of the lesser omentum. Posterior to the ridge, a small opening should be present. The opening is usually very small indeed, and may be sealed, but it can be enlarged to receive one finger. Do not scratch around without guidance. If the opening is found easily, slide the index finger through it. The finger has entered the epiploic foramen also known as the foramen of Winslow, or the opening into the lesser sac, which it is. Keep the left index finger in the opening while the right hand enters the opening made previously in the greater omentum. All being well, the finger and hand will meet behind the stomach because the index finger has entered the lesser sac through its natural opening, while the right hand has entered by an artificial opening created for that purpose. Thus it can be seen that the lesser sac is an extension behind the stomach of the main peritoneal cavity.

ITEM 17-14. To expose the pancreas, further enlarge the artificial opening into the lesser sac by cutting the greater omentum parallel to the stomach. Retract the stomach. The pancreas, lying deep to peritoneum of the posterior wall of the lesser sac, will now be in a good view.

ITEM 17-15. Keep one hand on the body of the pancreas now exposed, and with the other hand flip the transverse colon superiorly to expose once more the infracolic compartment. Place a finger on each part of the pancreas related to this compartment. You realize, of course, that this compartment is part of the greater sac, so you have demonstrated that the pancreas is related not just to the lesser sac, but also to the greater sac.

FACTS TO NOTE

1. Peritoneum is on the posterior surface of the stomach as well as on its anterior surface. Thus, if the stomach perforates through its anterior surface its contents will spill into the supracolic compartment of the greater sac. In contrast to this, if the stomach perforates through its posterior wall, its contents will still enter peritoneal cavity but, in this instance, a confined part of the cavity, the lesser sac.

2. The pancreas is separated from the stomach by two layers of peritoneum and the cavity of the lesser sac.

3. The pancreas is related to greater and lesser sacs, both of which may receive abnormal seepage of pancreatic juices.

The Spleen

It is not easy to get hold of the spleen because it lies deep; i.e., it is essentially a posterior structure, just anterior to the ninth, tenth, and eleventh ribs, but separated from them by the diaphragm and the left pleural cavity. It is almost entirely invested in peritoneum (Fig. 17-5) so it is mobile in the cadaver and much more so in the living. Surrounded by peritoneum, it lies in a sort of cleft between the left kidney and stomach (Fig. 17-5). As a result of embalming and of storing the body in the supine position, the peritoneal cavity between spleen, kidney, stomach, and diaphragm is frequently obliterated by adhesions.

ITEM 17-16. To mobilize the spleen, stand on the *right* side of the cadaver. Then, at the level of the stomach, slide the *right* hand deep to the left costal margin and, keeping the knuckles of the hand on the parietal peritoneum of the diaphragm, push the hand posteriorly. Almost certainly, your fingertips will touch a smooth surface, roughly oval in shape, measuring some 12 cm. by 7 cm.—the spleen. In many corpses, you must proceed until the wrist is level with the costal margin. In brief, go deep to get the spleen. Once you have identified the spleen, grasp it between fingers and thumb (Fig. 17-5). The fingers are in the peritoneal cavity between spleen and the left kidney, while the thumb is

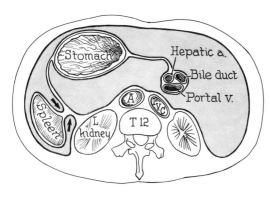

Figure 17-5. The spleen can be grasped by the fingers and thumb, represented here by arrows. Also note the interval between peritoneum covering the portal vein anteriorly and the inferior vena cava posteriorly. The interval is the only natural opening connecting the greater and lesser sacs. In life it scarcely admits one finger. The pancreas is not shown.

in the cavity between spleen and stomach. Between the fingers and thumb are two layers of peritoneum and between those layers are the vascular structures proceeding to and from the spleen and forming a pedicle (Fig. 17-5). More than likely you will tear peritoneum. Be as gentle as possible, for there will be a further opportunity to see this important vascular structure in its anatomic position. Meantime, as you consider the position of the spleen, it will become apparent to you why on some occasions it is necessary for the surgeon to reach the spleen through the thoracic cage as well as through the abdominal wall, using what he calls a thoracoabdominal approach.

Peritoneum in the Male Pelvis

The urinary bladder should be an immediate landmark, but very often in the cadaver it is empty and contracted into a hard lump immediately behind the symphysis pubis.*

ITEM 17-17. In the midline slide a finger posteriorly from the superior surface of the bladder. It will slip into a recess between the posterior surface, also known as the base of the bladder, and the rectum. It may be that the small bowel and possibly the sigmoid colon lie in this rectovesical pouch. If so, they must be pulled clear. Now move the fingers in the rectovesical pouch to each side for a short distance and feel through peritoneum the seminal vesicle, the ampulla of the ductus deferens, and the ureter. Only a small part of bladder is directly related to the rectum.

From the rectovesical pouch, trace the peritoneal surface out of the pelvis to the right and then to the left. In each instance the fingers will trail into the lowermost limits of the paracolic gutters.

Peritoneum Between the Bladder and Umbilicus

Three slightly prominent ridges of peritoneum may be traced from the umbilicus to the region of the bladder. The central one, called the median umbilical ligament, lies upon the remnant of the urachus, an embryologic structure connecting the bladder to the allantois. Hollow in the embryo, the urachus usually becomes fibrous, but sometimes it remains patent. What would lead you to suspect that the urachus was patent? It may remain patent throughout its length, or else for only a short distance, somewhere between bladder and umbilicus.

The other two ridges of peritoneum are the right and left lateral umbilical ligaments, passing from the lateral aspect of the bladder to the

---

*It is quite easy to catheterize the cadaver before embalming and to install 300 cc. of fluid into the bladder. Such a preliminary procedure makes it much easier to identify the bladder at this present stage of dissection.

umbilicus. In each ligament are the remains of an umbilical artery, which was a branch of the internal iliac artery and which brought blood *from* the fetus to the umbilical cord and thence to the placenta.

The Falciform Ligament

Identify the falciform ligament. Pay particular attention to its free edge, which was attached to the umbilicus before you cut it in dissecting the anterior abdominal wall. In this free edge, a fibrous strand is present. The strand, the ligamentum teres (round ligament), is all that remains of the one and only blood route *to* the fetus, namely the umbilical vein. That the vein is often patent in the adult has already been noted (p. 68).

REVIEW

A partial review of the fetal circulation is warranted. The umbilicus is a major landmark surrounding the vascular structures connecting the circulation of the fetus with the placenta. Two arteries, the umbilical arteries, bring blood *from* the fetus to the placenta, and one vein, the umbilical vein, conveys freshly oxygenated blood from the placenta *to* the fetal circulation. The arteries are branches of the internal iliac arteries. The umbilical vein enters the substance of the liver and ends by joining the portal circulation. An embryologic vessel, the ductus venosus, links the latter to the inferior vena cava (see p. 53).

PERITONEUM IN THE FEMALE PELVIS

Midline Structures

From behind the symphysis pubis to the anterior aspect of the sacrum in the midline there are four organs related to peritoneum, the bladder, uterus, vagina, and rectum.

ITEM 17-18. Identify the bladder (it will most likely be a hard lump behind the symphysis pubis) and then, proceeding posteriorly, move onto the vesical (bladder) surface of the uterus, over the fundus uteri, and onto the intestinal surface. It is inevitable that as the fingers continue inferiorly over the intestinal surface of the uterus, their tips will come to rest in a recess of peritoneum between vagina anteriorly and rectum posteriorly; they are in the rectovaginal pouch or recess. This pouch is accessible from the posterior fornix of the vagina as well as from the rectum.

Lateral Structures

ITEM 17-19. Grasp the body of the uterus with the index finger and thumb of each hand. Next slide each hand laterally toward the lateral edge of the uterus. Soon each finger and thumb leaving the uterus will be separated by two layers of peritoneum. Now drag the finger and thumb toward the free edge where the two surfaces of peritoneum become continuous with each other. The tubular structure felt in the free edge is the uterine tube. Trace it laterally to its fimbriae and identify the ovary.

What you have demonstrated is this: The layers of peritoneum, one on the vesical and the other on the intestinal surface of the uterus, meet at the lateral edges of the uterus to form the right and left broad ligaments. Consequently, each broad ligament is a fold of peritoneum extending from the side of the uterus to the pelvic wall. Each broad ligament becomes more shallow as one proceeds from the edge of the uterus to the brim of the pelvis. Soon the ligament disappears entirely, and the peritoneum of each of its surfaces merges imperceptibly with the rest of the peritoneum. Within the free edge of each broad ligament lies a uterine tube, and on the dorsal surface of each ligament rests an ovary. The part of the broad ligament adjacent to the uterine tube is called the mesosalpinx (*meso* from mesentery, *salpinx* meaning tube); the peritoneum that moors the ovary to the dorsal surface of the broad ligament is termed the mesovarium. The principle of the peritoneal cavity is maintained despite the somewhat unusual arrangement of these structures in relation to the ligament.

QUADRANTS

It does not require much thought to realize that such an extensive region as the abdomen must be subdivided in some way to give some precision to clinical descriptions of such things as the site of a pain or the location of a swelling (*mass* is the clinical term for swelling). For this purpose, several methods of subdividing the abdominal wall into nine regions have been described and they are illustrated in most anatomic and surgical texts. In practice, however, and that is what matters most, many clinicians simply divide the abdomen into quadrants. A vertical line at the linea alba crossed by a horizontal line at the umbilicus divides the anterior abdominal wall into right and left halves, each with an upper and lower quadrant. Thus the doctor may record, for example, that a mass is present in the right lower quadrant. Although the subdivision of the abdominal wall into nine exact regions by means of precise lines giving clearly defined areas has been largely abandoned, the names

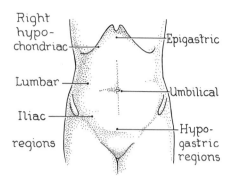

Figure 17-6. For clinical purposes the abdomen is usually divided into four quadrants, but the terms given here are still widely used.

of the nine regions are still included in the clinical vocabulary. For this reason, Figure 17-6 illustrates where these regions lie so that the student will not be caught unawares when he is asked to examine, for example, the epigastrium.

Disposition and Surface Marking of the Viscera

Disposition means the relative position of parts, and the student is now to divide the abdomen into quadrants in order to study the position of the various organs in each quadrant. During such a study he must bear constantly in mind the fact that this is a cadaver, and that, in the living, the disposition or relative position of many of the parts or organs will almost certainly be very different.

ITEM 17-20. To divide the abdomen, tie a string around it at the level of the umbilicus. Do not tie the string too tight. Then attach another piece of string between the xiphoid process at the sternum and the symphysis pubis at the pelvis. The quadrants are now visible and their underlying contents can be found. Identify the organs in each quadrant.

PALPABLE ORGANS

Preclinical students are confused by the term "palpable." Confusion arises when the student reads, for example, that the cecum is palpable in the right lower quadrant of the abdomen, yet he cannot identify the cecum on examining his own abdomen or his colleague's. Most of the abdominal organs are, in fact, so soft that they cannot be identified. There are exceptions, as we shall relate, but the following statement in general is correct. If an abdominal organ can actually be identified by palpation, the apprentice must consider it diseased until he establishes the truth. In other words, "palpable," used both anatomically and clinically, means "can be palpated;" it does not necessarily mean "can actually be felt." Thus, in the report of the physical examination of a healthy individual the majority of abdominal organs would be checked off as "not palpable."

Now, the exceptions: Both kidneys are sometimes palpable. The descending colon and sigmoid colon are palpable when they contain solid feces. The cecum is palpable when it is distended with gas. It must be pointed out, however, that before any decision is reached as to whether an organ is or is not palpable, the thickness of the abdominal wall and the relaxation of the abdominal musculature must be taken into account.

Finally, to this list of exceptions one must add the uterus and the ovaries. Depending on the thickness of fat, the degree of muscular relaxation, and the age of the woman, the uterus can almost always be palpated on bimanual examination (p. 190). Moreover, a clinician experienced in pelvic examination can usually palpate one or even both ovaries.

EXERCISES

1. If the cadaver is a female, imagine that she had complained of a mass palpable in the right lower quadrant. Examine and name the anatomic organs and structures you find in this quadrant. Each one of them could be the site of the mass, and your future studies, both in pathology and in clinical medicine, will help you to make a correct diagnosis.

2. Suppose your patient had complained of a mass in the left hypochondrium. In what organs might this mass be? Look and see.

3. In Chapter 1, brief mention was made of a problem of referred pain; pain from the organs of the chest can be referred to the anterior abdominal wall. With this information in mind, here is the third problem: Imagine your patient had complained of pain in the epigastrium. What organs might be responsible for this pain? Name the organs in the region, examine them, and do not forget to add the organs in the chest to your list.

4. Without becoming concerned about or involved in either the pathology or the clinical aspects, which will be taught in time in a proper setting, examine the abdomen now, quadrant by quadrant. When you can name fluently the organs and structures in each of these quadrants, you have mastered one of the first principles of abdominal diagnosis.

In the next chapter the student will proceed to remove abdominal viscera. In doing so, he will have a further opportunity to review the topographic anatomy of the abdominal organs.

Chapter 18

The Inguinal Canal

The medical student may as well know here and now that the anatomy of the inguinal canal is the most controversial subject in surgical anatomy, for nearly every surgeon who operates upon hernias has his own personal concept of the anatomy of the canal. For the beginner this is a sad state of affairs, especially since most surgeons and anatomists are agreed upon the basic anatomy of the canal while they disagree about detail. Accordingly, here the student is presented the basic anatomy, without which he will never understand controversial detail.

The term *canal* misleads the beginner, who expects to see a well-formed passageway with geometric sides like the Panama Canal. Instead, in each inguinal region he finds an oblique cleft barely equal to half a finger length. Under these circumstances the terms of description (anterior wall, posterior wall, roof, and floor) seem inappropriate, but, of course, they are used in a very broad descriptive sense. Perhaps boundaries would be a better word to use for the limits of the canal. Be that as it may, the inguinal canal, like any other anatomic structure or region, is best described by reference to the anatomic directions, i.e., superior, anterior, and so on, as is done here.

GENERAL DESCRIPTION OF THE CANAL

Each canal is approximately 4 cm. long, but its length varies. Get out a ruler and see what is meant by 4 cm. in length. The canal ends superficially at the superficial inguinal ring, found in the external oblique aponeurosis superolateral to the pubic tubercle. The canal itself lies immediately superior to the medial half of the inguinal ligament. At the other end of the canal is the deep inguinal ring in the transversalis fascia; this ring is seen best of all from within the abdomen. The surface marking of this ring is 1 cm. above the midinguinal point. Within the canal lies the spermatic cord, which consists of the vas deferens, testicular vessels, lymphatics, autonomic nerves, and, in addition, the ilioinguinal nerve. The vas joins the rest of the reproductive system, but the neurovascular and lymphatic structures proceed to the posterior abdominal wall.

98

Coverings

From the deep inguinal ring onward through the canal and into the scrotum, the spermatic cord and testis obtain investments of fascia. These investments, ultimately three in number, are spoken of as the first, second, and third coverings of the testis and cord, and they relate precisely to three planes of the anterior abdominal wall, namely the transversalis fascia, the internal oblique muscle, and the external oblique aponeurosis. The student will observe in his dissection that the third covering is present around the spermatic cord only after the cord is *beyond* the inguinal canal. To think otherwise is a common mistake.

Inguinal Canal in the Infant

The deep inguinal ring is deep to (i.e., posterior to) the superficial inguinal ring. In other words, the superficial inguinal ring is superimposed on the deep inguinal ring. Thus, if length is the criterion, there is little or no inguinal canal in the infant.

Inguinal Canal in the Female

The absence of a somewhat bulky spermatic cord means that the canal is narrower in the female. In place of the spermatic cord is the round ligament of the uterus, a strap of fibrous tissue which extends from the uterus through the inguinal canal to the labium majus.

DISSECTION OF INGUINAL CANAL

There are three stages to this dissection, and they are:
1. Exploration of the deep ring
2. Exploration of the superficial ring
3. Opening the canal

If you are not familiar with the following bony landmarks, please identify them now, because they are essential in understanding the anatomy of the canal.
1. Symphysis pubis
2. Pubic crest
3. Pubic tubercle
4. Pectineal line
5. Anterior superior iliac spine

Exploration of the Deep Ring

The anterior abdominal wall has already been reflected. If you have not slit it in the midline, do so now—strictly in the midline—from the umbilicus to the symphysis pubis. This procedure makes the wall over the iliac region easier to manipulate.

ITEM 18-1. This first procedure requires patience. Very gently peel peritoneum off the transversalis fascia on the abdominal wall in the vicinity of the deep inguinal ring. Be careful not to peel off transversalis fascia with peritoneum. A dimple of peritoneum is usually a clue to the site of the ring in the cadaver. In a good cadaver with vessels well-filled, the dissector will find that the testicular vessels meet the vas deferens to form the spermatic cord in the vicinity of the inguinal ring, but outside the peritoneum. Reflect the peritoneum to the brim of the pelvis.

ITEM 18-2. The second procedure must also be done with care. Seek help if you are in the slightest difficulty. The vas deferens and vessels, as they come together, are obscured by extraperitoneal tissue. Gently clear away the tissue around them until they are clearly seen. While a partner holds the abdominal wall fairly firmly, trace the vas and the vessels toward the deep inguinal ring. At this stage it is necessary to point out that "ring" is a misleading term. The deep inguinal ring is merely the beginning of the evagination of transversalis fascia, which continues as the internal spermatic fascia, the first covering of the cord. Therefore, the margins of the ring are inconspicuous. Note that you are approaching the ring from an abdominal aspect. Explore the ring with the blunt end of a probe. Then cautiously explore further for a short distance along the surface of the vas deferens to demonstrate without a doubt that the pocket of transversalis fascia does exist. This pocket, in fact, extends right down into the scrotum to contain the testis, but cannot be followed this far in the present dissection. Finally, with the probe still in the pocket of the transversalis fascia, identify the inferior epigastric vessels medial to the deep inguinal ring.

Exploration of the Superficial Ring

Return to the region of the superficial ring. The layer of fascia covering the cord just beyond the ring is the external spermatic fascia. It is very delicate, like fine lace, and masks the boundary of the superficial inguinal ring to which it is adherent.

ITEM 18-3. Carefully grasp the fascia with two pairs of forceps, just beyond the ring. Incise the fascia, remembering it is as thin as paper, and then carefully extend your incision toward the superficial ring. Examine the ring.

SUPERFICIAL INGUINAL RING

The superficial inguinal ring is merely an opening in the external oblique aponeurosis that allows the passage of the spermatic cord. It is often described as triangular, but it may be round and consequently may fit snugly around the spermatic cord. The edges of the ring, spoken of as crura (*crura* is the plural of *crus*), cannot be clearly seen until the external spermatic fascia is removed. But each crus of the ring can be felt, and that is what matters most to the diagnostician, who can invaginate the skin of the scrotum in a particular way with the tip of a finger to palpate the ring immediately lateral to the pubic tubercle.

ITEM 18-4. Opening the Inguinal Canal

Observe the oblique direction and the parallel arrangement of the fibers of the external oblique aponeurosis. Insert the point of scissors deep to the apex of the ring and slit the aponeurosis in the line of its fibers to open the inguinal canal (Fig. 18-1). Reflect the aponeurosis to each side and open the canal wide. In doing so, you will come upon the ilioinguinal nerve upon the surface of the cord structures in the canal. The second covering of the spermatic cord is now in view and is recognizable by strands of muscle fibers, usually a pale pinkish brown in the cadaver. This covering is the cremasteric fascia, and the muscle fibers belong to the cremaster muscle.

However, the inguinal canal is not yet completely open because the deep inguinal ring is still hidden from view by the lowermost fibers of the internal oblique. If your specimen is normal you can confirm this fact. Identify the position of the deep inguinal ring in relation to the lowermost fibers of the internal oblique.

That the canal is not yet open is really an academic argument. The only advantage of drawing attention to it is to impress upon the student the relationship of the internal oblique muscle fibers to the spermatic cord. The lowermost fibers of the internal oblique arise from the inguinal ligament anterior to the deep inguinal ring. From there, proceeding medially, they lie superior to the spermatic cord. Then, becoming aponeurotic, the fibers blend with the anterior aspect of the rectus sheath. Check this on your specimen and see that the muscle fibers of the internal oblique form part of the anterior wall of the inguinal canal and also of the so-called roof.

Yet to be examined are the posterior wall, the floor of the canal, and the internal spermatic fascia after the cremasteric fascia has been opened. Examine now the posterior wall of the inguinal canal (Fig. 18-2). In most anatomic specimens it will be possible to identify the lowermost edge of the internal oblique muscle. Do so but do not be disappointed if it is inconspicuous, because sometimes the muscle fibers are poorly developed and are short in length. From the canal side, place the index

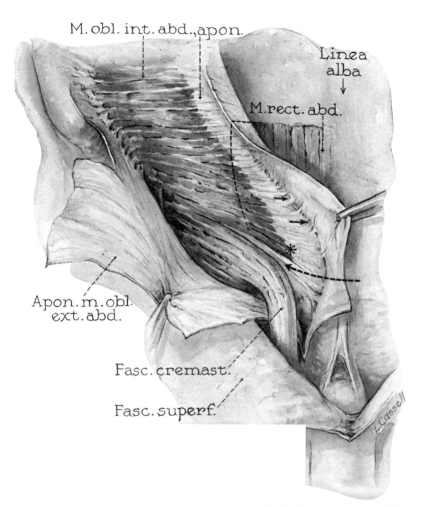

M. obl. int. abd., apon.

Linea alba

M. rect. abd.

*

Apon. m. obl. ext. abd.

Fasc. cremast.

Fasc. superf.

L. Cassell

Figure 18-1. Common type of internal oblique abdominal muscle layering. The internal oblique muscle, its aponeurosis, and the cremasteric fibers are shown. A small cleft, apparent when the cord is drawn downward, sets off an "aponeurotic inguinal falx" (above arrow at*). The line of junction of the aponeuroses of the oblique muscles lies well to the medial side of the lateral border of the rectus muscle (the latter at dotted line). (From B. J. Anson: Atlas of Human Anatomy. 2nd ed. Philadelphia, W. B. Saunders Co., 1963.

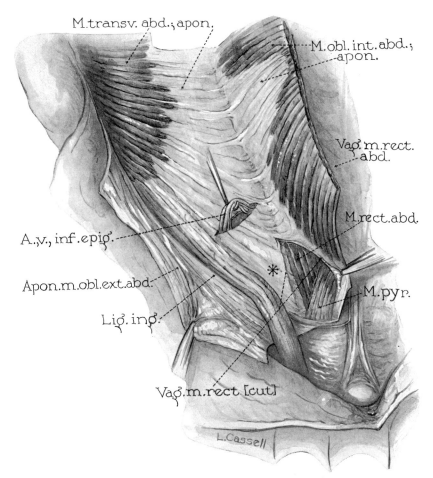

Figure 18-2. In this dissection the internal oblique muscle has been reflected and the inferior epigastric vessels exposed from the canal. Where is the deep ring? (From B. J. Anson: Atlas of Human Anatomy. 2nd ed. Philadelphia, W. B. Saunders Co., 1963.)

finger of one hand on the posterior wall of the inguinal canal immediately inferior to the lowermost edge of the internal oblique, which you have just identified. Keep the finger there. Now return to the abdominal aspect of the inguinal region to the vicinity of the deep ring where you identified inferior epigastric vessels. Adjacent to the inferior epigastric vessels, more so on their medial side, you can identify the transversalis fascia because it is thicker here than elsewhere. Put the index finger of the other hand on the transversalis fascia in this area. If you have followed the instructions successfully, then you will have between your index fingers part of the posterior wall of the inguinal canal; that part is formed by the transversalis fascia. Examine the attachment of transversalis fascia to the pectineal line. Examine also the pectineal ligament.

The floor of the inguinal canal is essentially the medial part of the inguinal ligament, which at this point curves posteriorly, forming the lacunar ligament. Note that a part of the medial end of the inguinal ligament is incorporated in the inferior crus of the superficial ring. Pull the inferior leaf of the external oblique aponeurosis downward and dissect along the inguinal ligament medially, toward the pubic tubercle to expose the lacunar ligament and to show how it curves posteriorly to become continuous with the pectineal ligament.

The final step in the dissection is to open the cremasteric fascia and to identify the internal spermatic fascia within the inguinal canal. Do this, and, by putting gentle tension on the internal spermatic fascia, identify the deep inguinal ring from its canal side.

REVIEW OF THE INGUINAL CANAL

1. The anterior wall is made up of:
     The opening of the superficial inguinal ring
     The external oblique aponeurosis
     The lowermost fibers of the internal oblique muscle arising from the inguinal ligament.
2. The posterior wall is made up of:
     The deep inguinal ring
     Transversalis fascia
3. The floor of the canal is inguinal ligament and its lacunar extension.
4. The roof is the horizontal fibers of the internal oblique.
5. Within the canal lies the spermatic cord having two coverings of fascia, internal spermatic fascia and cremasteric fascia. The ilioinguinal nerve is also a content. (The third covering, the external spermatic fascia, is not obtained until these structures have left the canal.)
     Read an account of the development and descent of the testis.

INTRODUCTION TO INGUINAL HERNIAE*

Restore the peritoneum to the abdominal wall. Then, in the region of the posterior wall of the inguinal canal, either medial or lateral to the inferior epigastric vessels, gently push the peritoneum anteriorly into the canal. You may be able to create only a dimple of peritoneum or quite a pocket. In either case, you have created the beginning of an inguinal hernia. The nomenclature of a hernia is detailed under Femoral Hernia (p. 106).

It is recommended that a member of staff prepare a demonstration of an inguinal hernia. It is a rare occasion when no cadaver in the laboratory has one, and seeing a practical demonstration is really the best way to understand the anatomy of inguinal hernias.

THE FEMORAL RING

The description here, in line with the work of McVay, will not agree with what is said in nearly every anatomy book and many surgical texts.

Normally the femoral ring does not exist. Furthermore, when it does exist, it has *four* boundaries, lateral, posterior, anterior, and medial; its so-called transverse diameter is 5 to 16 mm., so it is very small.

The boundaries define a potential opening from the abdomen into a very small potential space, the femoral canal, in the uppermost region of the thigh, medial to the femoral vein. The canal is a frequent site of hernia, which may increase to such a size as to be visible in the uppermost region of the thigh.

Examination of the Boundaries of the Femoral Ring

ITEM 18-5. The Lateral Boundary of the Ring

At the pelvic brim, identify the external iliac vein and trace it distally toward the inguinal region, where it changes its name to femoral vein; this is simply a change of name, without any change of direction. Until you are familiar with the other boundaries of the ring, do nothing more than identify the vein close to where it disappears into the thigh. At this point, the vein is a lateral relation of the site of the femoral ring.

ITEM 18-6. The Posterior Boundary of the Ring

From the vein, move slightly posteriorly and medially on to the body

---

*An abdominal hernia is a defect in the normal musculoaponeurotic and fascial continuity of the abdominal wall or the respiratory or pelvic diaphragms, either congenital or acquired, which permits the egress of any structures other than those that normally pass through the parietes. McVay.

of the pubis. In the cadaver the periosteum of the body of the pubis is glistening white and easily recognized. Check on the pelvis of a skeleton precisely where this is.

ITEM 18-7. The Anterior Boundary of the Ring

This boundary is the inguinal ligament just lateral to its lacunar part and cannot be seen from the abdominal aspect. Do not dissect toward it yet.

ITEM 18-8. The Medial Boundary of the Ring

While your partner holds the anterior abdominal wall taut in its usual position, look, from the abdominal aspect, at the region just above the pubic bone and examine the transversalis fascia as it attaches to the pectineal line. The medial area of this fascia is often thickened and may be reinforced by an aponeurotic expansion from the edge of the rectus abdominis sheath. It is the edge of this thickening and expansion that is the medial boundary of the femoral ring. Trace the transversalis fascia toward the site of the ring.

Confirm for yourself that you cannot see the lacunar part of the inguinal ligament or the inguinal ligament itself from your present viewpoint within the abdomen and at the present stage of the dissection.

ITEM 18-9. To enter the femoral canal push the tip of your little finger—gently—medial to the femoral vein, inferiorly toward the thigh. Your finger, having enlarged the femoral ring, is now in the femoral canal. In the canal you can feel anteriorly the inguinal ligament as a rigid structure, horizontal in disposition. But it is not until you have distended the canal further with the finger and directed the tip of the finger medially that you can feel the distinct edge of the lacunar ligament.

Creation of a Femoral Hernia

ITEM 18-10. Restore peritoneum over the pocket you just created when you pushed the tip of your finger into the femoral canal. Push the peritoneum into the canal, so creating a hernia. Clinically, this pocket of peritoneum is spoken of as a sac, and where the sac begins, i.e., the edge of the opening into the sac, is termed the "neck" of the sac. Coverings are the layers of tissue the sac obtains as it increases in size and progresses in a particular direction. In this instance, while the sac progresses inferiorly, posterior to the inguinal ligament, and lateral to the lacunar ligament, the covering is the transversalis fascia. The sac usually contains the small bowel or omentum. Often the urinary bladder may accompany the hernia, but not as a content of the sac. Do not be misled by the solid nature of the bladder in the cadaver. In life it can, in fact, slide into the femoral canal on the medial aspect of the peritoneal sac.

Now you are free to explore the region more extensively. By examining the region from the abdomen and from the inguinal canal, confirm the proximity of the femoral canal to the inguinal region.

Chapter 19

Introduction to Evisceration

While you remove the viscera take note of the following:

(1) Arteries. Pay attention to the arteries and, in doing so, perceive that there are autonomic nerves on their surfaces. In life, arteries are identified principally by their pulsation. Here you can identify them only by their reddish white color.

(2) Lymphatics. Give special consideration to the lymphatics because they cannot be adequately demonstrated in the cadaver, yet they are so important in the spread of cancer.

(3) Veins. Veins too must be observed. In life, their blood drains to the liver. They are bluish brown in a cadaver.

(4) Relationships. As you mobilize each organ, note the relationships of the organ to the peritoneal cavity and adjacent parts and of its blood vessels to neighboring organs and structures. For example, on both left and right sides, blood vessels crossing to the colon cling momentarily to the ureters; surgical techniques are planned to avoid damage to such structures.

(5) Function.

(6) Methods of physical examination.

Arteries

The arteries have a basic pattern related to the embryology of the gut (Fig. 19-1). The abdominal part of the foregut includes the abdominal esophagus, stomach, and proximal half of the duodenum; derivatives of the foregut are the liver, gallbladder, and pancreas; the

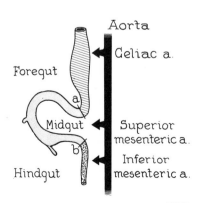

Figure 19-1. Diagram to show the divisions of the gut in the abdomen of the embryo and the artery supplying each division: a, middle of second part of duodenum; b, distal part of transverse colon. See also Figure 20-1.

spleen is derived from the dorsal mesogastrium. All of these structures are supplied by branches of the celiac artery. The midgut includes the distal half of the duodenum, the small bowel, and the large bowel as far as the splenic flexure. All of the structures in the midgut are supplied by the superior mesenteric artery and its branches. The hindgut includes the descending colon, sigmoid colon, and rectum, all supplied by the inferior mesenteric artery and its branches.

Lymphatic Drainage

The lymphatic drainage of viscera has a basic pattern that corresponds to the arterial pattern. In describing this correspondence, it is usually said that the lymph vessels accompany the arteries, but note that the lymph flow is opposite in direction to the flow of blood. Accordingly, it follows that if you know the arterial pattern, then, in essence, you know the lymphatic field.

The beginning of the lymphatic drainage is found in the wall of the organ, in collections of lymphoid tissue, which are microscopic except in the terminal ileum, where macroscopic collections can be seen with the naked eye. The drainage is from an extensive area and includes the esophagus, the stomach, the vermiform appendix, and the rectum. From these and other abdominal organs, the lymph vessels proceed, traveling centrally alongside the arteries toward the abdominal aorta. Ultimately, from the lymphatic fields emerge several lymphatic trunks, which join the lower end of the thoracic duct on the posterior abdominal wall, close to the vertebral column. Then the duct, ascending through the thorax anterior to the column, ultimately joins the venous circulation in the neck.

Now, as you come to the study of the upper abdominal organs, is the time to review in more detail their lymphatic drainage, using the principle set out in the previous paragraph. You will find that the lymphatic drainage of the proximal part of the duodenum corresponds to the celiac artery and its duodenal branches, while lymphatic drainage of its distal part corresponds to the superior mesenteric artery and its branches. In other words, this divergent lymphatic drainage of the duodenum fits in with the embryology of the gut. A similar divergence occurs in the region of the splenic flexure. Why?

Apart from the microscopic and macroscopic collections of lymph tissue mentioned in a previous paragraph, studded along the lymphatic pathways are innumerable lymph nodes with efferent and afferent vessels. Such nodes are usually named according to the nearest major artery, e.g., the superior mesenteric nodes, or perhaps according to the nearest organ or part of an organ, e.g., the pyloric nodes of the stomach.

In the lymphatic field of the large bowel, a simple pattern of lymph nodes is present: the paracolic (*para* means beside), intermediate colic, and terminal colic nodes are recognized, the first group lying along side the colon, the second group halfway along the arteries, and the third group either where the superior mesenteric or the inferior mesenteric arteries arise from the aorta. A similar but less definite arrangement exists in the mesentery of the small bowel, where lymph vessels and nodes abound.

Lymph nodes throughout the body play a defensive role in both local and systemic infections. Accordingly, in children, abdominal pain following a sore throat may be attributed to swelling of the mesenteric lymph nodes. Lymph nodes are significant also in the spread of cancer; a surgeon, finding that cancer of an abdominal organ has spread into the lymphatic system, surmises that the outlook, or the prognosis, is less favorable than if this spread had not occurred.

Veins

The venous blood from the gastrointestinal tract, including the abdominal esophagus, the vermiform appendix, and the rectum, as well as the blood from the pancreas and spleen, drains to the liver. This widespread system of drainage, which begins in microscopic venous plexuses in the walls of the organs and ends in the sinusoids (microscopic venous spaces) of the liver, is referred to as the portal system for the following reason: This system finally drains into one large vein, the portal vein, so named because it enters the liver at the porta hepatis, the gateway of the liver. (At this point the student often jumps to a wrong conclusion, so it is worth stressing here that the portal system ends in the substance of the liver.) From the porta hepatis another set of venous radicals drain from the liver into the inferior vena cava. With these facts in mind, you understand why a patient with infectious disease of the bowel sometimes gets a secondary infection in his liver (liver abscess) or, more commonly, why cancer of the digestive tract spreads to the liver (metastasis).

Autonomic Nervous System

The autonomic nervous system plays an important part in the function of the alimentary system. However, there is space for only certain basic facts here.

The sympathetic supply to the alimentary system stems from the thoracolumbar outflow and reaches the entire alimentary system, including vessels of the abdomen.

The parasympathetic system consists of two parts, cranial and sacral, usually put together as the craniosacral outflow. The cranial part, represented by the vagus nerves, innervates the alimentary system as far as the splenic flexure of the colon. The sacral part, which includes the colic nerves, is responsible for the rest.

In terms of embryology, the sympathetic distribution is to the entire gut system. The cranial outflow (parasympathetic) innervates only the fore- and midgut, while the sacral outflow (also parasympathetic) is responsible for hindgut innervation.

In addition to sympathetic and parasympathetic fibers, there are afferent fibers upon the surface of blood vessels. *Afferent* denotes that these fibers are sensory, returning to the central nervous system. Their peripheral nerve endings (that is, their endings in the walls of the viscera) do not respond in the same way that nerve endings in the skin do. Thus, after the surgeon has cut through the abdominal wall, anesthetized by a local anesthetic (not by a general anesthetic, which lulls the mind), he can manipulate the small bowel, even cut it or burn it with a cauterizing instrument, without the patient experiencing pain. In contrast to the painlessness of these stimuli, distention of the bowel causes pain, a pain the patient finds difficult to describe for it is vague, yet is real, sometimes very real.

Function

While you are dissecting an organ, give some thought to its function. In the early days of your dissection, you will obviously have some difficulty in relating function to structure. However, your knowledge of function will deepen as your studies in other disciplines expand. Then you will be able to, and you must, establish a concept of organ function. After all, it is usually a disorder of function that leads ultimately to the diagnosis of a disease of structure.

Physical Examination

It is a doctor's responsibility to examine patients. It will be yours one day. Therefore, while you are dissecting not just the abdominal viscera but other organs too, you must become acquainted with the usual methods of clinical examination. All forms of physical examination, with or without instruments, depend upon a knowledge of basic anatomy for their success. Methods of examination are found in *Anatomy* (E. Gardner, D. J. Gray, and R. O'Rahilly).

Chapter 20

Evisceration: Appendix, Colon, Jejunum, and Ileum

ITEM 20-1. Identify the vermiform appendix, if it is present.

VERMIFORM APPENDIX

Merely to glance at this organ is not enough; you must study it in depth because it is so often a site of infection (appendicitis).

Location of the Appendix in Relation to the Cecum

The vermiform appendix is attached to the cecum. Thus the location of the appendix depends upon the location of the cecum. To give a very rare and extreme example: If the cecum is on the *left* side of the body, and this can occur, the appendix will be there too.

Sometimes the cecum is close to the liver (subhepatic); if this is so, of course, the vermiform appendix would not be in its "usual" location. This unusual arrangement is noted frequently in infants and children. In contrast to a location high in the abdomen, the cecum may droop over the pelvic brim. Again the location of the appendix will be unusual. Indeed, Barclay found that in 30 unselected examples, the base of the appendix lay somewhere within a circle 7 inches in diameter. The center of the circle was at the junction of the lateral and middle third of a line between the umbilicus and the right anterior superior iliac spine.

Direction of the Appendix

Likening the vermiform appendix to the hand of clock is useful in describing its numerous possible positions. If you can imagine that the clock is tilted so that it faces superiorly as well as anteriorly, you will gain a better impression of the true direction of the appendix. At the 11 or 12 o'clock position, the appendix is retrocecal or retrocolic (*retro* means behind), and this is by far the commonest position (64 per cent). At 4 o'clock the appendix is in the pelvis (32 per cent). Any other position of the clock may be adopted by the appendix. Perhaps the other position to comment upon is 6 o'clock (2 per cent), because the tip of the appendix may then be related to the peritoneum of the anterior abdominal wall, but note how rarely this occurs.

ITEM 20-2.   Position of the Vermiform Appendix

What is the position of the appendix in your cadaver? To find it, identify one of the three teniae coli, three isolated straps on the surface of the colon and cecum. Trace the tenia inferiorly. Inevitably you will arrive at the base of the appendix. On what aspect of the cecum is the base? How long is the appendix in your specimen? Does it have a mesentery? Does the cecum have a mesentery?

If the appendix is not retrocecal, imagine that it is. Anterior to a retrocecal appendix are the cecum and its contents. Next lies the omentum and perhaps the small bowel* and its contents. For demonstration purposes, place these structures superficial to the cecum. Next, replace the anterior abdominal musculature. Then visualize in position several inches of fat and, last, skin. Estimate the depth of the appendix from the skin surface. Now you can see why the diagnosis of inflammation of the appendix is difficult.

Perhaps the appendix in your cadaver is pelvic in position. If it is, and even if it is not, answer this question: In what ways is the appendix palpable other than through the abdominal wall? The answer is the second footnote on this page.†

Relationships of the Appendix

In addition to cecum and peritoneal cavity, the appendix may be related to the muscles psoas and obturator internus, the right ureter and bladder, the rectum, the right ovary and uterine tube, and often the terminal ileum, a relationship frequently forgotten. The wide variety of clinical signs, symptoms, and diagnostic tests for appendicitis depends greatly on these possible relationships. Therefore the existence of a vermiform appendix must always be borne in mind after the dissector has stripped out the bowel and peritoneum to expose these adjacent structures.

Vessels of the Appendix

ITEM 20-3.   Identify the appendicular artery. Check its source. Also identify the vein, but do not delay.

One point more. To stress the anatomy of the vermiform appendix is wise; to ignore the rest of the gut is foolish. That you have not as yet heard of diseases of some of the other abdominal organs does not confer

---

*Usually the cecum is directly related to the anterior abdominal wall. Rarely does the small bowel lie between them.

†Answer to the question. A pelvic appendix is palpable per vaginam or per rectum. This means that between the doctor's finger and the appendix lie the wall of the rectum or vagina, the peritoneal cavity, and perhaps the small bowel. Therefore the doctor cannot expect to feel the appendix as distinctly as he can feel a pencil on his desk. Unfortunately, the pelvic tissues on the cadaver do not yield enough for a proper pelvic examination to be performed. Nevertheless, this will be done when the perineum is dissected.

upon them an immunity to disease. Every organ of the body may be stricken. Therefore, your present need is a great awakening to the total content of the human frame as preparation for the study of disease. Proceed to examine the rest of the gut.

THE COLON

ITEM 20-4. Identify the teniae coli, (translated the term means bands of the colon), sacculations (pouches between the teniae), and appendices epiploicae (tabs of fat), and quickly reidentify the cecum, ascending colon, hepatic flexure, transverse colon, splenic flexure, descending colon, and sigmoid. Appendices epiploicae are more significant than one realizes. Often an extension of the lumen of the colon enters the substance of an appendix. The extension is termed a diverticulum. The presence of many diverticula is referred to as diverticulosis, which may lead to several clinical conditions requiring treatment.

Continuity of the Colon

In removing the colon, take note that its parts belong to one continuous tube. This aspect of anatomy usually escapes the beginner, who is more concerned with the nomenclature of the various parts. The continuity of the colon is illustrated perhaps best of all when a barium enema is administered through the anal orifice; on a fluorescent screen the radiopaque fluid can be seen flowing into the rectum, sigmoid, and descending, transverse, and ascending colon, as far as the cecum. A different type of illustration is the effect of obstruction, i.e., narrowing of the lumen, of the sigmoid colon. Gas and feces accumulate proximal to the obstruction until even the cecum, the most proximal part of the colon, becomes distended with gas and fluid. Such distention gives rise to discomfort; accordingly, an astute clinician, examining a patient for discomfort in the right lower quadrant of the abdomen and detecting the distended cecum, will establish as quickly as possible the condition of the lower bowel. With these comments in mind, proceed with the removal of the whole colon, beginning with the sigmoid.

ITEM 20-5. The Sigmoid Colon and its Mesentery

Identify the sigmoid colon. What is its relationship to the urinary bladder or to the uterus?

THE SIGMOID COLON

The length of the sigmoid colon varies from 40 to 90 cm., which accounts for some of the difficulty a student has in applying standard anatomic descriptions to his specimen. If the sigmoid is long, it will have a slack mesentery, which can easily be identified. The root of this mesentery, i.e., its attachment, is shaped like an inverted V. The lateral limb of the Λ lies along the brim of the pelvis while the medial limb descends in front of the sacrum. Behind the peritoneum, i.e., retroperitoneal, at the apex of the Λ lies the left ureter. Identify this mesentery, recognize the apex just referred to, and expose, for a short distance, the ureter at this apex. Observe the degree of mobility of the sigmoid.

In marked contrast to the freely movable sigmoid colon just described, in your specimen there may be little or no mesentery. Under these circumstances the sigmoid colon is plastered onto the pelvic brim and the front of the sacrum by peritoneum and is relatively immobile. Then the sigmoid colon will be closely related to the major vessels in the area as well as to the left ureter. Identify the ureter.

There are no precise points at which the sigmoid colon begins and ends. For descriptive purposes, it begins at the brim of the pelvis, really at the first evidence of a mesocolon. The end, usually at the level of the body of the third~sacral~vertebra, is where each of the three teniae coli spread out and merge as one longitudinal layer of fibers continuing on to surround the rectum; in other words, the end of the teniae coli indicates the junction of sigmoid and rectum.

The rectosigmoid junction is a flexure that is accentuated when the body is upright; when the shoulders are in a position lower than the buttocks (in the Trendelenburg position for example) the flexure is undone, especially if the sigmoid is mobile. The junction is estimated as 15 cm. from the anal orifice, inferior to the sacral promontory, a readily identified bony landmark on pelvic examination.

EXAMINATION OF THE SIGMOID COLON (SIGMOIDOSCOPY)

The medical student must learn here, now, and forever that the internal surface, or mucosa, of the sigmoid colon can be seen by the naked eye with the aid of an instrument called a sigmoidoscope (see also p. 210, sigmoidoscopy). Also, the mucosa of the rectum can be seen with the aid of a proctoscope.

Approximately 66 per cent of tumors of the large intestine are within sight; 54 per cent of these occur in the rectum and are therefore within the reach of the finger; 12 per cent occur at the rectosigmoid junction and can be seen with a sigmoidoscope. Therefore, in every disorder of the lower bowel, proctoscopy and sigmoidoscopy are imperative.

Rectal digital examination (Fig. 30-1). perhaps even more important (and simpler) than sigmoidoscopy, is dealt with on p. 188.

ITEM 20-6. Mobilization of the Sigmoid

Remembering that peritoneum is as thin as paper, incise the peritoneum of the left paracolic gutter parallel to the descending colon and down to the pelvic brim. Mobilize the inferior end of the descending colon from the wall and raise it medially. Be sure you are in the correct plane of cleavage, otherwise posterior abdominal wall structures will remain adherent to peritoneum. Eventually the lower bowel will be free enough for you to identify the branches of the inferior mesenteric artery approaching the bowel.

To mobilize the bowel even more, judiciously make a vertical incision into peritoneum covering the abdominal aorta. This procedure should expose the inferior mesenteric artery, whose origin from the aorta you will find deep to the third part of the duodenum. Clear the artery from its origin toward its branches until its continuation, the superior rectal artery, is clearly identified. Preserve this artery but cut the colic vessels proceeding to the sigmoid and descending colon. In a crude fashion, the sigmoid colon has now been mobilized.

Tie string twice around the sigmoid junction, proximal to the superior rectal artery. Cut the bowel across between the two ties. The double ties prevent undue leakage of bowel contents.

COLIC NERVES

In mobilizing the sigmoid and descending colon you were unaware of the colic nerves, which ascend from the pelvis (the anterior aspect of the sacrum) superiorly and to the left to reach those organs. En route, the nerves cross the branches of the inferior mesenteric artery.

Do _not_ search for the colic nerves—meticulous dissection is essential to display them—but know of their existence, for they supply parasympathetic innervation to the descending colon and sigmoid. The same innervation to the rectum reaches that organ within the pelvis.

In review, note that the parasympathetic supply to the hindgut arises within the pelvis, whereas the supply to the foregut and midgut (Fig. 19-1) comes from the cranium through the vagus nerves. Thus, the proximal part of the colon gains its parasympathetic supply from one source while the distal part gains it from another. This dichotomy, which is said to occur in the region of the splenic flexure, is believed to explain why the distribution of referred pain is different in lesions of the proximal and distal parts of the large bowel.

A very convincing example of the unity of the autonomic nervous system is the gastrocolic reflex. The entry of food into the stomach induces in the colon a peristalsis which precedes evacuation of the bowel. This example of the unity of the autonomic nervous system is certainly very convincingly demonstrated to the nursing mother who has just tidied her baby for its feed.

ITEM 20-7.   Descending Colon

Strip up the descending colon as far as the splenic flexure (the left colic flexure). Where does the flexure lie in relation to the spleen, left kidney, pancreas, and stomach? Note how the terminal inches of the transverse colon lie anterior to the first few inches of the descending colon. A similar overlap occurs at the right colic flexure (hepatic flexure) and complicates the interpretation of barium enema radiographs. For practical reasons, it is easier for you to mobilize the terminal ileum, cecum, and ascending colon *now*, before you mobilize the transverse colon.

ITEM 20-8.   Terminal Ileum, Cecum, and Ascending Colon

Cut delicately into the peritoneum of the right paracolic gutter from the level of the hepatic flexure (right colic flexure) of the colon to the pelvic brim. Raise the ascending colon and cecum toward the midline. Take care not to raise also posterior abdominal wall structures, especially the right ureter, as the right colic and ileocolic arteries come into your field of view. Raise the bowel far enough to identify the origin of these vessels from the superior mesenteric artery. Peritoneum is, of course, elevated and may easily be torn.

Tie string twice around the terminal ileum. Cut the organ between the ties. To fully mobilize the organ, the arteries you have just identified will have to be cut.

The cecum and the ascending, descending, and sigmoid colon are now released from the posterior wall. Identify and cut the blood vessels. The final step is to mobilize and release the transverse colon, which involves cutting the mesocolon and the middle colic artery, now to be done.

TRANSVERSE COLON

Before removing the transverse colon, note how it droops across the abdomen from the hepatic to the splenic flexure. Indeed, in life, the middle of the transverse colon may lie as low as the pubic symphysis. It follows that both the transverse mesocolon and the middle colic artery slope downward. Diagrams showing this artery like a television antenna are very misleading to the unwary student.

ITEM 20-9.   Removal of the Transverse Colon

If the liver is obstructing your approach to the hepatic flexure, ask a member of the staff to remove a segment of liver.

Grasp the hepatic flexure and, by snipping peritoneum with scissors, not too deeply, raise the colon gently anteriorly to expose the second part of the duodenum and the head of the pancreas. The first inches of the transverse colon are directly related to these other two structures. The transverse mesocolon will now become more obvious.

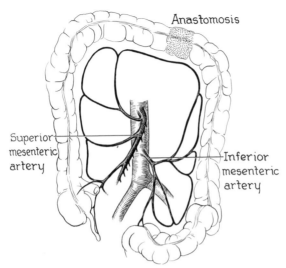

Figure 20-1.   The superior mesenteric artery supplies a large part of the large bowel, the entire small bowel, and part of the duodenum. The branches to the small bowel are indicated here by stumps. The inferior mesenteric artery supplies the descending colon, the sigmoid colon, and the rectum. The marginal artery is clearly shown.

Cut it, but not too close to the colon. You will cut the middle colic artery. Continue to cut the mesocolon until finally the transverse colon lies free. Remove the colon from the cadaver and examine the marginal artery.

ITEM 20-10.   The Marginal Artery (Fig. 20-1)

Identify the blood vessels going to the colon and you will find that there is an anastomosis that runs parallel to the margin of the colon and links the branches of the superior mesenteric artery with the branches from the inferior mesenteric artery. The marginal artery is an important artery of supply; its existence permits many extensive operative procedures to be done.

ITEM 20-11.   Ileocecal Junction

Tie two strings around the middle of the ascending colon. Cut the bowel between the ties.

Take the cecum to a sink, *not* a washbasin; open it and wash out its contents. Examine not only the orifice of the terminal ileum but also the orifice of the vermiform appendix.

ILEOCECAL VALVE

There is a degree of control over the terminal ileum that permits regulation of the passage of ileal contents into the cecum and that keeps this process in harmony with the digestive activity of the rest of the alimentary system.

As you can see, there is no obvious valve mechanism within this orifice, comparable, say, to the valves of the heart. Accordingly there is debate concerning how the structures act as a valve and how efficient, or competent, the valve is.

Pressure changes in the cecum reflect pressure changes elsewhere in the colon. It is believed that as pressure rises in the cecum the lips of the ileocecal valve are pressed together so that reflux of cecal contents into the ileum is prevented. This is true sometimes, and, when it is true, there is a real danger that a rising pressure will eventually rupture the cecum; obviously there are times when surgical intervention cannot be delayed. On the other hand, there are instances of reflux of cecal contents into the ileum occurring with very little pressure rise in the cecum. These findings together, therefore, lead to the present concept that the ileocecal valve may remain competent or become incompetent for reasons that are not clearly understood. The competence of the valve is revealed either during a barium enema examination or as a result of pathologic changes in the colon.

BOWEL CONTENTS

This very simple point, that the alimentary tract has contents, is largely overlooked by the medical student until he is in his clinical years, when he learns, sometimes quite unexpectedly, that examination of feces is a basic requirement, that the passing of gas (flatus) from the large bowel is a significant clinical sign, that the dark shadows of gas on an abdominal radiograph can serve a diagnostic purpose, and so on; in a word, he learns that gas, feces, and fluid are important matters in a clinical investigation.

RECTUM AND ANAL CANAL

For practical purposes, the rectum and the anal canal are dissected with the pelvis. They are mentioned here so that you do not divorce them entirely from the colon, which you have just dissected. The colon, rectum, and anal canal function as a unit. The function of these organs with reference to bowel habits will be discussed by your clinical tutors.

SMALL BOWEL

ITEM 20-12.   Identify the duodenojejunal flexure. Note the acute angle between the fourth part of the duodenum, which ascends, and the jejunum, whose first inch or two descends inferiorly and anteriorly as well as to the left.

ITEM 20-13.   Seek the suspensory muscle of the duodenum. Do not delay over this structure, for in the cadaver it is difficult to identify. To find it elevate the remaining portion of the transverse mesocolon and pull the duodenojejunal flexure gently inferiorly and anteriorly as well as to the left. The ridge of peritoneum from the flexure toward the midline overlies the suspensory muscle of the duodenum; the ridge is more obvious at operation, and is known to surgeons as the ligament of Treitz.

DIFFERENCES BETWEEN THE JEJUNUM AND ILEUM

The jejunum and ileum are parts of a continuous tube. The change from one to the other is gradual; only the proximal and distal parts of this continuous tube show distinctly different features. The jejunum is wider and thicker; its arterial arcades are not close to the bowel wall, and therefore the vasa recta are long. There is usually less fat in the mesentery. During digestion the lymphatics are more readily seen.

It follows that the ileum is narrower and feels thinner; its arterial arcades are closer to the bowel wall, and therefore the vasa recta are short. There is usually fat in considerable quantity in the mesentery, especially close to the terminal ileum.

The thick feel of the jejunum is due to the presence of circular folds of mucous membrane within the bowel. These folds, termed valvulae conniventes, or plicae circulares, and sometimes called the valves of Kerckring, project into the lumen of the bowel and are most plentiful in the proximal part of the small bowel. You will have the opportunity to see these folds later in the dissection, and to appreciate how they increase the surface of the mucous membrane for the purposes of digestion and absorption.

ITEM 20-14.   Identify the arterial arcades of the mesentery by cleaning away sufficient peritoneum from a proximal and distal portion of the mesentery. Note the difference in the lengths of the vasa recta.

ITEM 20-15.   Tie string twice around the first 2 inches of the jejunum. Cut the bowel between the string.

ITEM 20-16.   Cut the mesentery of the small bowel as in Figure 17-2. Remove the small bowel from the cadaver.

FUNCTION OF THE SMALL BOWEL

In life, the small intestine is more than the short, firm rubberlike tube you have just removed. In life, indeed, the small intestine measures 6 to 7 meters from the duodenojejunal flexure to the ileocecal junction, a length that is more than three times the height of the average man. It may distend to twice its girth under certain circumstances and shrink to half its girth in starvation. Above all, however, it is the site of an amount of biochemical activity that is difficult to envisage and a type of activity that is impossible to comprehend without a knowledge of biochemistry. The anatomy of the small bowel, concerned as it is with digestion and absorption, is indeed a study of the living cell.

BLOOD SUPPLY OF THE MIDGUT

The metabolic activity of the small bowel could not take place without a profuse blood supply. You have already seen the extent of the superior mesenteric tree. Figure 19-1 shows that this artery is in fact the artery to the midgut, which includes not just the small intestine but much of the large intestine as well. It is not generally realized that the superior mesenteric artery is virtually an end artery, meaning that its anastomosis with either the celiac tree or the inferior mesenteric arterial tree is poor (Cokkinis 1961). Thus, when the superior mesenteric artery is occluded at its origin from the aorta and the occlusion involves the middle colic artery as well, then not only is the small bowel deprived of its arterial supply but the large bowel is too, as far as the middle of the transverse colon. If such an arterial occlusion is not cleared rapidly, the affected gut will perish (infarction) with a tragic result.

PERISTALSIS

Peristalsis may be defined as a series of multiple contractions producing a wave that passes along all or part of the small bowel. Normal peristalsis produces regular low-pitched sounds when elicited with a stethoscope. When the small bowel is obstructed there is interference with the downward passage of its contents. Then peristalsis may be very vigorous with high-pitched sounds (called borborygmi) and intermittent rushes which can be easily heard by auscultation of the abdomen. In the later stages of obstruction visible peristalsis (seen through the abdominal wall) may be encountered. The absence of bowel sounds may be normal after an intraabdominal operative procedure or, in other instances, may be an ominous sign of peritonitis, or some other serious entity. Oral intake is usually restricted until normal peristalsis resumes.

Chapter 21

Esophagus, Stomach, Lesser Sac, and Pylorus

The junction of the esophagus and stomach is of particular interest because of disorders which can occur at the junction to impair ingestion. The junction, spoken of sometimes as the cardia (the opening of the stomach near the heart), is called more often the cardioesophageal (also esophagocardiac and esophagogastric) junction. It is self-evident that fluids and solids pass easily from the esophagus into the stomach in the healthy individual, and yet belching and vomiting can also occur with relative ease. In addition, regurgitation of gastric juice onto the vulnerable esophageal mucosa is normally prevented. The factors controlling the junction are not clearly understood (p. 127).

ITEM 21-1. The cardioesophageal junction lies posterior to the left lobe of the liver, and is obscured from view by the left triangular ligament of the liver. To expose the junction, depress the liver lobe sufficiently to expose the ligament extending toward and blending imperceptibly with the peritoneum of the under surface of the diaphragm. The ligament is in fact a peritoneal structure. Cut it. During a surgical operation the next procedure would be to retract the liver and to keep it clear of the operating field with the aid of a metal retractor. But, in the cadaver, to get an adequate view of the esophagus we must remove the left lobe of the liver. To do so, cut into the liver, carefully, so as not to damage the lesser omentum. Cut as close to the falciform ligament as possible. As you approach the posterior aspect of the lobe, be careful where you direct the point of the knife.

Note that in order to expose the esophagus and diaphragm more fully a surgeon would now cut the lesser omentum. But, at our present stage of dissection, this would spoil the lesser omentum. Accordingly, turn now to a study of the gross anatomy of the stomach and the lesser sac. When this study is complete you can destroy the lesser omentum and return to the exposure of the esophagus.

ITEM 21-2. Identify the landmarks of the stomach.

THE STOMACH*

Surely since the days of William Beaumont (1785-1853) and his patient, Alexis St. Martin, no organ has been the subject of more investi-

---

Gaster, hence the adjective *gastric.*

gation, clinical and experimental, than the stomach. Attention today is focused upon the histology and physiology of the stomach, so it is upon those subjects the student must concentrate his attention. Nevertheless, there are some anatomic points to be stressed:

(1) The shape and degree of distention of a healthy stomach vary markedly. That the greater curvature may lie at the level of the pelvic brim is but one example.

(2) The peritoneum covers the posterior as well as the anterior surface of the stomach.

(3) Externally, one cannot distinguish the body of the stomach from the pyloric antrum.

(4) The position of the pylorus may be indicated quite often on the external surface by a groove in which the prepyloric vein is found.

(5) The pylorus is palpable.

(6) The pylorus has a vertical range of movement of 2 to 3 cm. Rarely, therefore, is it on a level with the first lumbar vertebra (the level of the anatomic transpyloric plane).

(7) The muscle fibers of the stomach are: outer layer, longitudinal; intermediate layer, circular; and inner layer, oblique. The oblique layer is really in the shape of an inverted U, the curve of the ∩ riding upon the cardiac notch. The limbs of the ∩ descend along the lesser curvature on each side of the magenstrasse.*

(8) The mucous membrane of the body of the stomach is in the form of loose folds, or rugosities, whereas that of the antrum is more adherent to the submucous layers, and therefore is less rugose.

(9) On a radiograph of the stomach, there is usually a radiolucent area at the fundus of the stomach. This is an air bubble that is a useful radiographic landmark.

Read an account of the histology of the stomach and also of its lymphatic drainage.

ITEM 21-3.   Further Exploration of the Lesser Sac

The lesser sac is an extension of the main part of the peritoneal cavity and lies posterior to the stomach. Reidentify the epiploic foramen, which connects the greater and lesser sacs, and the artificial opening into the sac that you made when you cut the greater omentum (p. 90).

To open the lesser sac more widely it is necessary to cut across the stomach halfway between its cardiac and pyloric ends. Do so, and extend the cut into the lesser omentum toward the liver. In cutting the stomach in this fashion you will inevitably cut the arterial anastomosis between the left and right gastroepiploic arteries parallel to the greater curvature

---

*The magenstrasse is the strip of smooth mucous membrane deep to the lesser curvature of the stomach. On each edge of the strip a fold of mucosa occurs and creates the magenstrasse, believed to convey at least fluids, if not solids, from the cardia to the pylorus. Not much emphasis is put upon the magenstrasse today, except that it is a common site of ulceration.

and a similar anastomosis between the left and right gastric arteries along the lesser curvature. In addition, remember that the accompanying veins, not usually well seen in a cadaver, will also be cut, as well as lymphatics and autonomic nerve fibers.

Retract the antrum, i.e., the distal part of the stomach, to the right and the body of the stomach, i.e., its proximal part, to the left. The lesser sac is now wide open and you can see peritoneum on the abdominal surface of the pancreas and other structures, to be identified. In passing, examine the mucosa both in the body and the antrum of the stomach. Postmortem autolysis more than likely has destroyed their normal appearance.

ITEM 21-4. Lesser Sac and Spleen

Slip the fingers (preferably of the left hand, while you stand on the right hand side of the body) posterior to the stomach and to the left — gently, because peritoneum in the cadaver tears easily — and you will reach the spleen. Now establish the relationship of the spleen by grasping it between fingers and thumb of the right hand as shown in Figure 17-5.

The peritoneum between spleen and stomach is the gastrosplenic ligament, which you should identify, whereas the peritoneum between the spleen and the left kidney is the lienorenal ligament (*lien*—spleen). You should be able to get the fingers of the left hand on to the hilum of the spleen, so demonstrating the left lateral extent of the lesser sac. (Fig. 17-5).

ITEM 21-5. Upper Recess of the Lesser Sac

Next identify through the peritoneum the celiac artery on the aorta, nearly in the midline, just superior to the neck of the pancreas.

You should be able to slide a finger superiorly on the right side of the celiac artery into a recess behind the liver. This recess is termed the upper recess of the lesser sac. Don't waste time, for the anatomy is easy although the instructions may seem complex; ask for a demonstration, if need be.

The area of the liver anterior to the recess you have just explored is called the caudate lobe. At its inferior limit you will notice a projection of liver substance, called the caudate process. The caudate process lies superior to the epiploic foramen.*

ITEM 21-6. With scissors, trim away the left portion of the lesser omentum by cutting it close to the lesser curvature; in doing so the left gastric artery will be exposed. Then trim away the attachment of this part of the omentum to the liver. If the pyloric antrum and the remainder of the omentum are held well over to the right you should have a good view of the origin of the celiac artery and its branches.

---

*The caudate lobe of the liver was so-called because of the taillike appearance of the caudate process (*cauda* — tail).

Celiac Artery and Branches

You have already identified the celiac artery. Now you must consider its branches, the hepatic, the splenic, and the left gastric arteries. Be alert for possible arterial variations, for there are many such possibilities in this region of the abdomen.

ITEM 21-7. Identify all three arteries in relation to peritoneum, and establish their relationship to the lesser sac (Figure 21-1).

ITEM 21-8. Left Gastric Artery

From the celiac artery, the left gastric artery ascends to the left and can be seen through peritoneum. Soon it turns inferiorly (the bend in the artery is abreast of the cardioesophageal junction) to reach the lesser curvature of the stomach. Pull on the stomach to demonstrate the artery through peritoneum. The cut end of the artery may be noted between the two layers of the lesser omentum.

ITEM 21-9. Splenic Artery

Mark the celiac artery, then grasp the spleen and pull it firmly to the left as well as anteriorly. This maneuver should raise a ridge of peritoneum immediately superior to and parallel to the pancreas and extending from the celiac artery. Trace the artery up to the hilum of the spleen.

To identify the left gastroepiploic and the short gastric arteries, have one partner pull the body of the stomach superiorly. This procedure ought to put tension on the gastrosplenic ligament in which the short gastric arteries and the left gastroepiploic artery lie.

ITEM 21-10. Hepatic Artery

Pull the pyloric antrum of the stomach to the right and you should observe a conspicuous ridge in the peritoneum from the region of the celiac artery to the margin of the lesser omentum. Deep to the ridge lies the hepatic artery.

Before you tear away peritoneum to expose these arteries more clearly, consider for a moment their relationship to peritoneum. These arteries, in their relationship to the peritoneum, exemplify the principle stated on p. 80 that nothing passes through the peritoneal cavity. Before you advance further, make sure you appreciate this point with the aid of Figure 21-1.

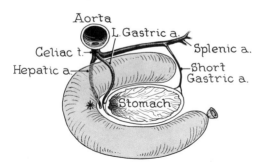

Figure 21-1. By bending an inflated long, thin balloon one can create a greater and lesser sac. The stomach fits into the cleft, as illustrated. The branches of the celiac artery travel posterior to, inferior to, and superior to the lesser sac to reach their destination. The asterisk inside the balloon indicates the free edge of the lesser omentum. See also Figure 17-5.

ITEM 21-11. Now remove peritoneum to expose the three branches of the celiac artery and their branches. Look out for variations. With the aid of diagrams, establish the arterial supply to the stomach.

ITEM 21-12. Resume dissection of the lower end of the esophagus. A helpful procedure is to cut away the left costal margin and the anterior half of the left diaphragm. This procedure is possible if the thorax has already been dissected and the arrangement of the diaphragm investigated.

ITEM 21-13. It is your purpose now to show the following points concerning the esophagus.

(1) Its relationship to peritoneum, hence the peritoneal cavity
(2) Its arterial supply from the left gastric artery
(3) Its venous drainage to the left gastric vein
(4) Its relationship to the vagus nerves
(5) The phrenicoesophageal ligament
(6) The esophageal opening in the diaphragm

To expose (2), (3), (4), (5), and (6), it is necessary to strip off peritoneum from the esophagus. Do so now to expose (2) and (3).

THE VENOUS DRAINAGE OF THE LOWER END OF THE ESOPHAGUS

Essentially, the veins in the area you have just dissected have a pattern similar to the arteries you have just identified. No doubt, while cleaning the arteries you destroyed or mutilated their accompanying veins.

One vein requires special mention, namely the left gastric vein, for it drains not just its particular territory on the stomach but also the lower end of the esophagus. The left gastric vein joins the portal vein. Now if the blood flow from any part of the body is obstructed, the veins of that part will become engorged while the venous pressure rises. The portal vein is no exception. Therefore, when it is obstructed, all the veins whose blood drains ultimately into it will eventually become congested (portal hypertension). In severe portal hypertension the esophageal veins become distended like varicose veins of the leg. Hence distended esophageal veins are called esophageal varices. They are highly significant because they may rupture, causing a profound, and probably fatal, hemorrhage.

ITEM 21-14. The exposure of the vagus nerves from below the diaphragm is very difficult in a cadaver because the different tissues look and feel alike. Therefore, do not attempt to expose them until you have mobilized the vagus nerves above the diaphragm, even though the usual surgical approach to the vagus nerves in this region is from the abdominal aspect. If the thorax has already been dissected, you will then have removed pleura from the esophagus and exposed the esophageal plexus of nerves. From the inferior edge of this plexus emerge the strands of the vagus nerves, which you identified, leaving the thorax through the esophageal hiatus in the diaphragm. Let one partner pull gently on the left vagus nerve in the thorax while you pull the stomach and esophagus inferiorly. Clean away peritoneum and extraperitoneal tissue, probably the phrenicoesophageal ligament, and you should see the vagus nerve on the anterior aspect of the esophagus.

Do likewise with the right vagus nerve, which you will find by twisting the esophagus to expose its posterior surface, where the right vagus nerve now lies. This nerve, unlike the left one, may not be closely applied to the esophagus, but may be lying free in the space between the esophagus and the aorta.

Each vagus nerve may consist of more than one strand. During vagotomy, a surgical procedure adopted in the treatment of duodenal ulcer to reduce the secretion of gastric juice, it is essential for the surgeon to recognize the variations of the vagus nerve. It is not necessary for you to do so at this level of instruction, but you should possess the following information:

Each vagus nerve divides into two components. The right vagus has a small gastric branch to the stomach and a large branch to the celiac plexus. The left vagus has a large gastric branch and a smaller branch to the liver, gallbladder, pylorus, and pyloric canal. To reach the canal, this last branch, often a plexus of nerves, travels in the lesser omentum, which you have already destroyed. You will have observed, no doubt, that the right vagus nerve passed onto the posterior surface of the stomach and that the left vagus nerve was distributed to the anterior surface of the stomach. Hence there is a change in terminology, and instead of referring to right and left vagus nerves we refer to posterior and anterior gastric nerves.

Do not be dismayed if the dissection is untidy. It is nearly impossible for the undergraduate to cut and reflect neatly cadaveric peritoneum or fascia. Tags of tissue are an inevitable consequence of his dissection in this difficult region of the abdomen.

ITEM 21-15.   To expose the esophageal hiatus, remove as much peritoneum as possible to mobilize the esophagus. In doing so you will come upon fascia filling the gap between the esophagus and the margins of the diaphragmatic opening. This fascia, called the phrenicoesophageal ligament, is a surgical landmark in operative procedures in this region.

ITEM 21-16.   Continue to remove peritoneum and fascia until the right crus of the diaphragm is exposed. It is in this crus of the diaphragm that the esophageal opening is most commonly found. Examine the slinglike arrangement of the right crus over the cardiac notch.

THE CARDIOESOPHAGEAL JUNCTION

Acid indigestion and similar complaints are now so frequently investigated by radiology that the factors controlling the movement of contents into and out of the stomach merit considerable attention. However, only a brief synopsis of the present concepts of the functional anatomy of the cardioesophageal junction is given here.

It is generally believed that the efficiency of the junction depends upon intrinsic and extrinsic factors. The extrinsic factors have been considered more important during this past decade because an intrinsic sphincter had not been demonstrated. Recent work, however, reveals that an intrinsic sphincter may well exist (Zaino et al., 1963).

The intrinsic factors operative at the lower end of the esophagus are:

(1) circular smooth muscle fibers, reinforced by additional muscle bundles irregular in shape, size, and direction (Zaino et al.).

(2) the esophageal mucosa and its underlying lamina muscularis mucosae (the muscle layer of the mucosa).

(3) the oblique fibers of the stomach, a third layer of fibers that straddle the cardiac notch.

The extrinsic factors are: (1) the phrenicoesophageal fascia (also called ligament), (2) the angle at which the esophagus joins the stomach, and (3) the crus of the diaphragm wherein lies the esophageal hiatus. The diaphragmatic fibers do not fit snugly around the esophagus, nor do they fit tightly into the cardiac notch. Moreover, while it is true that the hiatus is usually in the right crus of the diaphragm, frequently muscle slips from the left crus lie along the boundaries of the hiatus.

ITEM 21-17. Explore the lower end of the esophagus with an index finger inserted into its lumen from the body of the stomach. Press around and test how patulous the hiatus may be. The portion of the esophagus within the confines of the hiatus is spoken of as the vestibule by radiologists.

ITEM 21-18. The pylorus

Slit the right portion of the stomach longitudinally, i.e., proceeding from the pyloric antrum to the pyloric canal as far as the pylorus. Note that the pyloric canal is distinct from and proximal to the pylorus. The latter is recognizable by its easily identified sphincter of muscle. Slit the pylorus. No doubt you will slit the first part of the duodenum too.

PYLORUS

One reason for paying attention to the pylorus is the fairly common occurrence of congenital pyloric stenosis (stenosis means narrowing). In this condition the narrowing of the lumen of the pylorus is due to both hypertrophy and contraction of the pyloric musculature. As a result, emptying of the stomach is delayed; vomiting occurs and may require surgery. If this is so, the operative procedure is to slit the musculature but not the mucosa of the pylorus. That the pylorus is palpable and that visible peristalsis of the stomach may be seen through the anterior abdominal wall of the infant are physical signs noted in this condition.

Chapter 22

The Region of the Head of the Pancreas

Because the duodenum, the head of the pancreas, the bile duct, and the portal vein, (as well as the major arteries in this area) are so intimately related to each other that one cannot be dissected without disturbing the other, the following order is recommended to demonstrate the anatomy of these structures to best advantage. It will become obvious that further consideration will be necessary in order to gain a total concept of each organ, structure, and system. The methods of dissection are based upon standard surgical procedures.

Structures posterior to the head of the pancreas:
Bile duct
Portal vein
Inferior vena cava
Structures superior to the head of the pancreas:
Biliary ducts
Portal vein
Hepatic artery
The duodenum

STRUCTURES POSTERIOR TO THE HEAD OF THE PANCREAS

The Bile Duct

ITEM 22-1. This duct may be exposed by displacing the second part of the duodenum. If the liver in your specimen obstructs your approach in the procedure, ask a staff member to remove a large segment of the liver to allow you to proceed. Then make a vertical incision, cautiously, into what remains of the peritoneum between the right kidney and the duodenum (the removal of the transverse colon may have destroyed much of the peritoneum in this area). Next roll the duodenum over to the left and somewhat inferiorly. The posterior surface of the head of the pancreas should come into view almost immediately, and you should have no difficulty in identifying the bile duct, which is invariably stained green in the cadaver. In the process of your exposure of the duct you will certainly meet pancreaticoduodenal arteries, and you will inadvertently destroy some veins. In a surgical operative procedure similar to what you are now doing, such vessels must be managed with great care by the surgeon because otherwise the operative field may be flooded with blood, but you are at liberty to ignore them in dissecting a cadaver.

Portal Vein

ITEM 22-2. If your specimen will yield sufficiently, continue to displace the duodenum and head of the pancreas anteriorly and to the left, until you expose the portal vein posterior to the neck of the pancreas. If all goes well you will finally expose at least two veins joining to form the portal vein, namely the splenic vein from the left and the superior mesenteric vein from an inferior direction; often the inferior mesenteric vein joins here too.

Return, for the moment, to the origin of the superior mesenteric artery and, on its right, identify the superior mesenteric vein. By blunt dissection with an index finger, maneuver the finger along the vein posterior to the neck of the pancreas and anterior to a portion of the pancreas called the uncinate process. Maneuver your index finger superiorly until the superior mesenteric vein and its continuation, the portal vein, are sufficiently free.

Inferior Vena Cava

ITEM 22-3. Return to the anterior surface of the right kidney and identify on its anteromedial aspect a part of the inferior vena cava.

Note the proximity of the head of the pancreas, the bile duct, and portal vein to the inferior vena cava, relationships of real significance in surgery. For example, it is in this area that the portal vein may be connected to the inferior vena cava (portacaval anastomosis) in order to reduce the venous engorgement of the portal system. See p. 125, Esophageal Varices.

Pancreatic Duct

The principal pancreatic duct extends throughout the length of the gland from the tail, where the duct begins, into the head, where the duct terminates. The main pancreatic duct terminates in several ways, all of them in association with the bile duct. The relationship of the two ducts is important clinically, and that is why it is mentioned here. In a cadaver, however, it is easier to demonstrate the association of the pancreatic duct and the bile duct once the pancreas has been removed.

STRUCTURES SUPERIOR TO THE HEAD OF THE PANCREAS IN THE FREE EDGE OF THE LESSER OMENTUM

ITEM 22-4. Identify the right portion of the lesser omentum (the lesser omentum was cut when the stomach was divided). Reidentify the right margin of the lesser omentum. It is the ridge you palpated immediately anterior to the epiploic foramen.

The procedure now is to remove peritoneum to expose the hepatic artery, the portal vein, and the biliary ducts, all of them, as they lie in the lesser omentum. Begin with the hepatic artery and trace it to the porta hepatis. Expect variations, and take note of the cystic artery.

ITEM 22-5. To expose the cystic duct, let one partner pull the liver and gallbladder superiorly. At the same time, another partner pulls the first part of the duodenum inferiorly and to the left. The edge of the lesser omentum and the structures therein should appear tense. Now, from the gallbladder, follow the cystic duct to the point where it joins the common hepatic duct, at the beginning of the bile duct. Look out for the cystic artery, so variable in position.

Having identified the termination of the common hepatic duct, trace it proximally (i.e., toward the liver) to where it begins. The common hepatic duct begins where the right and left hepatic ducts conjoin. If you cannot identify the right and left hepatic ducts overlapped by the lips of the porta hepatis, they can be identified later, once the liver has been removed.

ITEM 22-6. Establish the continuity of the extrahepatic bile system from the portal hepatis to the duodenum. Note that the portal vein lies posterior to both the hepatic artery and the biliary ducts, the artery is on the left, and the ducts are to the right, anterior to the portal vein.

BILIARY SYSTEM

The gallbladder and the rest of the biliary system must not be passed over lightly, for they are a common center of clinical problems ranging from atresia of the bile duct, discovered at birth, to a small cancer, occurring at the ampulla, in a much older age group. In both instances, jaundice is the result of obstruction of the free flow of bile into the duodenum.

The basic anatomy of the biliary system is easily understood. Only certain anatomic facts that seem to escape the student are discussed here.

In life, the gallbladder is *not* the thick-walled, shrunken, deep green organ you see in the cadaver. Instead, it is a relatively thin-walled organ, bluish green in color; it may distend to such a size and become so firm that its fundus is palpable through the anterior abdominal wall at the level of the ninth costal cartilage.

In the erect position, the fundus of the gallbladder is at a lower level than its neck. Therefore, do not misinterpret diagrams showing the gallbladder sticking up like a toadstool from the forest floor. When the gallbladder contents are infected by bacteria the fundus of the gall-bladder is like a cesspool and is the more common site of rupture.

At the neck of the gallbladder a dilatation (Hartmann's pouch) is commonly seen.

The bile duct, on a radiograph, is superimposed upon the transverse processes of L1 and 2. The commencement of the right ureter occupies the same position. Both are tubular structures likely to be obstructed by stones. It follows that radiographs of this region can only be interpreted correctly by taking the complete medical history into consideration.

The student of gross anatomy tends to recognize only the more obvious parts of the biliary system and to ignore the microscopic parts in the liver substance. Both parts, microscopic and macroscopic, are important in the pathology of the biliary system.

The system begins with microscopic bile canaliculi between the liver cells. These canaliculi join to form bile ductules, which emerge from the microscopic lobules of liver tissue. Ultimately, the ductules join the tributaries of the right and left hepatic ducts that emerge from the liver at the porta hepatis. Thus, the biliary system may be divided into an intrahepatic part (*intra*—within) that we have just briefly described and an extrahepatic part (*extra*-outside) to be described next.

The right and left hepatic ducts lie horizontally between the lips of the porta hepatis. In the embalmed liver, those lips are usually conspicuous, overshadowing the hepatic ducts. Once the liver of your cadaver is removed, you should carve away sufficient liver from around the porta to expose these hepatic ducts as they join together to form the common hepatic duct. In passing, it is of value to comment upon the size of the hepatic ducts, the volume of bile they transmit, and their location. Both ducts are explored by a surgeon investigating obstructive jaundice.

To continue, the common hepatic duct, after it is joined by the cystic duct, is renamed the bile duct, which finally opens into the duodenum.

Offshoots of the main biliary pathway are the cystic duct and gall-bladder. A common error is to believe that bile reaches the gallbladder directly from the liver. Of course it does not; bile reaches the gallbladder from the hepatic duct via the cystic duct. The gallbladder is simply a reservoir for bile, but, in addition, it concentrates bile and adds mucus as well as regulating the flow of bile into the duodenum during digestion.

The Bile Duct

For descriptive purposes five parts of the bile duct are recognized:
1. The supraduodenal part, in the lesser omentum
2. The *retro-* (behind) or *para-* (beside) duodenal part alongside the first part of the duodenum
3. The pancreatic part, posterior to or perhaps partially or totally embedded in the head of the pancreas
4. The mural part, within the wall of the duodenum
5. The ampullary part, the cavity of a papilla that projects into the lumen of the duodenum

ITEM 22-7. Identify the first three descriptive parts of the bile duct. Then, identify the fifth part: make a longitudinal incision into the second part of the duodenum throughout the length of its convex border. Open the duodenum widely and, with a damp cloth, remove any debris. If a papilla is not visible on first inspection, insert a needle and inject water into the bile duct. Some water will emerge into the duodenum to reveal the position of the papilla.

Exploration of the mural part, i.e., the fourth descriptive part of the bile duct, is to be left until the pancreatic duct is exposed.

Note: To some readers, it may seem pedantic to describe in five parts a structure that is only 7.5 cm. long, but each single part can be involved in a disease process, and the careful surgeon must examine each part to establish a final diagnosis of one of the causes of obstructive jaundice; this is the one region of the body where the price of success is precision.

Jaundice

In discussing the anatomy of the extrahepatic biliary system it is inevitable that jaundice be mentioned. By definition, jaundice is a clinical condition characterized by an excess of bilirubin in the blood and the deposition of bile pigment in the skin and mucous membranes, causing the characteristic yellow appearance of the patient's skin. Bili-rubin, a breakdown product of red blood cells, is excreted by the biliary

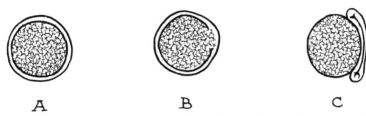

Figure 22-1. Three ways to block a tube. *A.* Stone lodged in the lumen. *B.* Growth from the wall of the tube. *C.* Pressure from without the tube.

system. One, and only one, of the causes of jaundice is obstruction of the flow of bile from the liver to the duodenum (obstructive jaundice), the obstruction occurring somewhere in the extrahepatic biliary system, which includes, mark you, the right and left hepatic ducts. There are several other causes of jaundice to be classified and discussed in detail by your clinical instructors.

Obstruction of a Hollow Organ

This applied anatomy topic is dealt with here because the biliary system is most suitable for it. A tube may be blocked in three ways (Fig. 22-1): (1) obstruction in the lumen, e.g., gallstone; (2) obstruction of the lumen by growth from the wall, e.g., cancer of the wall of the bile duct; and (3) narrowing of the lumen by pressure from without, e.g., cancer of the head of the pancreas. In other hollow tubular organs, similar conditions occur.

THE DUODENUM

In reviewing the anatomy of the duodenum, observe the following points:

First Part

The first part of the duodenum passes posteriorly almost at right angles to the pylorus (Fig. 22-2). This angle, frequently unnoticed, is of some importance because it means that there is a precise part of the duodenal wall upon which stomach contents are ejected from the pylorus. The first part of the duodenum is mobile because it is almost entirely surrounded by peritoneum. The gallbladder is apposed to the first part of the duodenum, but of course, the peritoneal cavity separates them.

With this fact in mind, take a second look at anatomic and surgical illustrations of this region; normally the duodenal cap (p. 88) touches the inferior surface of the liver *across* the peritoneal cavity. Knowledge of

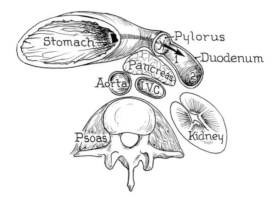

Figure 22-2. The first part of the duodenum proceeds posteriorly and so makes an angle with the stomach. The black arrow indicates the principal direction of stomach contents leaving the stomach through the pylorus.

the proximity of the gallbladder to the duodenum is necessary in order to understand how a false passage, known as a fistula, may develop between the fundus of the gallbladder and the duodenum after inflammation and adhesions have obliterated the peritoneal cavity between them. In like fashion, a fistula may also occur between gallbladder and transverse colon. In both instances, gallstones may pass directly from the gallbladder into the other organ.

Second Part

For descriptive purposes, the second part of the duodenum is divided by the attachment of the mesocolon into a supracolic and infracolic part. Often the transverse colon is directly related to the duodenum. In other words, the mesocolon may not extend far to the right. Recall the arrangement in your specimen before you removed the transverse colon.

Third part

This part crosses anterior to the vertebral column. Refer to p. 89 and recall how far forward the bodies of the vertebrae project. Look at the lumbar vertebrae of a skeleton. Then it will be easy to understand how a blow to the abdomen can damage the third part of the duodenum. The superior mesenteric vessels cross this part of the duodenum at right angles.

Fourth Part

Around the area of the duodenojejunal flexure various minor peritoneal recesses occur. Rarely are these recesses seen in a cadaver, but they are frequently illustrated to perfection in anatomic texts. You do *not* need to learn the anatomic details of these recesses, but you must know of their existence. Sometimes a loop of bowel may herniate into one of them and become strangulated. The clinical diagnosis of this condition, an internal hernia, tests the acumen of the clinician. The anatomic diagnosis can be made accurately only at operation. When a surgeon suspects that a loop of bowel has become strangulated in this manner he will not delay operation.

Read an account of the duodenum and the head of the pancreas.

Chapter 23

The Liver, Pancreas, and Spleen

REMOVAL OF THE LIVER AND ADNEXA

The structures to be severed are the inferior vena cava (above and below the liver), and the peritoneal ligaments between the liver and diaphragm. In addition, to release the pancreas, the hepatic artery and splenic artery must be cut, the duodenum mobilized in the region of the duodenojejunal flexure, and the spleen detached from the proximal part of the stomach. If all goes well, liver, pancreas, duodenum, and spleen will be removed together. Proceed as follows.

ITEM 23-1. If a better exposure of the superior aspect of the liver is needed, remove the right costal margin and trim an inch off the diaphragm. This maneuver is possible only if the thorax has already been dissected.

ITEM 23-2. (1) Begin with inferior vena cava. Identify and cut it just above the right renal vein. (2) Pull the diaphragm superiorly and the liver inferiorly to expose one layer of the coronary ligament and the right triangular ligament. Slit these with a knife. (3) If you can (it is often impossible in a cadaver), expose the other layer of the coronary ligament between the liver and the right kidney, and slit it. (4) The left triangular ligament was cut when the esophagus was exposed. (5) Pull the liver forward and the remaining peritoneal attachments between liver and body wall will tear quite easily. The liver should be quite free now. If not, consult with an instructor.

ITEM 23-3. (1) Close to the celiac artery cut the splenic and the hepatic artery. (2) Mobilize the duodenojejunal flexure. (3) Cut the gastrosplenic ligaments between the spleen and stomach. It should now be possible to remove the liver, pancreas, duodenum, and spleen from the cadaver. If there is difficulty consult an instructor.

THE LIVER

In keeping with the progress in medical knowledge in our time, less and less attention is being paid to the surfaces, borders, grooves, impressions, and indentions of the cadaveric liver, while interest is centering upon the internal segmental anatomy of the liver, especially in the surgical patient. Therefore, while it is a challenge of intellect to identify markings on an isolated liver, it is more practical to adopt the present more common approach, to visualize the liver in situ and to describe it as having visceral and diaphragmatic surfaces.

The visceral surface is related primarily to the peritoneal cavity and is separated by the cavity from the following structures, in order from left to right: (1) the esophagus, stomach, and lesser omentum; (2) the lesser sac, posterior to the lesser omentum, which separates the liver from the pancreas; (3) the pylorus and first part of the duodenum; and (4) the transverse colon and right colic (hepatic) flexure, posterior to which is the right kidney.

Two structures are related directly to the visceral surface of the liver, the gallbladder and right suprarenal gland.

It is the extent of the diaphragmatic surface the student does not immediately comprehend. This surface fits into the dome of the diaphragm, but is separated from the diaphragm by the peritoneal cavity (see Subphrenic Spaces, p. 89). In one area, between the coronary ligaments, the liver and diaphragm are not separated by the peritoneal cavity; they are separated only by a thin layer of areolar tissue. This, the so-called bare area of the liver, is no different from similar areas on other organs. Wherever peritoneum is reflected in order to maintain the continuity of its surface (p. 80) bare areas occur. The significance of the bare area of the liver is that only the diaphragm separates the liver from the pleural cavity.

The dome shape of the diaphragm is worth mentioning again. Because of its relationship to this dome, the superior aspect of the liver is well within the thoracic cage and may reach the level of the fourth costal cartilage. It follows that the liver is related just beyond the diaphragm to the pleural cavities and, on the right, to the depths of the right costodiaphragmatic recess. A knife plunged into the rib cage over the flank would probably pass through the pleural cavity twice, transfix the lung, cross the peritoneal cavity, and enter the liver.

Physical Examination of the Liver

The one edge or border of the liver the medical student must know of is the one that is roughly parallel to the right costal margin and demarcates the diaphragmatic from the visceral surface anteriorly. When the consistency of the liver substance is altered by disease, this edge is usually palpable. Indeed, one of the fundamental procedures in a physical examination is to determine whether or not the liver edge is palpable and, if it is, to decide why.

Segments of the Liver

Obviously the falciform ligament divides the liver into two parts, but this obvious external division does not correspond with an internal division revealed by modern research. The true plane of division, based upon the distribution of vessels and ducts, is about 2 inches to the right of the falciform ligament. The plane is vertical, and it cuts the liver through the bed of the gallbladder and extends posteriorly and to the left toward the vertically disposed inferior vena cava. As a result the caudate and quadrate lobes of the liver are part of the left surgical lobe, whereas the right surgical lobe does not extend as far to the left as the falciform ligament. Additional smaller subsegments are identifiable. The segmental arrangement of the liver is the basis of modern liver surgery.

EXPLORATION OF THE PANCREAS

ITEM 23-4. Identify the gross features of the pancreas. You have already identified the head of the pancreas, confined by the duodenum, and the neck of the pancreas, behind which lie the superior mesenteric vessels and portal vein; the rest of the pancreas is termed the body, and it tapers somewhat to a tail touching the hilum of the spleen. Review the peritoneal relationships of the pancreas, pp. 81 and 91.

ITEM 23-5. To find the pancreatic duct, identify the posterior surface of the pancreas. This is best done by laying the liver and adnexa on a flat surface so that their posterior aspects are exposed. Identify the bile duct and trace it toward the duodenum by carefully snipping away adjacent pancreatic tissue. Proceed carefully in the neighborhood of the termination of the bile duct, where the termination of the pancreatic duct will be found. The pancreatic duct usually joins the bile duct from an inferior direction. Once you have found the main pancreatic duct, proceed to expose it by dissecting for several inches toward the tail of the pancreas. You may come across an accessory pancreatic duct leaving the main duct and heading toward the superior aspect of the second part of the duodenum. The presence of an accessory pancreatic duct means that there is an alternative route for pancreatic juice if the main duct is obstructed.

ITEM 23-6. Intramural and ampullary parts of both the bile duct and the pancreatic duct can be exposed properly only by meticulous dissection under magnification. Nevertheless, attempt to expose them by threading a plastic thread, or some blunt slender object, into (1) the bile duct and (2) the pancreatic duct. With a very sharp knife or razor blade, slit the lumen of each duct, continuing through the duodenal wall and the ampulla. Try to observe precisely where and how the bile and pancreatic ducts conjoin.

Read an account of the termination of the bile and pancreatic ducts. The ampulla is still frequently referred to as the ampulla of Vater, the sphincter of muscle within the papilla as the sphincter of Oddi, and the sphincter at the lower end of the bile duct as the sphincter of Boyden.

CLINICAL EXAMINATION OF THE PANCREAS

The pancreas, slung across the posterior abdominal wall, may seem remote. Nevertheless, clues about its functions can be gleaned by indirect methods. Its two main functions are the production of enzymes and insulin. The deficiency of enzyme production is revealed in the quality and quantity of feces; in cystic fibrosis, for example, the stool is slimy, bulky, and offensive, and is described clinically as a fatty stool. In another instance, derangement of enzyme production leads to an accumulation of the enzymes in the blood, thence the urine.

Insulin production is estimated by the level of the blood sugar. In summary, therefore, examination of the feces, urine, and blood gives valuable evidence about the state of the pancreas. Finally, radiographic studies of the duodenum with the aid of barium may reveal distortions of the normal shape of the head of the pancreas. Thus the pancreas can be "examined," remote though it seems to be from the anterior abdominal wall.

THE SPLEEN

The spleen was considered in relation to the peritoneal cavity on p. 92. Here your attention is drawn to two other aspects of clinical importance, namely the spleen as an organ of the hematopoietic system and palpation of the spleen.

It is difficult for a student in the gross anatomy laboratory to visualize the key role played by the spleen in the normal function of the hematopoietic system. Not only does the spleen take part in the destruction of blood cells and, to a lesser extent, the production of blood cells, but it also plays a large part in the immunologic responses of the body. When blood destruction by the spleen is of a degree to endanger life, then splenectomy must be considered, and once you have seen clinicians contemplating the removal of a spleen, you will realize the balance of power held by the spleen in the government of the hematopoietic system. Therefore, in time, you must study that system and the role played by the spleen.

In doing so include a review of the embryology of the spleen. Why? Because accessory spleens are not uncommon. An accessory spleen is a small rounded mass of splenic tissue remote from the main organ; it is believed that after splenectomy accessory spleens may assume the function of the definitive spleen and so perpetuate the blood disorder. Therefore, accessory spleens must be sought for and removed by a surgeon performing splenectomy.

Look for accessory spleens in your specimen. One or two can often be found at the hilum of the definitive spleen.

Palpation of the Spleen

What is meant by palpation of the spleen is very confusing to the student. First of all, normally a spleen is not palpable. If it is palpable, then it must be considered abnormal until proven otherwise. It is generally held that the spleen must increase in size by at least one third before it is palpable.

Confusion arises in the student's mind when he reads in anatomic and clinical textbooks that the spleen is palpable at the left costal margin. What is meant, really, is that this is the quadrant of abdomen that the clinician would palpate to see if the spleen is or is not palpable. If the spleen is actually felt at the left costal margin, then it is abnormal in size, and the clinician must discover why. There is an exact technique for seeking the spleen by palpation to be learned at the bedside from your clinical instructors. Meanwhile, revise your knowledge of the location of the normal spleen. Where does the spleen normally lie?

ITEM 23-7. Detach the spleen from the other abdominal viscera. Replace the spleen in its normal position adjacent to the left kidney. Note the proximity of kidney to spleen. A palpable mass in the left flank may not be spleen; it may be kidney. Observe the notches on the anterior border of the spleen; their presence may help to establish that a palpable mass in the left flank or the left upper quadrant is, in fact, the spleen.

Chapter 24

Posterior Abdominal Wall

Introduction

This wall consists of a protruding central zone of vertical extent, and, on each side, a receding area quadrilateral in shape (Figs. 17-3 and 17-5).

The central zone consists of longitudinal structures, the lumbar spine, the right and left sympathetic trunks, the abdominal aorta, and the inferior vena cava; the right and left crura of the diaphragm are attached to the lumbar spine; deep to the right crus lies the cisterna chyli and the beginning of the thoracic duct. Lateral to each crus lies the psoas major, but this muscle is best included in the topographic anatomy of the lateral area.

Two muscles form the background of each lateral area, the psoas major covered on its abdominal surface by the psoas fascia and, lateral to the psoas, the quadratus lumborum. Related to these muscles are some of the branches of the lumbar plexus emerging from the psoas fascia to cross the quadratus lumborum in a horizontal direction. The prominent feature of each lateral area, however, is a kidney embedded in fat and invested in fascia; a suprarenal (adrenal) gland rests on the upper pole of the kidney while the ureter arises at the anteromedial aspect.

In approaching the dissection of this region the following points are important:

(1) You have come through the peritoneal cavity. Therefore, one layer of peritoneum covers, to some extent, all the structures you will encounter. No doubt this posterior layer of peritoneum has already been mutilated in your dissection so far. Nevertheless, you must recall the existence of peritoneum, for it is a landmark in surgical operations upon structures of this region when the transperitoneal route is used.

(2) It is not always necessary to open the peritoneal cavity to reach the posterior abdominal wall structures. It is possible to reach the region through an incision extending across the flank and the lateral aspect of the posterior abdominal wall. Then peritoneum is peeled back, so to speak, to displace the peritoneal cavity, which remains intact. This approach is called extraperitoneal or retroperitoneal, and is particularly useful if the surgeon wishes to avoid contamination of the peritoneal cavity. The extraperitoneal approach is commonly used in surgical procedures on the kidney and also in the removal of the lumbar sympathetic chain (sympathectomy) and in the drainage of pus collected in psoas major (psoas abscess).

(3) The posterior abdominal wall is not a flat surface. The central

140

vertical part of the wall projects anteriorly (Figs. 17-3 and 17-5). On each side of this central projection the wall recedes rapidly and then gradually turns anteriorly to join the flank. In other words, the central part is like a steep mountain range between two broad valleys.

Accordingly, the exact anatomic position of structures related to the wall cannot be portrayed accurately in illustrations unless the artist is extremely skilled in revealing the third dimension. In this region there is not only height and breadth; there is also depth. The kidneys, for example, face laterally as well as anteriorly; the pancreas, molded to the rise and fall of the posterior abdominal wall, is rather like an elongated S in shape; the duodenum conforms to the contours of this region so that the first part of it lies anterior to the second part, creating the duodenal bulb or cap appearance seen on radiographs.

Now that you appreciate the rise and fall of the posterior abdominal wall you can see how blunt trauma upon the anterior abdominal wall (e.g., the impact of a steering wheel) can damage the pancreas, duodenum, and aorta, as a result of the compressive force between the injuring object and the vertebral column.

Proceed now to dissect the central zone of the posterior abdominal wall.

ITEM 24-1. Identify the abdominal aorta—a cardinal feature of the posterior abdominal wall. Observe the entire abdominal aorta, from its point of entry into the abdomen behind the median arcuate ligament of the diaphragm down to its bifurcation into the right and left common iliac arteries. Consider its branches, which may be divided into two groups: group 1 is central and unpaired; group 2 is lateral and paired.

In the first group, the celiac artery, superior mesenteric artery, and inferior mesenteric artery arise from the anterior aspect of the aorta while the median sacral artery arises from the *posterior* aspect just above the bifurcation. In the second group are the phrenic arteries, suprarenal arteries, renal arteries, gonadal arteries, and lumbar arteries.

Now reconsider the abdominal aorta as a whole and take note of the precise location of the renal arteries. Aortic aneurysm occurs most commonly distal to the origins of the renal arteries. If an aneurysm extends proximally to involve the origins of the renal arteries, or more proximal still, beyond the diaphragm, into the thorax, then the surgical treatment of the aneurysm is greatly complicated. Distally, an aneurysm may extend into both common iliac arteries.

ITEM 24-2. Exercise

In an intact specimen, what structures lie anterior to the abdominal aorta? What structures lie posterior to the abdominal aorta? What structures lie on each side?

What organs and structures are supplied by the branches of the aorta between the renal arteries and the aortic bifurcation? In an operative procedure on the abdominal aorta, these anatomic structures must be taken into consideration.

ITEM 24-3.   Search for lesser arteries to the kidneys arising at unusual locations on the aorta. Such vessels are termed aberrant or anomalous renal arteries. Their significance will be dealt with later.

THE ABDOMINAL AORTA

The extent to which the aorta, a huge vessel pounding with blood, can now be successfully operated upon is one of the most impressive surgical developments in your lifetime. To aid your understanding of these developments you must conceive the aorta as an entire structure, as a conduit extending from the heart to the aortic bifurcation, and supplying blood by branches to all the peripheral regions of the body. For descriptive purposes, however, it is certainly useful to divide the vessel into ascending aorta and arch, descending thoracic aorta, and descending abdominal aorta, with which you are now concerned.

That the abdominal aorta, a posterior abdominal wall structure, is not remote from the *anterior* abdominal wall is worth stressing again. Its pulsations are usually readily palpable although small bowel and omentum separate the vessel from the wall. Furthermore, in a person of slender build the pulsations may be transmitted through the intervening structures to the anterior abdominal wall to a degree that they can be seen. They may be seen or felt above and to the left of the umbilicus (an unreliable landmark); that abdominal aortic aneurysms usually present in this region, i.e., to the left, is a well recognized clinical fact.

The abdominal aorta has been described as a "veritable floodgate" for blood flowing to the lower part of the body. When the vessel is occluded, the blood flow to distal regions may be reduced to such a degree that death (gangrene) of the lower limbs is inevitable; acute occlusion without immediate operative intervention is fatal.

However, in chronic occlusion of the abdominal aorta, collateral vessels transmit blood to the distal parts. One of the more obvious vessels that can maintain a collateral supply is the inferior mesenteric artery. It supplies blood to the pelvic organs, which are also supplied by blood from branches of the internal iliac artery. In event of an occlusion in the aorta distal to the origin of the inferior mesenteric artery and proximal to the origin of the internal iliac artery, blood may be transmitted via the inferior mesenteric artery to the branches of the internal iliac artery so that blood ultimately reaches distal parts. Obviously there must be a reversal of the normal direction of blood flow in some of the collateral channels. There are other examples of the collateral supply, which you will be able to identify in the course of your dissection.

The study of the collateral blood supply is a fascinating anatomic exercise, but even more fascinating are the hemodynamics of the vascular tree, which must be carefully considered and planned for in any surgical procedure. What changes would you expect in the distribution of blood if the abdominal aorta is occluded deliberately by a clamp for a surgical procedure, or as a result of an acute pathologic process (e.g., embolism)? Would the arterial pulses of the upper and lower limbs be the same? What changes would occur in the venous pressure proximal and distal to the arterial obstruction?

The regions supplied by branches of the abdominal aorta are all perfectly obvious. Not so obvious, but nevertheless of critical importance, are the vessels that supply the spinal cord. Because these vessels travel along the nerve roots to reach the cord they are described as radicular. Thus, although they are out of sight, the radicular arteries are never out of the surgeon's mind, particularly when he must cut branches to mobilize a long segment of the aorta to remove an aneurysm. Because the spinal cord ends at the level of the second lumbar vertebra (i.e., about the level of the superior mesenteric artery) it is plain that secondary damage to the cord is more likely to occur in operations upon the more proximal part of the aorta. Even so, a blood supply to the spinal cord must always be maintained because death of cord tissue (infarction) is practically irreversible.

In summary, we have described — (1) the surface anatomy of the abdominal aorta, (2) the commanding position of the aorta in the blood supply to the lower part of the body, (3) the collateral circulation, (4) the hemodynamics, and (5) a critical supply of blood to the spinal cord. Proceed now to study briefly the aortic lymph nodes and sympathetic plexuses before you remove the abdominal aorta. Briefly, we say, not because they are unimportant, but because their dissection, requiring time, is not usually very successful.

ITEM 24-4. The Aortic Autonomic Plexuses

Identify and observe the continuity of these plexuses in the following locations.

(1) Around the celiac artery, where they are known as the celiac plexus.

(2) On the anterior surface of the aorta between the celiac artery and the aortic bifurcation. This plexus is known as the aortic plexus.

(3) At the bifurcation of the aorta, where they are known as the superior hypogastric plexus.

ITEM 24-5. The Celiac Plexus and Ganglions

In addition to the plexus, in a good specimen, the right and left celiac ganglia can be identified. Each ganglion is an irregularly shaped flat structure about the size of a thumbnail, just lateral to the celiac plexus and medial to the hilum of the suprarenal gland. The right celiac ganglion is posterior to the inferior vena cava and will not be seen unless you displace that vessel laterally.

On each side, observe the splanchnic nerves piercing the crus of the diaphragm to join the celiac ganglion and plexus. To do this easily, if the thorax has already been dissected, one partner should pull gently on one of the splanchnic nerves in the thorax. Then the dissector, observing the abdominal aspect of the crus of the diaphragm, pulls the celiac ganglion and plexus inferiorly. The splanchnic nerve will be observed piercing the crus. It is sufficient to identify one nerve in order to grasp the principle involved. There are in fact greater and lesser splanchnic nerves on each side.

CELIAC PLEXUS AND PANCREAS

The proximity of the celiac plexus and the left celiac ganglion to the pancreas accounts, in part at least, for the drop in blood pressure and severe back pain that occurs in pancreatitis. Discussion of this clinical condition is out of place here. The condition is mentioned merely to emphasize an important anatomic relationship, easily overlooked in an interrupted sequence of dissection.

THE SUPERIOR HYPOGASTRIC PLEXUS

The superior hypogastric plexus is a solitary network centrally located at the bifurcation of the abdominal aorta. Inferiorly, the plexus divides into right and left hypogastric nerves, to be found entering the true pelvis at the pelvic brim; each nerve there spreads out into a right or left inferior hypogastric plexus. Note that, in contrast to the solitary superior hypogastric plexus, there are, indeed, two inferior hypogastric plexuses. The latter are often referred to as the right and left pelvic plexuses. Discussion of the alternative names for the superior hypogastric plexus follows now.

The superior hypogastric plexus is sometimes resected in the management of pain of the pelvic region. That several different names are applied to this same plexus leads to confusion. The official anatomic nomenclature is *superior hypogastric plexus*, but often, among clinicians, the plexus is called *the* hypogastric plexus, or more commonly, the presacral nerve. However, as you can see on your specimen, the plexus has several strands, so it is not really a nerve, in addition, it is not located anterior to the sacrum. It lies anterior to the common iliac arteries and the left common iliac vein. Be that as it may, there seems no doubt that surgical resection of the superior hypogastric plexus will continue to be called presacral neurectomy.

In resecting the abdominal aorta, including its bifurcation, the superior hypogastric plexus is also removed. In some male patients (the percentage is difficult to assess) a distressing symptom, failure of ejaculation, occurs postoperatively. The cause of this failure is attributed to the removal of the superior hypogastric plexus.

PARAAORTIC LYMPH NODES

The paraaortic lymph nodes lie beside the aorta, and drain lymph from very extensive territories. Of these, probably the most important from a clinical diagnostic point of view is the lymphatic drainage of the testes. If you understand the embryology of the testes and how the testes develop on the posterior abdominal wall before they migrate to the scrotum, then you will understand why the arterial venous and lymphatic vessels of the testes are connected to the vessels of the posterior abdominal wall. Hence the lymph from each testis drains ultimately into the paraaortic lymph nodes.

Sometimes the first evidence of an undetected malignancy in a testis is the swelling of the paraaortic lymph nodes into which the cancer cells have spread and multiplied (metastasis). It follows, therefore, that in any investigation of an obscure mass of the posterior abdominal wall in a male, the doctor must exclude cancer of one or other of the testes.

In some surgical circles, as part of the treatment of cancer of the testis, in order to minimize the possibility of spread of the disease throughout the body, the surgeon will remove the paraaortic lymph nodes, an operation called paraaortic lymphadenectomy.

ITEM 24-6. Exploration of the Saddle (or Carina) of the Aortic Bifurcation

Slit the left side of the aorta as far inferiorly as the bifurcation. Clean out all debris. Examine the internal lining of the aorta and the orifices of the major branches. The lining should be smooth and should gleam when moist. The orifices should be flush with the aortic wall.

Separate the cut edges to see the orifices of the right and left common iliac arteries and the saddle or carina, which lies between them. Sometimes a long clot of blood may straddle the saddle to completely obstruct blood flow to both lower extremities. This condition is spoken of as saddle embolus.

ITEM 24-7. The Inferior Vena Cava

Identify the inferior vena cava lying to the right of the aorta. Superiorly, you may have already cut the vein in removing the liver. Inferiorly, the vein begins where the right and left common iliac veins conjoin. Observe that the right common iliac artery lies transversely anterior to the left common iliac vein. Also note that the right common iliac artery slants across the right common iliac vein and the beginning of the inferior vena cava. You may also be able to observe that the right and left internal iliac arteries lie transversely across the external iliac veins. Some authorities consider that disease of these arteries lying transversely across veins may obstruct the flow of blood and create venous congestion of the limb involved.

ITEM 24-8. Identify the veins joining the inferior vena cava, and remember the hepatic veins buried in the substance of the liver. Note whether the left renal vein passes anterior or posterior to the aorta. In general, the veins joining the inferior vena cava correspond to the arteries leaving the aorta, except that the left gonadal vein and the left suprarenal vein join the left renal vein and not the inferior vena cava.

INFERIOR VENA CAVA

Although for descriptive purposes we refer to the beginning and end of the inferior vena cava, it is much more practical to look upon this great vein as part of the entire venous system from the feet to the heart. The continuity of this system becomes all too obvious when the blood in the deep veins of the calf clots (deep vein thrombosis) and fragments of dislodged clot (emboli) are swept in the venous return, not just to the right side of the heart, but beyond, into the lungs.

The site and size of the inferior vena cava suggest that profound congestion of the lower part of the body would occur if the vein was blocked. Curiously, this is not so. Accordingly, in the management of persistent pulmonary emboli from the lower limbs, from the pelvis, or from the inferior vena cava itself, the inferior vena cava is sometimes deliberately tied. Venous congestion does not necessarily follow, and venous return is maintained via alternative collateral venous systems.

ITEM 24-9.   Identification of the Lumbar Sympathetic Trunks

To embark on a search for the ganglia of these trunks with preconceived ideas will waste time. There is a remarkable variation in the thickness and length of each trunk and in the number of ganglia.

Look for the ganglia on the vertebral column along the medial border of the psoas muscle. On the left side the ganglia are to the left of the aorta, while on the right they lie posterior to the inferior vena cava.

ITEM 24-10.   Examination of One Ganglion

Select a well-formed ganglion and examine its connections. They connect the lumbar sympathetic trunk to the preaortic plexuses and are named lumbar splanchnic nerves. Usually there are four on each side. The most inferior one joins the superior hypogastric plexus.

Scratch away sufficient psoas muscle to expose the adjacent ventral ramus of a lumbar spinal nerve. Without too much difficulty you should see one or two strands connecting the sympathetic ganglion to the nerve. Such rami communicantes are important in that they transmit most of the sympathetic fibers destined to control the caliber of arterial vessels in the lower limb. Here, then, is an example of how autonomic nerve fibers reach their destination by using somatic nerves as an intermediate crosswalk. These rami communicantes are also destroyed when the surgeon performs a lumbar sympathectomy to improve the caliber of arterial vessels in the limb.

The anatomy of the vertebral column is dealt with in Chapter 26. Psoas major and the lumbar plexus are dealt with when the lower limb is dissected.

ITEM 24-11.   The Cisterna Chyli

At the medial margin of the right crus of the diaphragm, retract the psoas major to the right and identify the cisterna chyli.

Review

Return to the introduction at the beginning of this chapter. It will serve equally well as a review.

Chapter 25

The Lateral Region of the Posterior Abdominal Wall

The Urinary Tract

Anatomic dissection is of necessity a process of disintegration; done region by region, it is inevitable the continuity of each system encountered is broken. Thus it is a real possibility that the student will be left with a thousand pieces, so to speak, like the mirror in *Richard III*, "dashed to a thousand slivers." If this is so, then the student will likely have difficulty in grasping the main principles of the diagnosis and management of systemic disease. In no system of the body is this possibility more real than in the urinary system. Accordingly, study thoroughly a diagram of the urinary tract and see the continuity of the urinary system from the kidneys to the pot.

For descriptive purposes, the urinary tract is divided into an upper and lower tract. The former includes kidneys and ureters, while the latter includes the bladder and the entire male or female urethra. (The female urethra is very short in comparison to the male urethra.) At the present stage of your dissection, you are concerned only with the upper urinary tract. The lower urinary tract is dissected later. Even so, even now, you must establish their continuity in your mind.

THE NEPHRON

A million or more individual nephrons are the functional units of the kidney; each nephron is measured in microns and can only be examined under magnification. The nephron, by a complex process of filtration and osmosis, produces urine and so plays a key role, a vital role, in maintaining in balance the water and electrolytes of the entire body. Today, renal research concentrates heavily upon the nephron, its anatomy and function. Accordingly, in the dissection of your cadaver in the gross anatomy laboratory, you must look upon each kidney as a house of many nephrons.

It is as well, however, to leave the functional aspects of the tract until you have received some basic instruction in physiology and biochemistry because of the complex changes occurring as urine passes through the component parts of the nephron.

PALPATION OF EACH KIDNEY

The kidneys are exceptions to the general rule that, in the living, abdominal organs cannot be felt unless their texture has been altered by disease. Sometimes the lower end of the kidney, the right kidney especially, can be held between the fingertips of one hand pressing anteriorly into the lumbar region and of the other hand pressing into the loin while the patient is relaxed. Precise instruction in the method of physical examination of the kidney is the responsibility of your clinical tutors, who will also be responsible for teaching you how to detect the abnormal kidney. At the present time, merely observe carefully the position of each kidney in relation to the body wall. What is the surface marking of each kidney?

Peritoneum

The relationship of kidney to peritoneum was described previously, but it is worth stressing again that the kidney and the ureter are immediately deep to the peritoneum covering the posterior abdominal wall. Examine these relationships.

ITEM 25-1.   Observe that each kidney is related to an infracolic compartment. Therefore each kidney is related to small bowel across the peritoneal cavity. Recall that the right kidney was separated from the liver by the hepatorenal recess and that the left kidney was separated from the stomach by the lesser sac. The colon is related directly to each kidney, the second part of the duodenum to the right kidney, and the pancreas to the left kidney. What is the relationship of spleen to left kidney?

ITEM 25-2.   Make a vertical incision into the peritoneum over the anterior surface of each kidney—boldly, but with care—down to the actual surface of the kidney. Peel back the edges of the incision to expose the kidney. Compare the level of the lower pole of each kidney. Which kidney is lower? Name the precise direction to which this exposed surface of the kidney faces. Recall, or reread, the introductory description of the posterior abdominal wall (p. 140).

ITEM 25-3. Identify the cut edge of peritoneum and a second edge belonging to the anterior layer of the renal fascia, known to clinicians as the fascia of Gerota. Establish that to reach the kidney you proceeded through peritoneum, renal fascia, and fat, called the perirenal fat (also called perinephric fat).

ITEM 25-4. Kidneys to Pleural Cavities

Make sure you have exposed fully the anterior surface of the kidney by removing sufficient perirenal fat. Then, standing on the right side of the corpse, place the fingertips of the left hand in the right posterior costodiaphragmatic recess of the right pleural cavity. Manipulate the right kidney with your right hand and establish the relationship of the kidney to the pleural cavity. Do likewise on the left side. What is the relationship of kidney to pleural cavity?

ITEM 25-5. Pararenal fat. *Para* means beside or nearby. The following demonstration is not always clear in a cadaver; in any event, it need not be a precise dissection. But posterior and lateral to the renal capsule (identified in Item 25-3) lies a layer of fat that may be considerable. This is the pararenal fat, separated from the actual kidney by the renal fascia, which encloses the perirenal fat (*peri*—around). The essential fact is that each kidney is surrounded by layers of fat.

RENAL FAT AND FASCIA

Renal fat is important as a site of infection (perirenal abscess). Perirenal abscess is a serious complication of infection, usually of the kidney, the infection spreading from the actual kidney into the surrounding fat but never crossing the midline to the opposite side because of the attachments of renal fascia. A patient with perirenal abscess is dangerously ill.

ITEM 25-6. Mobilize the kidney (i.e., remove the kidney from its bed of fat). Do not cut the renal artery, vein, or ureter. In mobilizing the kidney, note that the suprarenal gland lies undisturbed. Thus it is possible to remove either the kidney or the gland without disturbing the other organ. The fact that a kidney is easily removed from its bed of fat and fascia is of considerable surgical importance.

ITEM 25-7. The thin fibrous connective tissue capsule you observe upon the surface of the kidney may be stripped easily. See if the capsules of the kidneys of your cadaver strip easily. Stripping is a part of some surgical procedures as well as an essential part of the examination of a kidney at autopsy.

ITEM 25-8. Identify the Renal Artery, Vein, and Ureter

Be sure the kidney is mobile and clear of its fat. Identify the renal pedicle, an assembly of vessels, ureter, lymphatics, and nerves proceeding to or from the kidney. On the medial border of the kidney is a slight vertical cleft, the hilus, (hilus and hilum are synonyms) beyond which, i.e., in the kidney, is the renal sinus. Through the hilus into the sinus pass renal arteries and nerves, while the lymphatics, veins, and ureter emerge. Manipulate the kidney and clean away fat and fascia until the principal structures of the pedicle are clearly seen. The anatomy of the renal pedicle has always been important in surgical procedures upon the kidney (e.g., nephrectomy, removal of kidney). Today, however, the anatomy of the pedicle is even more important because of the development of human kidney transplantation, which requires the careful removal of the donor's kidney and its connection to the internal iliac vessels and bladder of the recipient. How many arteries and veins can you see in each renal pedicle? Are the ureters solitary or duplicated? Be on the lookout for aberrant segmental arteries.

ITEM 25-9.   The Ureter

Lift the kidney clear of fat and gently pull it out of the abdomen. This maneuver lifts the ureter clear of the posterior abdominal wall. In doing so, observe how blood vessels cross anterior to the ureter, i.e., between the ureter and peritoneum, and then how the ureter crosses anterior to the iliac vessels.

Trace the ureters to the brim of the pelvis, but no further. The ureters have special relationships in the pelvis best seen by a different approach. Most of the upper urinary tract is now apparent.

THE KIDNEYS

Without kidneys to remove toxic products of protein digestion from the blood as well as to regulate the water content of the body, death is inevitable unless the help of an artificial mechanical kidney is available to the victim. It must be stressed, however, that with only one kidney (or even half a kidney) life may still go on as normal until, perhaps, a disorder of renal function draws attention to the solitary kidney and so to the precarious life of the patient. It follows that in considering any operative procedure on one kidney, the presence or absence of the other kidney and its functional capacity are foremost thoughts in the surgeon's mind. Thus the embryology and physiology of the kidneys and ureters require your careful attention. It is clear from the literature on the kidneys that, in our present time, renal function is of prime importance, but it will always be true that a knowledge of structure aids the comprehension of complex function. Accordingly, you will soon open each kidney to expose its gross internal structure (Fig. 25-1).

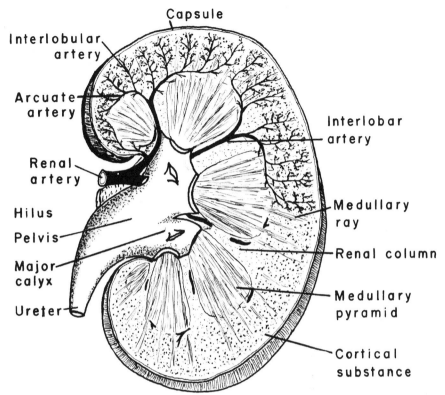

Figure 25-1. Diagram of the human kidney, sectioned vertically. The arterial supply is indicated in the upper half of the kidney only. (From C. R. Leeson and T. S. Leeson: Histology. Philadelphia. W. B. Saunders Co., 1966.)

SEGMENTAL ARTERIES

When the abdominal aorta was examined you were asked to look out for aberrant renal arteries arising from the aorta. Aberrant arteries are also called accessory arteries, but, on the basis of work by Graves (1954), such arteries are best called aberrant segmental arteries because each is distributed solely to a segment of renal tissue. In the next stage of dissection you will expose the typical segmental arteries branching from the renal artery in the pedicle or within the hilum. Meantime note that segmental arteries are end arteries. Therefore, if a segmental artery is tied and divided, a segment of renal tissue will inevitably perish. It follows, then, that to sever a segmental renal artery is a grave surgical decision.

ITEM 25-10. Cut any aberrant segmental arteries present. Cut the definitive renal artery and vein on each side. Observe the difference in length between the right and left renal veins. Note the short length of the right renal vein and how close it is to the inferior vena cava, and realize how exact the technique of ligaturing that renal vein must be.

ITEM 25-11.   Exploration for Segmental Arteries

On one kidney only (the other one is to be kept for an exploration of the ureter), by blunt dissection, using the closed and open scissors technique, trace the renal artery into the substance of the kidney. With the aid of Figure 183.1, *Grant's Atlas of Anatomy*, see if you can identify the segmental arteries. Note how the apical and lower segments of the kidney include the entire thickness of the kidney, whereas the posterior segment is posterior only, and the so-called upper and middle segments are anterior only. If you can demonstrate to some extent that segmentation does occur you will have achieved your objective.

ITEM 25-12.   The Ureter

The dilated upper end of the ureter is called the pelvis of the ureter, and the junction of the ureter and pelvis is called the pelviureteric junction. At this junction the lumen of the ureter is narrower than elsewhere (similar narrowing is said to occur in the ureter at the pelvic brim and occurs also at the ureterovesical junction). In your specimen it may be that the pelviureteric junction is related to an aberrant segmental artery.

Pare away carefully the anterior lip of the kidney to expose more and more of the pelvis. Persist until you see the pelvis dividing into two, possibly three, parts. Each of these divisions is called a major calix, but you must realize that major calices are not always identifiable as separate parts.

Now select one major calix and remove carefully sufficient renal tissue to the point where this major calix divides into several minor calices.

Then open the pelvis, major calix, and one or two minor calices to expose the tip of a renal pyramid, upon which the cup-shaped end of a minor calix fits. The cup-shaped end explains the use of the word calix, for the latin word for cup is *calix*.

ITEM 25-13.   Section of Kidney

With a sharp knife make a section of kidney, cutting through the minor calix you have just exposed, the major calices, and the ureteric pelvis (Fig. 25-1). Identify the gross features of the kidney's structure.

Review

The anatomy of each kidney has been dealt with under the following headings: position and surface marking, relationship to peritoneum and to the adjacent pleural cavity, renal fat and fascia, internal structure and segmentation, and blood supply.

Read a brief account of the embryology of the kidney, and finally, dwell heavily upon its physiology.

THE SUPRARENAL GLANDS

Before proceeding to study the ureters, it is opportune to comment upon the suprarenal (adrenal) glands. Each suprarenal gland is related to the superior pole of a kidney, but the gland is separated from the kidney by a layer of fascia which permits independent removal of either organ. Often, in an embalmed cadaver, it is difficult to isolate with ease the adrenal glands from surrounding fat because postmortem autolysis has largely obliterated the gland and has also led to its fusion with the surrounding fat. Make some attempt to isolate each gland, noting its intimate connection to the adjacent celiac ganglion, the many small arteries reaching the cortex of the gland, and the solitary principal vein emerging from the hilus of the gland and joining either the inferior vena cava or the renal vein. Then read an account of the gross anatomy, embryology, and histology of the gland.

The degree to which the function of this pair of glands has been investigated is a measure of the vast amount of medical research that has developed in your lifetime. Not so long ago, obliteration of the cortex of the suprarenal glands meant death was inevitable. Nowadays, when the cortex of both suprarenal glands is obliterated, life may be prolonged by the use of synthetic cortical extracts. Accordingly, both suprarenal glands may be removed surgically for therapeutic reasons, e.g., in the treatment of tumors.

URETERS

Apart from their all-important function, conveying urine from each kidney to the bladder, there are a few other pertinent facts concerning each ureter.

The ureter is a muscular structure, and, in life, waves of muscular contractions (peristalsis) produce a wormlike movement along it, milking urine toward the bladder. The musculature of the ureter is the subject of much discussion today.

The violent contractions precipitated in the musculature of a ureter by the presence of a stone, known clinically as a calculus, in the lumen of the ureter, may produce such waves of pain, known as colic, that the patient is in need of immediate medical aid. Thus it comes about that a knowledge of the pharmacologic action of drugs upon the muscles and upon the mind is essential to the physician, and he must also be aware of the segmental nerve supply of the ureter. What is the nerve supply of the ureter? Look it up in a textbook.

The position of the ureter with reference to the vertebral column was mentioned previously, but it is worth mentioning again: the ureters lie anterior to the tips of the transverse processes of the lower four lumbar vertebrae and enter the pelvis medial to the sacroiliac joints.

It may be many years before you assume full responsibility for a surgical procedure. Nevertheless, as a practicing physician you must be aware of the concern all surgeons have, whatever the procedure, for the safety of the ureters. What organs or structures lie in relationship to the right, and the left ureter? A surgeon, isolating the right colic artery for example, while operating upon the ascending colon, is concerned lest he inadvertently damage the right ureter. Likewise, a surgeon operating upon the left ureter is concerned about the left colic vessels close by. In the pelvis the same principles apply, especially in the female pelvis. Accordingly, from this point of view, you should take a second look at the relations, especially the anterior relations, of both ureters, and their particular relationship to the peritoneal cavity.

Finally, the arterial blood is supplied to the ureter by branches from the renal, gonadal, and internal iliac arteries, and by vesical arteries. These branches form an anastomosis in the fat and fascia around the ureter; stripping off this fascia diminishes the blood supply to the ureter, a fact the surgeon bears in mind when he mobilizes the ureter for transplantation.

Review

Reconsider the anatomy of the ureter and review its relationship to peritoneum and adjacent structures, musculature and lumen, segmental nerve supply, and blood supply. The pelvic part of the ureter and the ureterovesical junction will be explored more fully at a later stage.

Read a brief account of the embryology of the ureter.

Do *not* cut the ureters at this stage. Simply place the kidneys and ureters so that they are clear of the dissector's field.

The Muscles and Significant Fascia of the Posterior Abdominal Wall

Two muscles on each side are to be considered; they are quadratus lumborum and psoas major. The former is not greatly significant, except that it is encountered in the extraperitoneal surgical approach to the kidney. Then the muscle must be retracted medially or even be cut to gain an adequate exposure of the kidney. The psoas muscle is important clinically because (1) its fascia determines the direction of the spread of pus from a diseased part of the vertebral column and (2) its muscular contractions influence the vertebral column and the tilt of the pelvis, as well as the hip joint.

Psoas Fascia

Observe how, medially, the fascia is attached to the vertebral column, leaving gaps occupied by neurovascular structures; superiorly it is attached to the medial arcuate ligament; laterally it is continuous with transversalis fascia on the anterior aspect of quadratus lumborum; inferiorly the fascia is continuous with fascia iliaca. Observe particularly, however, that the combined psoas and iliacus fascia pass deep to the inguinal ligament.

ITEM 25-14.   The Routes of Pus from the Vertebral Column

Make a vertical slit in the psoas fascia. Confirm the adherence of the fascia to the column. Raise the lateral flap and by finger dissection demonstrate a plane of cleavage that proceeds laterally to the region of the lumbar triangle.

Continue blunt dissection in an inferior direction toward the anterior superior iliac spine. The plane of cleavage is now between iliacus muscle and the iliacus fascia. Confirm that a mass at the periphery of the lower abdominal quadrant could be an accumulation of pus deep to iliacus fascia.

Then, if you have not already done so, slit the psoas fascia inferiorly as far as the inguinal ligament. Now, slip an index finger into the plane of cleavage and burrow toward the lower limb to demonstrate that the plane of cleavage exists inferior to the inguinal ligament. Thus, a mass in the groin could be a collection of pus deep to the psoas fascia. Finally, establish in your mind the continuity of this plane of cleavage from the body of the twelfth thoracic vertebra to the thigh.

ITEM 25-15.   Strip away all fascia to expose clearly the quadratus lumborum and observe its lateral edge. Restore the kidney and establish as best you can the relationship of kidney to that edge and to psoas major.

Chapter 26

Division of the Vertebral Column

This important step is necessary to mobilize the pelvis and lower limbs and thereby give easier access to the perineum. Then, if the method of making a median sagittal section of the pelvis is followed (p. 167)—and it is strongly recommended—each lower limb is free. Experience has shown that when the lower limb is free and can be rolled over with ease its dissection is easier, quicker, and more readily comprehensible.

INTRODUCTION TO THE VERTEBRAL COLUMN

For centuries "backbone" has been used as a figure of speech to illuminate the strength and position of a central figure without whom an organization could not fulfill its purpose. Why that metaphor has stood the test of time becomes immediately apparent when injury or disease strikes the vertebral column. Then, it is also apparent that sound structure is the backbone of good function.

In describing the structure of the column, the fact that it is an entire structure and functions as such must not be lost sight of, although it is extremely useful to consider the column as a series of segments. A segment consists of two adjacent vertebrae and their joints and ligaments, and the corresponding segments of paravertebral muscles. In addition to the concept of segments, however, there are specific regions, cervical, thoracic, lumbar, and sacrococcygeal. Each region has a characteristic curvature and other characteristic features, but it must be stressed again that the vertebral column functions as a whole and that segments and regions are only parts of the entire structure.

ITEM 26-1.   On a skeleton (or with two adjacent disarticulated vertebrae), identify the following features and relate them to each other with the aid of Figure 26-1. On each vertebra the features are the body, two pedicles, two lamina, two transverse processes, and a spinous process; in addition, the superior and inferior pair of articular processes are noteworthy.

Articulate the vertebrae and visualize the following ligaments (Fig. 26-1): supraspinous and interspinous ligaments, the bilateral ligamentum flavum, the capsules of the apophyseal joints, the posterior and

156

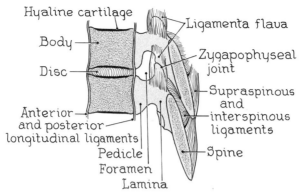

Figure 26-1. Median section of two vertebrae to show the ligaments. The zygapophyseal (sometimes shortened to apophyseal) joint is between the inferior articular facet of the vertebra above with a reciprocal facet on the vertebra below. (*Apophysis* is from a Greek word meaning offshoot. Zyg- is from the greek word *zygon*, meaning yoke; used here, zyg- indicates a junction.)

anterior longitudinal ligaments, and the intervertebral disc. Consult the section "The Vertebrae and the Vertebral Column" in *Grant's Atlas of Anatomy*. You will observe, for instance, that the ligamentum flavum is attached not to the margins of the laminae but to their internal surfaces.

The main functions ascribed to the vertebral column are support, movement, and protection, and, on examining the vertebral column of a skeleton, it is easy to see the parts responsible for each of these functions.

(1) Support is the function of the intervertebral disc and the vertebral bodies. Discs must be kept clearly in mind when the vertebral column is studied on a skeleton. Discs account for a quarter of the total length of an intact column. The structure of a disc is studied in detail in the course of dissection. At this stage, however, you must recognize that degeneration of one disc, narrowing the interval between two adjacent vertebrae, will alter the mechanics of the entire column.

Observe how the vertebrae become progressively more sturdy from the base of the skull to the sacrum; the height of each body increases so that a lumbar body is about twice as tall as a cervical body; the width and depth of each vertebra also increases, but to a lesser degree. Furthermore, there is a corresponding increase in the dimensions of each disc as the shape of each disc is adapted to suit the relationship of one vertebra to another in the transition from one curvature to the next. All these increases are in keeping with the apparent need to transmit progressively increasing weight to the pelvis.

A section of the body of a vertebra reveals an interesting and perhaps unexpected finding. The bone within is cancellous in type and is composed of exquisitely delicate lamellae; externally there is but a mere coat of compact bone. Closer inspection of a cut surface reveals that the stronger lamellae are vertically disposed; this is in keeping with the basic function of the vertebral body, namely support and the transmission of weight.

(2) Only a limited amount of movement is possible in each of the synovial joints between vertebrae and in each intervertebral disc. It is the accumulation of many such small movements that produces the obvious flexibility of the entire column. This summation of movement may be conceived as a vertical integration of movement to distinguish it from the horizontal integration of movement of a disc and its related synovial joints. With these two categories of movement in mind it is an obvious advantage to view the column as a mechanical construction and to apply basic engineering principles. It is certainly true that disc degeneration and disc narrowing affect both the vertical and horizontal integration of movements.

The movements of the column are flexion, extension, side flexion, and rotation. Those names are self-explanatory. It is the degree of movement in the different regions of the column that requires further consideration, and the principal features to be taken into account are (a) the apophyseal joints, (b) the rib cage, and (c) the elasticity of the discs.

In the cervical region all the movements just listed are possible, and they are enhanced by the movements occurring between the atlas and the axis and between the atlas and the base of the skull. The head and neck have a considerable range of movement, controlled to a fine degree, which is in keeping with the need to position accurately the organs of hearing, sight, and smell. In recent times it has become apparent that the range of flexion and extension of the cervical spine diminishes from the superior to the inferior half of the cervical region. Accordingly, the inferior half is likened to the handle of a whip and the superior half to the lash. Sudden changes of momentum produce the so-called whiplash injury, roughly at the midcervical region.

Thoracic movement is handicapped by the rib cage, so that all the basic movements are somewhat limited. Curiously, the apophyseal joints are designed to allow maximal rotation, as if to compensate for the limitation imposed by the rib cage. It is believed that maximal rotation occurs in the lower thoracic region.

In the lumbar region little rotation occurs, and examination of the apophyseal joints reveals why. Thus flexion and extension, as well as side flexion, are the principal movements of the lumbar spine. It is clear, however, that bending forward includes movement in the hip joints. An analysis of flexion of the lumbar spine must, therefore, take hip-joint flexion into account.

ITEM 26-2.   With these facts in mind, examine the apophyseal joints of the entire vertebral column. Look for differences in the size, shape, and direction of the articular facets and relate these differences to the movements possible in the three regions of the column.

(3) Protection of the spinal cord would seem to be the function of the short stout pedicles and the broad solid laminae with the projecting

spine as an additional defense. The vertebral canal is well and truly surrounded by bone, and, if you are examining a skeleton, you must remember the protection offered by tough ligaments, particularly the ligamentum flavum, filling in gaps between the vertebrae.

THE VERTEBRAL COLUMN AND ITS MUSCLES

The flexibility of the column is controlled by groups of muscles that are vertically disposed (therefore they are parallel to the column), as well as by obliquely disposed muscles swathed around the torso.

The muscles of the back are the principal extensors; the two rectus abdominis muscles are powerful flexors; the oblique fibers of the abdominal muscles act as rotators and their vertical fibers form part of the side flexor group, along with the appropriate rectus abdominis, quadratus lumborum, and erector spinae. Gravity, however, must be taken into account. Therefore it is more correct to say that the muscle groups have the specific actions that have just been outlined when they act against a resistance, which may, indeed, be gravity.

Because of the influence of gravity upon muscle action, it is true that when the trunk is bent forward from the upright position it is the extensor muscles that control the forward movement. Thus the vertebral column has been likened to a pole. As the pole topples slightly to one side, the contralateral muscles act strongly to prevent the pole's toppling over completely. It follows, then, that when the vertebral column is both in the normal upright position and moving, there is an ever-shifting balance of power between different muscle groups to steady the column and oppose the influence of gravity.

Segmental Innervation of the Paravertebral Muscles

That the paravertebral muscles are supplied in a segmental pattern by the posterior rami of the spinal nerves is of clinical importance. To understand why this is important requires clinical information beyond the scope of this text. One can say that an orthopedic surgeon, aware of the segmental innervation of the paravertebral muscles, can narrow down the field of his investigation to a particular unit or segment of the column and so reach an accurate diagnosis.

NAMING THE MUSCLES OF THE BACK

Conversing with clinicians, with orthopedic surgeons in particular, one realizes that the detailed nomenclature of these muscles, listed at length in most anatomic texts, is not used clinically. The entire muscle mass is referred to clinically by such names as: the spinal muscles, the extensors of the spine, erector spinae, or simply, muscles of the back. It is therefore obviously quite unnecessary for the preclinical student to study the nomenclature of the many components of the muscles of the back.

It is necessary, however, to have a knowledge of their function, for problems related to the muscles are common in general practice as well as in the specialized field of orthopedics. Therefore, do not skip lightly through the dissection of the muscles of the back, but observe their thickness, distribution, layering, and ligamentous or fibrous content, and, especially, consider their function. Realize that the stability and symmetry of the normal vertebral column depends not just upon the integrative activity of the several layers of longitudinal muscles on each side of the column, but also upon an equitable balance of activity between the right and left muscle groups. This activity, in turn, depends upon nerve supply to bring segment after segment of muscle into action, to a degree that varies, naturally, with the movement of the body as a whole. Thus, paralysis of the muscles of the back will not only lead to deformities of the vertebral column but will also limit, sometimes severely, even the simplest of movements of the entire body.

LAMINECTOMY

In the practice of medicine, abnormal structures within the vertebral canal are commonly exposed by a surgical procedure, laminectomy, which is the removal of one or more laminae. The procedure is adapted, in a crude way, to our purpose, which is to open the vertebral canal of a cadaver. To do so, the paravertebral muscles are dissected off the spinous processes and laminae. Then the spinous processes and laminae are removed.

ITEM 26-3. If flaps ABCD (Fig. 15-3) have not been created, remove as much skin as necessary to expose the lower half of the back, carefully, so that skin only is removed.

ITEM 26-4. Identify the lower end of each trapezius muscle (*Grant's Atlas of Anatomy*, Fig. 477). The trapezius muscles usually extend to the spinous process of the twelfth thoracic vertebra. Thus the trapezius muscle is a useful cadaveric landmark. Identify the lower border of each latissimus dorsi (*Grant's Atlas of Anatomy*, Fig. 477). Mobilize it. Observe the attachment of the muscle to the thoracolumbar (also known as lumbodorsal) fascia.

ITEM 26-5. On each side of the spinous processes T12 to S1 incise the thoracolumbar fascia. Peel the fascia laterally to reveal the longitudinal layers of the muscles of the back (*Grant's Atlas of Anatomy*, Fig. 479).

SUBPERIOSTEAL RESECTION OF MUSCLE

To reach a lamina, a surgeon must proceed beyond the mass of muscle you have just exposed. To do so he takes advantage of the strength of living periosteum and the relatively bloodless plane of cleavage between periosteum and actual bone. It is impossible to demonstrate the maneuver nicely in a cadaver. However, in order to have some awareness of the principle, proceed as follows:

ITEM 26-6. On each side, incise the vertebral muscles parallel to the spinous processes from T12 to S1.

ITEM 26-7. Identify the supraspinous ligament, between T12 and L5. Now, with a sharp broad chisel, just lateral to the ligament, begin to elevate the spinal muscles from each side of the spinous processes and from the laminae. The blade of the chisel moves in the subperiosteal plane so that muscle, together with periosteum is separated from bone. In spinal surgery there are special instruments to elevate muscle and periosteum. But persevere with your chisel until the spinal muscles on each side are retracted as far as the capsules of the intervertebral articulations between the levels T12 to L5.

ITEM 26-8. In a surgical procedure usually both laminae and the spinous process of one or two vertebra are removed. Section the laminae of L2 and 3 with an autopsy saw or strong bone forceps.

ITEM 26-9. To remove completely the bone you have just freed, it is necessary to cut supraspinous ligament, interspinous ligament, and the ligamentum flavum between adjacent laminae on each side. Do so with a knife sharp to the point, and be sure the point is always in view. Then no harm to underlying structures can occur.

ITEM 26-10. The vertebral canal is now open, and within it you see fat and thin-walled veins occupying the vertebral extradural (also called epidural) space. Deep to the fat is the dura mater. The epidural space extends as high as the base of the skull and as low as the sacral hiatus. Accordingly, in your present dissection you are seeing only a limited part of the entire space. The entire space has a capacity for 80–100 cc. fluid, in addition to the fat and veins already present.

VEINS OF THE VERTEBRAL COLUMN

In 1940 Batson, an anatomist, established the continuity of the longitudinal venous systems of the entire vertebral column. He did so by injecting a thin solution of radiopaque material into pelvic veins; radiographs demonstrated that the material spread through the venous systems of the entire column, even as far as the skull. This discovery must be in the forefront of your mind when you expose fragments of the various vertebral venous plexuses in the course of your dissection. It reveals not just an interesting aspect of the continuity of a system, but also a pathway for the spread of disease, with devastating result.

THE EPIDURAL (EXTRADURAL) SPACE

The development of anesthetic agents that are readily absorbed led to an increasing use of the vertebral epidural space to obtain spinal anesthesia. A select quantity of an appropriate agent is injected into the epidural space, where it can soak into the dural sheaths of the lowermost spinal nerves to reach the actual nerve fibers. The effect of the agent, which need not be analyzed in detail in this text, is to block primarily all ingoing (sensory) impulses and possibly outgoing (motor) nerve impulses in sensory and motor fibers, respectively. Thus the skin becomes numb to pain and the muscles may become powerless in the affected regions of the body.

The advantage of epidural anesthesia is that no agent is injected directly into the subarachnoid space, which is a space containing a special fluid, immediately adjacent not only to the spinal cord, but also to the brain stem and the brain itself. Thus, inadvertently, the vital centers could also be anesthetized, with death as a consequence. You will learn, however, that there are disadvantages with epidural anesthesia too. Meantime, concentrate upon the anatomy of the space, especially in the lumbar region, the usual site for epidural anesthesia. What structures are to be pierced to reach the space?

ITEM 26-11.   Immediately internal to the dura mater is a weblike membrane, the arachnoid; internal to the arachnoid is the subarachnoid space, full, in life, of cerebrospinal fluid, always abbreviated to C.S.F. The space is usually empty in a cadaver. Do not open the dura yet.

LUMBAR PUNCTURE (SPINAL TAP)

An absolute requirement in the examination of the central nervous system is a study of the cerebrospinal fluid, its nature and its pressure. An examination of this kind is achieved by introducing a special needle into the subarachnoid space. The site commonly chosen for this procedure is the lumbar region. That strict aseptic technique and other precautionary measures are necessary so as not to infect or damage the central nervous system will be made quite clear to you by your tutors in clinical medicine. For the moment, then, concentrate upon the anatomic facts of significance in lumbar puncture.

A lumbar puncture needle is usually inserted strictly in the midline through skin, supraspinous ligament, and interspinous ligament. At this point, the tip of the needle lies in the extradural space. Then, advancing, the needle tip punctures dura mater and arachnoid to enter the subarachnoid space.

Before you open the dura, obtain a needle at least 10 cm. long and insert it through the supraspinous and interspinous ligaments, forward into the extradural space, thence through dura mater. You will be aware of the needle tip puncturing the dura; you experience a sensation that can best be described vocally as a "plip." If a syringe and colored water are available, inject a few cubic centimeters so that you may establish the exact site of your puncture. There are several interspinous spaces still intact, so several students may attempt this procedure.

The Vertebral Column and Lumbar Puncture

The success or failure of a lumbar puncture in medical practice hinges, to a marked degree, upon the position of the vertebral column. In positioning the patient there are two anatomic points to bear in mind.

First, flexion of the column separates the spinous processes to their maximum. However, adopting the so-called "fetal" position (head flexed, hips and knees bent) does not necessarily achieve full flexion of the thoracolumbar spine because the neck may be long and supple and the hip joints easily bent. Only when shoulders are pulled toward the pelvis is full thoracolumbar flexion obtained.

Second, when one lies on one's side, the vertebral column, if it is normally mobile, adjusts to the shape of the supporting surface. Accordingly, a normal vertebral column will not be horizontal and symmetric unless that surface is flat and solid. Therefore, if a side-lying position is chosen for lumbar puncture, the surface on which the patient is to lie must be flat, horizontal, and solid.

ITEM 26-12.   Remove the remaining laminae, spinous processes, and attached ligaments from the level of T12 down and inferiorly with care, open the vertebral canal as far as S2 and 3.

ITEM 26-13.   In the region of S2, identify the lower end of the dura tapering to a tip from which a thin silvery strand, the filum terminale, continues inferiorly and finally ends at the coccyx.

ITEM 26-14.   Now that you have exposed the extradural space at the level of S2 and appreciate its depth you can, if you wish, expose the space as far inferiorly as the coccyx of your cadaver or, more rapidly, you can review the anatomy of the sacral hiatus on a skeleton. The hiatus is another route for the administration of epidural anesthesia, to the sacral nerves.

SACRAL HIATUS

The anesthetist who employs epidural anesthesia and makes use of the sacral hiatus, described as the sacral route, must be thoroughly aware of the anatomic variations of this opening. At this stage, however, all you need to know are the main features of the hiatus and all else will follow as your experience grows.

In an intact specimen the hiatus is "roofed" over by a fairly dense ligament, the sacrococcygeal ligament. Nevertheless, the hiatus may be identified by palpation and the sacral cornua and the superior margin of the hiatus are the bony landmarks to be sought. The tip of a needle, having passed through skin, the sacrococcygeal ligament, and the hiatus, is successfully placed in the sacral epidural space.

The anatomy of hiatus is by no means constant, whereas the anatomy of the lumbar spine is constant, and that is why the latter is preferred for epidural anesthesia.

ITEM 26-15. Proceed to open the subarachnoid space. About 1 inch superior to the lowermost end of the dura, incise the dura in the midline. In doing so, you will usually also incise the arachnoid, and enter the subarachnoid space. Put a finger into the subarachnoid space, push the fingertip inferiorly toward the end of the space, and confirm that the subarachnoid space ends where the dura ends, at S2.

ITEM 26-16. By means of two parallel incisions, one on each side, raise a rectangular flap of dura and retract it superiorly, until the lowermost end of the spinal cord, the conus medullaris, and the lower lumbar, sacral, and coccygeal nerve roots (collectively called cauda equina—meaning horse's tail) and the filum terminale are exposed. Trim away dura until you see clearly how these structures lie "free" in the subarachnoid space.

The anatomy of the extradural space and the subarachnoid space are dealt with in more detail on p. 162.

ITEM 26-17. Next, as your objective is to divide transversely the vertebral column, identify the anterior longitudinal ligament anterior to the disc between T12 and L1. Incise the ligament transversely. Look for evidence of disc degeneration and signs of change with age. Most cadavers are elderly and show some evidence of degenerative joint disease.

ITEM 26-18. With a sharp knife, cut transversely through the disc between T12 and L1. Then cut the posterior longitudinal ligament. At the same level, make sure you have cut all soft tissues, including the dura mater and cord.

ITEM 26-19. Only the paired intervertebral articulations remain to be disarticulated. If you find it difficult to disarticulate them, complete the separation with a saw. Then observe the remnants of their capsules.

THE INTERVERTEBRAL DISC

The anatomy of the intervertebral disc is of great practical concern to the orthopedist, for a disc lesion, popularly misnamed "slipped disc," is a very common medical problem. To state bluntly that an intervertebral disc consists of an annulus fibrosus and a nucleus pulposus, both between two cartilaginous plates, is to deny the very significant research into the structure and function of the disc, which is reported with great clarity in a monograph, *Lumbar Disc Lesions*, by Armstrong (1965).

At this stage, however, that brief description of the disc is enough to clarify what is meant by "slipped disc." Actually the entire disc does not slip. Instead, the posterior arc of annulus fibrosus degenerates and disintegrates, allowing some of the nucleus pulposus, which has also degenerated, to protrude toward the epidural space. The protrusion meets some resistance from the posterior longitudinal ligament. Commonly, therefore, the protrusion is more marked on one or other side of that ligament. The protrusion then exerts pressure in two directions: upon the main dural sheath (thence upon the cauda equina), and upon the the intervertebral foramina. Pressure of the latter type is more significant because of the relative immobility of the nerve roots in their sheath. As a result, the nerve roots are stretched to some extent by the protrusion; sensory roots are more readily affected than motor roots, and sensory symptoms, especially pain, appear.

ITEM 26-20. With these facts in mind, review the anatomy of the intervertebral disc you have just cut through. Identify the central nucleus pulposus, surrounded by its annulus fibrosus, and identify also the superior and inferior cartilaginous plates and the posterior longitudinal ligament. Finally, identify the dural sheath investing nerve roots. A more detailed study of this important region is done in the section titled lower limb.

Study the annulus fibrosus further and confirm that it consists of concentric lamellae, usually 10 to 12 in number. Also confirm that there is no sharp division between the annulus fibrosus and the nucleus pulposus. Observe how small the nucleus is relative to the total size of the disc.

REFERENCES

Armstrong, J. R.: Lumbar Disc Lesions, Pathogenesis and Treatment of Low Back Pain and Sciatica. Edinburgh, E. & S. Livingstone Ltd., 1965.

Barclay, A. E.: The Digestive Tract. London, Cambridge University Press, 1936.

Batson, O. V.: The function of the vertebral veins and their role in the spread of metastases. Annals of Surgery, *112*:138, 1940.

Cokkinis, A. J.: Intestinal ischaemia. Proceedings of the Royal Society of Medicine, *54*: 354, 1961.

Gardner, E., Gray, D. J., and O'Rahilly, R.: Anatomy. 2nd ed. Philadelphia, W. B. Saunders Co., 1963.

Graves, F. T.: The anatomy of the intrarenal arteries and its application to segmental resection of the kidney. British Journal of Surgery, *42*:132, 1954.

Leeson, C. R., and Leeson, T. S.: Histology. Philadelphia, W. B. Saunders Co., 1966.

Lockhart, R. D.: Living Anatomy. London, Faber & Faber Ltd., 1963.

Zaino, C., et al.: The Lower Esophageal Vestibular Complex. Springfield, Ill., Charles C Thomas, 1963.

PART 4

MALE AND FEMALE PELVIS

Part 4A   The Male Pelvis

THE MALE PELVIS

Read Chapter 34, The Bony Pelvis, and study Figures 34-1, 34-2, and 34-3 in Part 4B, Female Pelvis. Although the chapter and figures refer to the bony pelvis in the female, the basic facts concerning the anatomic orientation and the axis of the pelvic cavity apply also to the male.

Read Chapter 35, The External Genitalia.

The rectum and anal canal are described on p. 206.

The lower urinary tract is introduced on p. 223.

Chapter 27

Hemisection of the Male Pelvis and Perineum

The first step is to section what is left of the vertebral column. Using an autopsy saw with a broad blade, cut in the median sagittal plane any spinous processes still intact, and then the vertebral bodies to the level of the promontory. Complete the split with the aid of a hand saw. The second step is division of the pelvis in the following order.

ITEM 27-1.   Peel peritoneum off the anterior abdominal wall to open the retropubic space. Use a finger to dissect and explore the extent of the space between the bladder and the anterior half of the bony pelvis and related structures.

The Retropubic Space

This space is important for two reasons. First, its existence allows a surgeon to reach the bladder and prostate without going through the peritoneal cavity. Second, upon rupture of the anterolateral surface of the bladder (a surface not covered by peritoneum), or of the prostatic urethra, urine will enter the space, accumulate there, and spread beyond the space. Spread of urine in this fashion is spoken of clinically as extravasation.

"The seriousness of urinary extravasation has been known for a long time. When sterile urine permeates undrained tissue, it causes necrosis, sloughing, and suppuration, which, if untreated, obviously proves fatal. When urine is infected the toxic and necrotic action against the tissue is accelerated."*

*Prather, G. C.: Injuries of the bladder. *In* M. F. Campbell (ed.): Urology. 2nd Ed. Philadelphia, W. B. Saunders Co., 1963.

Prather reports that urine from the retropubic space may reach the region of the kidneys, the inguinal region through the inguinal canal, and even the gluteal region through the sciatic notch. It is wrong, therefore, to think of the retropubic space as having precise limits.

ITEM 27-2.   From now on, stay strictly in the midline, except when you cut the prostate. Using straight scissors with one sharp point, cut through the ventral aspect of the penis. The ventral aspect of the penis may be described as its inferior aspect. Insert the sharp point of the scissors into the urethra and so identify the urethra before you cut. It will be necessary to divide the scrotum while you continue dividing the ventral aspect of the penis as far posteriorly as the bulb. Divide the scrotum with a sharp blade.

The Mucous Membrane of the Male Urethra

The features of the mucous membrane are illustrated in *Grant's Atlas of Anatomy*, Figure 199.1, and they are discussed with reference to the passage of instruments on p. 173. Examine the mucous membrane before you divide the penis into right and left parts.

ITEM 27-3.   Depress the penis and make a sagittal cut into the suspensory ligaments of the penis anterior to the symphysis pubis. Carefully peel the penis off the inferior aspect of the symphysis pubis.

ITEM 27-4.   Slip a thin, strong Gigli saw inferior to the symphysis pubis, between the puboprostatic ligaments, and split the joint.

ITEM 27-5.   Divide the bladder strictly anteroposteriorly in the midline. To open the bladder of a cadaver, select a point on the superior surface central to the root of the urachus and the two ureterovesical junctions. Stick the closed points of straight scissors millimeter by millimeter through the bladder wall, until you reach the cavity of the bladder. Before withdrawing the scissors, open them and keep them open as you withdraw. The cavity becomes more obvious. It is worth emphasizing that the solid chunk of flesh, the usual form of the cadaveric bladder, bears not the slightest resemblance to the delicate texture of the bladder alive.

Of the genitourinary system, only the prostate and a portion of the urethra now need to be cut. Wait until you have divided the rectum and anal canal before doing so.

ITEM 27-6. Divide the sacrum. Complete division of the column and sacrum with a hand saw.

Fractures of the Pelvis

Once the symphysis pubis and the sacrum are split, you have a practical demonstration of the dangers of extensive fractures of the pelvis. The soft tissues are in peril when the pelvis is fractured in two places, especially if the fractures are diametrically opposite each other; the soft tissues cannot withstand the shearing forces that now exist. Which organs may be torn in pelvic fractures or fracture-dislocations involving either the sacroiliac joints or the symphysis pubis? In all fractures of the pelvis, damage to the soft parts must be suspected until the truth is established.

ITEM 27-7 Divide the rectum—a messy business if feces are present. Feces in a cadaver are sterile and are not a menace to your health, so persevere. Stay strictly in the midline as you approach the bladder; otherwise you will incise a vas and perhaps a seminal vesicle. Divide the anal canal.

ITEM 27-8. Do not swipe blindly with the knife. Identify the prostatic urethra and mark it with a probe inserted from within the bladder. Remain off center and make a cut to connect the cut through the bladder with that through the penis.

ITEM 27-9. At a deep sink, *not* a wash basin, flush away all debris and feces from the specimens.

This is not popular action with the laboratory attendants, but is necessary to make further study pleasant and tolerable.

The student can now complete the dissection of the gastrointestinal tract by studying the anatomy of the rectum and anal canal. Proceed to p. 206, where description of those structures begins.

Chapter 28

The Male Urethra

For descriptive purposes in anatomy, the urethra is divided into three parts, prostatic, membranous, and spongy, descriptive terms based on the location, not the structure, of the urethra.

For clinical purposes, however, the urethra is divided into two parts, posterior and anterior. The posterior urethra includes both the prostatic and the membranous parts; the anterior urethra refers to the spongy part. Furthermore, the anterior urethra is divided into penile and bulbar parts; the former is in the pendulous portion of the penis, and the latter is in the perineum (the bulbar part, therefore, does not include the membranous urethra).

ITEM 28-1. Identify both the posterior and anterior urethra. In life, few microorganisms exist in the posterior urethra, which is therefore said to be sterile, whereas many microorganisms exist in the anterior urethra. The microorganisms of the anterior urethra are foreign to the rest of the genitourinary system. Accordingly, in passing an instrument from the anterior urethra into the bladder, the danger of transporting infection into the bladder is real.

ITEM 28-2. Identify the prostatic and membranous parts of the urethra and the bulbar and penile parts of the spongy urethra.

The Prostatic Urethra (Figs. 28-1 and 28-2)

This part of the urethra is so named because it passes through the prostate. Enlargement of the prostate is common, especially in the elderly. Thus the prostatic urethra of your specimen is probably abnormal. If so, it will be narrower than usual, elongated, and sinuous, because one or more elevations of prostatic tissue protrude into the lumen. The normal prostatic urethra has an easily demonstrable lumen, is approximately 2.5 cm. long, and is essentially straight; one slight elevation (ridge), is normally present and is called the urethral crest. The prostatic urethra is beautifully illustrated in *Grant's Atlas of Anatomy*, Figure 208, and, perhaps, it is best understood on cross section (Fig. 28-2).

There is one indispensable fact concerning the prostatic urethra. It is the beginning of the final common pathway of urine from *both* kidneys. When that pathway is obstructed urine accumulates, first in the bladder, then in the ureters, and finally in the pelvis and calices of each

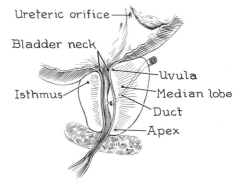

Figure 28-1. Sagittal section of the prostate to the left of the midline. The duct is the left ejaculatory duct opening on the left side of the colliculus of the urethral crest, which is not labeled (see Figure 28-2). The right ureteric orifice is labeled. The smooth area medial to it is the right half of the trigone. There are two orifices shown at the proximal end of the ejaculatory duct. Name them.

ureter. As distention of the calices proceeds, atrophy of kidney tissue continues until a mere shell of tissue remains. Thus, prostatic obstruction is one cause of bilateral hydroureter and hydronephrosis, from which death from renal failure is inevitable unless an early diagnosis is made and adequate treatment undertaken. With this vital fact in mind, examine in detail the prostatic urethra.

ITEM 28-3. Identify the base of the prostate adjoining the bladder, a region described as the bladder neck. Identify the uvula, which is a mound of prostatic tissue of varying height, posterior to and close to the internal urethral orifice. The uvula may enlarge and overhang the orifice. Acting like a ball valve, it then creates a bladder neck obstruction.

ITEM 28-4. Separate the cut edges of the gland to expose the lumen of the prostatic urethra. Separation is difficult in the cadaver, so it is not easy for the beginner to appreciate that, in life, the normal prostatic urethra is the most easily dilated part of the entire urethra. It can accommodate an instrument almost as thick as a finger (Fig. 28-3). Separate the edges and identify the urethral crest, and seek a rounded eminence toward the lower end of the crest. This eminence is called the colliculus, and it is a cardinal landmark in transurethral surgery of the prostate. Then identify the shallow channel, the prostatic sinus, on each side of the urethral crest.

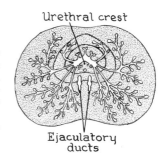

Figure 28-2. Schematic cross section of the prostate. The mucosal, submucosal, and principal components are arranged more or less concentrically around the lumen. Clinically, the first two components are considered to be one division and the principal component to be the other. (Adapted from C. R. Leeson and T. S. Leeson: Histology. Philadelphia. W. B. Saunders Co., 1966.)

ITEM 28-5. Several minute openings are present in the prostatic urethra. They can be seen with the naked eye, but ought to be examined under magnification. The easiest opening to find is the opening of the prostatic utricle, a solitary slit on the summit of the colliculus. The utricle is a cul-de-sac. Then, on each side of that opening is an even smaller slit, the opening of an ejaculatory duct. Students are usually surprised at the minute size of this orifice relative to the volume of an ejaculate. In addition, however, in each prostatic sinus there are 15 to 20 very very small orifices through which prostatic secretions emerge. The total volume of an ejaculate, 3 to 4 cc. in all, emerges through the ejaculatory orifices and the 30 to 40 orifices in the prostatic sinuses.

Infection in the prostatic urethra may spread in many directions. In addition to spreading throughout the prostate, infection may reach one or both seminal vesicles. Furthermore, via the two vasa, infection may involve the epididymis and both testes. Finally, infection reaching the bladder may ascend both ureters to involve the kidneys.

ITEM 28-6. Examine the membranous urethra just distal to the apex of the prostate. It is only about 1.5 cm. long and is surrounded by the sphincter urethrae muscle. This part of the urethra, in life, is the *least* mobile and the *least* dilatable, the opposite to one's findings in the cadaver. Except for the external urethral orifice, the membranous urethra is the narrowest part of the entire urethra.

ITEM 28-7. Examine the bulbar part of the spongy urethra. Note how it dilates to form the intrabulbar fossa. When the body is upright, the fossa lies at a lower level than the rest of the bulbar urethra. Accordingly, the fossa serves as a sump to receive the liquid products of inflammation. Observe also the relationship of the urethra to the spongy tissue of the penis; there is a substantial amount posterior to the bulbar urethra, but little or none anterosuperiorly. Finally, observe how the posterior wall of the bulbar urethra may, in some specimens, extend slightly more posterior than the orifice of the membranous urethra. Do not underestimate the importance of these facts; they will be referred to again when catheterization is discussed.

Injuries to the Bulbar Urethra

Kicks, blows, and falls astride a fence are ways in which serious damage may be done to the bulbar urethra, as well as to other parts. The clinical aspects do not need attention at this time. It is simply necessary for you to realize that the bulbar urethra, lying close to the body surface, is vulnerable. Examine your specimen.

ITEM 28-8. The Bulbourethral Glands

Two tiny glands, about 0.5 cm. in diameter, lie adjacent to the membranous urethra. From each gland a microscopic duct descends to open into the bulbar fossa. Do not waste time searching for these minute structures. They are, nevertheless, extremely significant when they harbor infection.

ITEM 28-9. Examine the penile urethra. On its roof, and, to some extent, on its floor, there are tiny flaps of mucous membrane. The recess, sheltered by each flap, is called a lacuna urethralis. On the dorsal aspect of the urethra, at the junction of the glans and the body of the penis, there is a more conspicuous fold, sometimes referred to as the valvule of the navicular fossa. About 1 cm. posterior to the valvule a smaller fold may be present; when it is present it forms a boundary of the lacuna magna. The significant fact is that the free edge of each of these folds is directed toward the external urethral orifice. Thus a lacuna may trap the tip of a very thin instrument or catheter. The urethral mucous membrane is studded with the orifices of many small glands, the urethral glands.

Finally, observe the expanded portion of the urethra, the fossa navicularis, within the glans.

The Passing of Instruments Along the Male Urethra

One of the most common clinical procedures is catheterization. The reasons for catheterization and the various types of catheters need not be described here. It is also frequently necessary to pass a viewing instrument (Fig. 28-3) to examine the internal aspect of the bladder and urethra, as well as for other procedures. Finally, it is sometimes necessary to pass a steel rod, known as a bougie, to dilate the urethra when it has been narrowed to a harmful degree by disease. For the

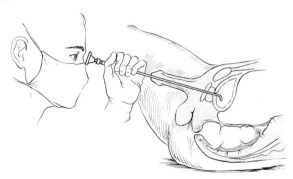

Figure 28-3. A cystoscope is a basic requirement in urology. In addition to the examination of the bladder and its orifices, surgical procedures are performed through the cystoscope with the aid of carefully designed instruments supported on steel rods that can be inserted along the barrel of the "scope." A catheter, inserted into each ureter through the "scope," is used to obtain a sample of urine from each kidney and to inject radiopaque fluid for retrograde pyelography.

success of all these procedures, knowledge of the anatomy of the urethra is absolutely necessary, and the relevant anatomy is listed now:

(1) The external urethral orifice is the narrowest part of the entire urethra. Therefore, if an instrument can pass through the meatus, it should pass along the rest of a normal urethra.

(2) The shape of the fossa navicularis, the formation of a valvule, and the presence of a lacuna magna may trap the tip of an instrument. Therefore the tip of the instrument is directed toward the floor of the fossa until the tip is beyond these anatomic landmarks.

(3) The penile urethra and the bulbar urethra lie at an acute angle when the penis is flaccid. Therefore, in instrumentation, the penile urethra must be raised to eliminate that angle. When this is done the entire urethra becomes J-shaped, a shape that is kept in mind in the design of the appropriate instruments.

(4) The bulbar fossa sometimes bulges posteriorly. Thus the tip of an instrument, held at an incorrect angle, may proceed posteriorly a few significant millimeters beyond the orifice of the membranous urethra. Pressure applied to the perineum or from the anal canal by the clinician's other hand may be sufficient to guide the tip easily into the orifice.

(5) The roof of the bulbar fossa is not substantial. Therefore, the possibility of thrusting the tip of an instrument through that roof is real.

(6) That the direction of the prostatic urethra is essentially vertical must be kept in mind while the tip of an instrument is being advanced through the prostatic urethra. The J shape of the entire urethra has already been referred to.

(7) The average urethra measures 20 cm. from the external to the internal urethral orifice.

In conclusion, it is stressed that the instrumentation of the male urethra is sometimes very difficult, especially when normal anatomy is distorted by disease. Nevertheless, a knowledge of the normal anatomy of the urethra will go a long way toward diminishing difficulty.

The Urine

So much valuable evidence about the state of the urinary system can be gotten from an examination of the urine that urinalysis is an absolute requirement in any physical examination. The clinician must know whether urine is being produced and, if so, whether it is being passed and in what amount. You realize that there is a difference between the production of urine, a function of the kidneys, and the passing of urine, the function of the urinary tract. The clinician is also interested in the frequency of micturition during the day (diurnal) and during the night (nocturnal frequency); the color and specific gravity of urine and other observations and tests you learn of first at the laboratory bench are equally important. It is necessary, then, for a medical student to study the function of the urinary system in depth, and not to concentrate solely on its structure.

Chapter 29

Fascial Layers of the Perineum

If you approach this dissection with preconceived ideas from reading accounts of the perineum, you may discover that your findings differ from your concept. The trouble arises because one particular layer of fascia, the external perineal fascia, is often ignored in descriptions of the fascial layers of the perineum.

The external perineal fascia is the posterior extension onto the perineum of the deep fascia of the penis (Fig. 29-1) and it plays a significant part in limiting the spread of pus or blood from the penis. The fascia is indeed significant, a significance that is brought forth with great clarity and brevity by Tobin and Benjamin (1944) in a paper introduced with interesting historical highlights. It is upon their paper that the dissection of the perineum presented here is based. Figure 29-1 shows the layers to be identified.

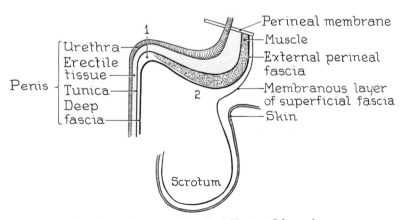

Figure 29-1. Diagram of the fascial layers of the perineum.

ITEM 29-1. Identify the corpus spongiosum, the erectile tissue surrounding the urethra, and identify, in particular, its thin outer envelope, the tunica, which is white in color.

ITEM 29-2. About halfway along the pendulous urethra, identify a well-defined sheet of fascia immediately external to the tunica. Define this fascia, which is the deep fascia of the penis (Buck's fascia). By gentle but deliberate blunt dissection, trace the fascia posteriorly, where it lies superficial, i.e., inferior, to a layer of muscle, the bulbocavernosus muscle. The fascia is robust and may be defined by blunt dissection as far posteriorly as the posterior aspect of the penile bulb. By further blunt dissection, explore the lateral extent of the fascia.

The fascia you have just demonstrated is obviously in continuity with the deep fascia of the penis, but on the perineum anatomists have renamed it the external perineal fascia (Fig. 29-1).

ITEM 29-3. Another easily identified layer of fascia is the membranous layer of the superficial fascia (Fig. 29-1). To identify it proceed from the skin of the perineum into the superficial fat. The membranous layer may not be immediately apparent, but with a little skillful dissection it should be easily demonstrated. By blunt dissection trace the membranous layer inferiorly toward the scrotum and anteriorly over the penis (where it is external to the deep fascia). It is usually possible to demonstrate how this layer of fascia extends superolaterally to become continuous with the membranous layer of the superficial fascia in the groin. See if you can establish that continuity.

Two Planes of Cleavage

The first plane of cleavage (1, Fig. 29-1) lies external to the tunica of the corpus spongiosum and internal to the deep fascia of the penis. Posteriorly, however, this plane of cleavage is between the bulbospongiosus muscle and the external perineal fascia. The second plane of cleavage (2, Fig. 29-1) is external to the deep fascia of the penis and its extension, the external perineal fascia, and internal to the membranous layer of superficial fascia.

Fluid extravasated into the first plane of cleavage will be confined to the region of the corpus and bulb, and will have similar outline. On the other hand, fluid extravasated into the second plane of cleavage can spread widely over the surface of the scrotum and the penis, and even onto the anterior abdominal wall.

The first plane of cleavage is the superficial perineal compartment (known also as a pouch, or interspace), which extends from the perineal membrane superiorly and to the external perineal fascia inferiorly (Fig. 29-1). The second plane of cleavage is called the superficial perineal fascial cleft. In many texts, however, the existence of the external perineal fascia is ignored. Then the term superficial perineal pouch is applied to the entire space between the perineal membrane and the membranous layer of the superficial fascia (Fig. 29-1).

Clearly it is important to see the real anatomy here and to appreciate that pus, blood, and possibly urine confined by the deep fascia of the penis and the external perineal fascia are less menacing to the health of a patient than urine immediately deep to the membranous layer of the superficial fascia. Once urine enters that plane of cleavage, it can spread widely with very serious results.

Chapter 30

The Male Reproductive System

There are two parts to the system, one producing sperm and the other producing a medium for the sperm.

In a normal male, sperm are formed in each testis, from where they proceed into an epididymis, thence through a vas deferens to an ejaculatory duct that opens into the prostatic urethra. It must be made clear that sperm are not formed in any other part of the reproductive system.

Some of the medium for sperm is supplied by both the epididymides. Most of it, however, is produced by the two seminal vesicles and the solitary prostate, which are sometimes referred to as auxiliary glands.

The objectives of the next dissection are to trace the pathway of sperm and to examine the auxiliary glands.

ITEM 30-1. The spermatic cord has already been exposed at the external (superficial) inguinal ring. Revise the coverings of the cord, then slit the scrotum to demonstrate how the coverings enclose the testis. It is reassuring to know that in a cadaver several additional coverings are often demonstrated. It is assumed that these are artifacts, the result of the toughening with embalming of delicate areolar tissue, which is not particularly obvious in the living body. Remove all layers until the tunica vaginalis of the testis is exposed.

ITEM 30-2. It may be a practical advantage to remove the testis from the scrotum. Then incise the tunica vaginalis. Open it wide to demonstrate that, in principle, it has the same design as peritoneum, namely a visceral layer and a parietal layer, with a potential cavity between. The recess between the testis and the epididymis is named the sinus of the tunica vaginalis.

TUNICA VAGINALIS

For reasons not clearly understood, fluid may accumulate in and distend the tunica vaginalis to a considerable size, a condition called hydrocele of the testis. Because of the location of the tunica in relation to the testis, the normal testis lies posterior when a hydrocele is present. Furthermore, the sinus of the tunica vaginalis between the testis and the epididymis may also be distended when a hydrocele is present so that those two structures are separated, but not completely.

There are varieties of hydrocele to be discussed by your clinical tutors. One important fact, however, is worth stressing now. The tunica vaginalis is an immediate relation of the testis; the hydrocele may be secondary to disease of the testis. Therefore, hydrocele of the testis must be considered serious until the health of the underlying testis is established.

ITEM 30-3. Retract the tunica widely. Examine the surface of both the testis and the epididymis for minute appendages. See *Grant's Atlas of Anatomy*, Figure 116. The appendages are minute, but they are of clinical significance.

ITEM 30-4. The tunica albuginea of the testis is the grayish-white coat seen through the visceral layer of the tunica vaginalis. The presence of this tough coat, which does not yield, explains why swelling of the testes in orchitis (inflammation of the testis) is so painful and so devastating to the cells producing sperm.

DISSECTION OF THE TESTIS AND EPIDIDYMIS

ITEM 30-5. Identify the head, body, and tail of the epididymis. Then carefully break through the tunica vaginalis between the upper pole of the testis and the head of the epididymis. By blunt dissection, expose some of the efferent ducts, 15 to 20 in number, that connect the rete testis to the head of the epididymis. *Rete testis* means a network of channels, and will be demonstrated next. Having identified the efferent ducts, make a longitudinal section of the testis — *do not* include the epididymis — to demonstrate the location of the rete testis in the mediastinum testis. At the same time, observe the incomplete septa that divide the testis into compartments, each compartment being occupied by a lobule of tubules. The tubules terminate in the rete testis. Thus sperm, formed in the tubules, reach the rete testis, from where they proceed through the efferent ducts to enter a solitary canal, the epididymis. Where the epididymis ends, the vas deferens begins.

ITEM 30-6. Trace the vas deferens into the spermatic cord. It will be necessary to separate the other longitudinal components of the cord, such as the testicular artery, a plexus of veins, and lymphatic vessels, which are not seen. Autonomic nerves are also present. The vas is easily recognized because it looks like and feels like a piece of cord. It is a very muscular structure and, in life, vigorous peristaltic waves propel sperm along its lumen.

VAS DEFERENS

The fact that the vas deferens is subcutaneous before it enters the superficial inguinal ring is of great practical importance. Palpation of the vas to assess its condition is an essential procedure in examination of the male reproductive system. Moreover, it is external to the ring that each vas may be sectioned to render a male sterile. Bilateral vasectomy is a simple enough procedure compared to bilateral ligation of the uterine tubes, which requires opening of the peritoneal cavity. Thus bilateral vasectomy has some advocates as a means of control of world population.

ITEM 30-7. Trace the vas through the inguinal canal. Review its relationships, e.g., to the inferior epigastric artery. Continue to trace the vas into the pelvis to the point where it lies superior to the ureter. To do this it will be necessary to reflect peritoneum medially.

ITEM 30-8. To expose the seminal vesicle, reflect peritoneum toward the midline. Close to the termination of the ureter and to the spot where the vas deferens crosses the ureter, the blunt end of the seminal vesicle will be found. The end may be obscured by fascia. Remove some of the fascia to reveal the vesicle—its characteristic lobulated appearance is unmistakable.

Do not remove too much fascia at this stage lest in doing so you destroy structures best seen by a perineal approach to this region.

Read an account of the lymphatic drainage, venous drainage, nerve supply, and arterial supply of the testis. The information is clearly given in major anatomy texts.

THE SEMINAL VESICLES

The combined secretions of the seminal vesicles provide the bulk of an ejaculate. The vesicles do not produce sperm, nor do they store sperm.

The size and shape of the seminal vesicles vary from man to man, and their fullness varies from time to time. Furthermore, the position of the seminal vesicles varies with the fullness of the bladder. A full bladder pushes the vesicles inferiorly so that they are more readily palpable per rectum. Therefore study the size, shape, position, and relationships with care when you expose each vesicle in the course of your dissection. In life, healthy seminal vesicles are soft. Therefore they are not actually palpable. See palpable organs, p. 96.

Posteriorly, each vesicle is separated by a sheet of fascia from the rectum, but, even so, the posterior surface of each vesicle is palpable per rectum (p. 188). Anteriorly the vesicles are related to the bladder and prostate, while the two vasa come to lie between the two vesicles (Fig. 30-1). The tip of each vesicle is related to a ureter; the tip is also subjacent to peritoneum, and is level with the ischial spine.

There are three basic surgical approaches to a seminal vesicle, (1) extraperitoneal — to some degree you have already demonstrated this route in your dissection (2) transperitoneal — rarely used and not advocated because of the possibility of infecting the peritoneum, but your specimen does show that this approach is possible, and (3) from the perineum — this route will be demonstrated by dissection (p. 183).

THE PROSTATE

The prostate is as important as the seminal vesicles in providing a medium for sperm. Furthermore, normal prostatic secretions are alkaline and play an important part in the neutralization of vaginal secretions and the success of fertilization. The prostate is a solid structure and is therefore actually palpable per rectum (Fig. 30-1).

Position

ITEM 30-9.   Note that the base of the prostate joins the bladder at the bladder neck where prostate and bladder have an intimate relationship. In fact, bundles of muscle fibers proceed without interruption between the two organs.

Appreciate that the position of the prostate will depend upon the fullness of the bladder. An inexperienced clinical student, examining the prostate of a patient with a full bladder, may assume the gland is enlarged when the gland is in fact normal in size. The full bladder has displaced the gland inferiorly so that it is more readily palpable.

In general, then, the gland lies posterior to the lower half of the symphysis pubis and anterior to the ampulla of the rectum. Confirm this on your specimen.

Shape

Shape depends primarily on the fullness of the gland and the age of the individual. Normally the gland has a fairly extensive posterior

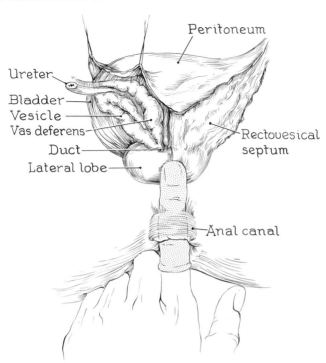

Peritoneum
Ureter
Bladder
Vesicle
Vas deferens
Duct
Lateral lobe
Rectovesical septum
Anal canal

Figure 30-1. Only the posterior surface of the prostate is palpable through the rectum. The wall of the rectum and the rectovesical septum separate the finger from the gland but the gland is easily recognized by its firm consistency. A final decision regarding the prostatic urethra must not be made until the urethra has been examined with either a urethroscope or a cystoscope.

surface, a narrow anterior border, a base joining the bladder, and an apex projecting inferiorly (Fig. 28-1).

Relationships

On your specimen, relationships are readily apparent. One relationship, often forgotten needs to be stressed—the pair of ejaculatory ducts traversing the substance of the gland to reach the colliculus of the prostatic urethra (Fig. 28-1). Clearly, removal of the prostate gland will render a male infertile because of retrograde ejaculation.

Subdivisions

Modern research shows the gland has two main divisions, inner and outer, centered upon the prostatic urethra (Fig. 28-2). However, the classic subdivisions, emphasized until recent times, are still useful for clinical purposes. On each side there is a lateral lobe. The lobes are connected anteriorly by a muscular, not a glandular, bridge, the isthmus prostatae. Identify the isthmus.

The glandular tissue, wedged between the ejaculatory ducts posteriorly and the urethra anteriorly, is named the median lobe. It lies inferior to the uvula, an eminence of varying size at the neck of the bladder. Identify the uvula vesicae and compare its size with other specimens.

The Median Lobe of the Prostate

This lobe may become sufficiently enlarged to obstruct the prostatic urethra. It is possible for this lobe to be enlarged while the rest of the prostate seems normal. Therefore, you must appreciate that accurate decisions about the condition of the median lobe can be made only after it has been inspected per urethram (Fig. 28-1).

Capsule and Sheath

The external surface of the prostate forms a capsule that contains a high percentage of muscle fibers as well as elastic fibers. The capsule is not easy to identify in the gross anatomy laboratory. From the capsule, septa of similar tissue pass into the depths of the gland to create ill-defined subdivisions in which lobules of glandular tissue are found.

More easily identifiable is the sheath, loosely woven and loosely fitting, with a plexus of veins embedded in it. There are, however, no veins in the prostatic sheath posteriorly, where the fascial sheath is avascular and blends with the rectovesical septum.

SEMINAL FLUID

Often it is essential to examine the seminal fluid. The methods of collecting a specimen and what is required in the report are described in detail in appropriate clinical texts.

Exercise

You, as a practicing physician, examine a patient's left testis and suspect he has a disease that could involve the entire reproductive system. Name the parts you would proceed to examine and how you would examine them.

Chapter 31

Perineal Approach to the Male Pelvis

Except in the removal of the anal canal and rectum, the perineal approach to the contents of the male pelvis is not commonly used by surgeons because the operative procedure is not easy and not without hazard. Nevertheless, on a median sagittal section of the pelvis of a cadaver, the approach is both easy to demonstrate and instructive.

It is best to demonstrate the rectovesical fascia first (Fig. 30-1).

ITEM 31-1. Gently mobilize the peritoneum between the bladder and the rectum and you will demonstrate a vertical sheet of fascia extending inferiorly between the genitourinary system and the rectum. The fascia is avascular and therefore provides an ideal plane of cleavage between the anterior group of pelvic organs and the rectum. Called the rectovesical fascia, it is also known clinically as the fascia of Denonvilliers. Demonstrate that inferiorly the fascia blends with the fascial sheath of the prostate.

ITEM 31-2. Return now to the perineum. Identify the external sphincter of the anal canal (Fig. 31-1). In a good cadaver, that sphincter is darker than the internal sphincter. Immediately external to the external sphincter the anal fascia must be identified. In life, the fascia is strong enough to be manipulated with forceps. Expose the anterior surface of the anal fascia by blunt dissection anterosuperiorly into the pelvis.

ITEM 31-3. Soon you will demonstrate muscle bundles of the external anal sphincter traveling anteriorly to join the perineal body. Stay strictly in the midline as you cut, for if you cut too far laterally you will cut the medial margin of levator ani. Pull the anal canal posteroinferiorly and cut the muscle bundles you have just demonstrated.

ITEM 31-4. If you proceed cautiously, you will demonstrate the rectourethralis muscles (there may be two, inferior and superior). Pull the rectum posteriorly and the bulb of the penis anteroinferiorly, and you will see the rectourethralis muscle extending from the rectum to the membranous urethra. Cut the rectourethralis muscles.

ITEM 31-5. The rectum and anal canal may now be pulled posteriorly and the genitourinary system anteriorly to open widely a plane of cleavage. Clearly neither the rectum and anal canal posteriorly nor the genitourinary system anteriorly has been unduly disturbed by this procedure.

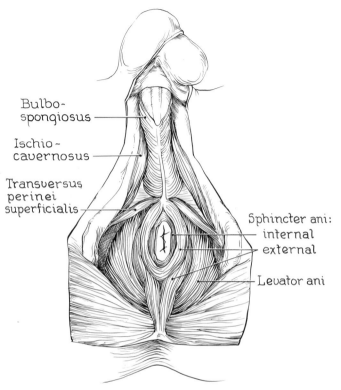

Bulbo-
spongiosus

Ischio-
cavernosus

Transversus
perinei
superficialis

Sphincter ani:
internal
external

Levator ani

Figure 31-1. The musculature of the male perineum. Posterior to the transversus perinei superficialis lies the inferior end of the plane of cleavage between the anal canal and rectum posteriorly and the genitourinary system anteriorly.

ITEM 31-6. The transversus perinei muscles (Fig. 31-1) are easily identified, useful landmarks to the surgeon using the perineal approach. The plane of cleavage you have just demonstrated lies posterior to the transversus perinei muscles. Accordingly, as long as the surgeon remains posterior to those slender but identifiable muscles, there is little chance of his entering inadvertently the urinary system.

From the midline proceed laterally and identify the transversus perinei muscle.

ITEM 31-7. Open up the gap between bladder and rectum and expose the entire seminal vesicle and the termination of the vas.

ITEM 31-8. By careful but deliberate blunt dissection (the tissues do not yield easily), seek the ejaculatory duct at the inferior ends of the vesicle and vas. The duct can be found entering the prostate.

The perineal approach you have just demonstrated may at times be used in the removal of the prostate, for example, or even removal of a seminal vesicle. Figure 193, in *Grant's Atlas of Anatomy*, however, demonstrates that the access to pelvic organs is limited, not only because of the bony frame of the pelvic outlet but also because of the proximity of the levatores ani forming the pelvic diaphragm.

Chapter 32

Sidewall of the Male Pelvis

The peritoneum has already been reflected to some extent in exposing the ureter, vas, and seminal vesicle. Now make sure that the peritoneum is sufficiently loose for you to pull the rectum and bladder medially in order to enter the interval between the viscera and the sidewall.

The dissection proceeds thus:

1. Demonstration of the pelvic splanchnic nerves
2. Examination of the parietal endopelvic fascia
3. Partial identification of obturator internus and levator ani
4. Levator ani
5. Demonstration of branches of the internal iliac artery and the sacral plexus

In this next dissection, be careful not to penetrate the parietal endopelvic fascia, a gray membranous thin sheet coating the sidewall of the pelvis.

ITEM 32-1.   To demonstrate, to some degree, the pelvic splanchnic nerves, pull the rectum medially and the bladder anteromedially and clean away areolar tissue between the lateral aspect of the rectum and the sidewall of the pelvis. Interconnected bundles of nerve fibers, traveling in a posteroanterior direction, usually emerge during the removal of this areolar tissue. The nerves are part of the pelvic splanchnic network and they are parasympathetic in function. They may be destroyed during removal of the rectum. It is suspected that their destruction is one factor in the explanation of retention of urine in the bladder after excision of the rectum.

ITEM 32-2.   To examine the parietal endopelvic fascia, proceed as follows: Slide a finger over the pelvic brim into the pelvic cavity. It is inevitable that you will slide onto a sheet of fascia, easily identified for it is light gray in color and has the appearance and tension of a delicate drumskin. Do not proceed if you are uncertain, because once this sheet of fascia is sundered its anatomy is difficult to reconstruct. By blunt dissection with the fingers, remove all loose tissue until you demonstrate how the parietal endopelvic fascia is continuous with the visceral endopelvic fascia on the bladder. Pull the bladder medially to demonstrate this fact.

In the gray parietal endopelvic fascia you will see condensed tissue, white in color, in contrast to the gray of the fascia as a whole. The tissue is in the shape of a letter Y lying on its side. The solitary limb is attached posteriorly to the ischial spine. Anteriorly, one stem proceeds to the posteroinferior edge of the body of the pubis while the other stem ascends to the brim of the pelvis to the vicinity of the obturator canal.

This peculiar Y-shaped formation is due to a combination of two tendinous arches, one for the levator ani and the other for the pelvic fascia. Posteriorly, the two arches merge in the solitary limb of the Y, while anteriorly they separate; the arcus tendineus of the levator ani ascends to the obturator canal; the arcus tendineus of the pelvic fascia continues anteriorly to the pubis.

It is not essential for the undergraduate to study the two arches in detail, but they are mentioned in both anatomic and surgical texts. It is much easier to understand what they are by seeing them than by reading about them without a specimen at hand.

Superior to the arcus tendineus of levator ani, some of the obturator internus muscle is visible through the parietal endopelvic fascia. Inferior and anterior to the same arcus, the visible muscle fibers belong to levator ani.

Levator ani is a bilateral structure. The levatores ani form an almost complete sheet across the cavity of the pelvis; together they are known as the pelvic diaphragm. The anatomy of each levator ani is difficult to comprehend from descriptions; it is without doubt the one structure that must be seen to be understood.

ITEM 32-3. To see the levator ani, carefully incise the parietal endopelvic fascia parallel to the arcus tendineus of the pelvic fascia. With care, remove as much of the fascia as possible to expose the underlying levator ani muscle. Observe how bundles of muscle fibers turn medially to the midline, where they would normally meet their fellows from the opposite side. Trace the puboprostatae fibers from the body of the pubis to a point *posterior* to the prostate (and thus anterior to the rectum).

ITEM 32-4. Displace the rectum medially and trace the remaining fibers in a dorsal direction to the posterior aspect of the anorectal junction and to the coccyx.

LEVATORES ANI

It must be stressed again that the anatomy of this pair of muscles must be learned from a specimen. The component parts of each muscle are well illustrated in atlases and textbooks, which should be consulted with a specimen in hand. The muscles forming the pelvic diaphragm will be referred to frequently, in obstetrics and gynecology especially, and in pelvic surgery in general.

Two aspects that present difficulty to the student are illustrated in Figure 45-1. Puborectalis is a component of the levator ani that meets its fellow of the opposite side posteriorly to the anorectal junction. The puborectalis is believed to be an integral part of the mechanism for the continence of feces.

The second aspect is the ease with which fibers of levator ani become part of the longitudinal coat of the anal canal. The key fact here is the oblique direction of the anal canal; the essentially horizontal fibers of levatores ani sweep naturally into place in the anal canal. Confusion arises when an illustration of a longitudinal section of the anal canal is interpreted as being in a vertical plane.

ITEM 32-5. To demonstrate the branches of the internal iliac artery, usually well illustrated in most texts and atlases, identify the common iliac artery and its major branches plus the accompanying veins.

Pursue the internal iliac artery into the pelvis and identify the origin of its many branches. Remember, variations of these origins are very common. In order to save time and to avoid prolonged debate, it is best to delay final identification of arteries until the gluteal region is dissected (p. 237). Use illustrations as a guide to the interpretation of your findings in your specimen. If need be, sacrifice without restraint the many veins in this region. Obviously in a surgical procedure veins cannot be treated with such abandon.

The rami of the sacral plexus are in close relationship with several branches of the internal iliac artery. *Grant's Atlas of Anatomy*, Figure 213, illustrates the essential facts. The rami are dealt with again when the lower limb is dissected.

THE PUDENDAL NERVE AND VESSELS

Dissection of these structures has barely begun. They have yet to be identified in the gluteal region, in the ischiorectal fossa, and on the perineum. Nevertheless your attention is drawn to them now, especially to the nerve. Local anesthesia of one side of the perineum may be obtained by anesthetizing the pudendal nerve in the vicinity of the ischial spine.

ITEM 32-6. Identify the ischial spine and the pudendal vessels and nerve.

The continuation of the pudendal vessels and nerve is studied most easily when the gluteal region is dissected and the ischiorectal fossa is cleared of fat.

Chapter 33

Pelvic Examination

It is the regular performance of simple clinical procedures such as digital examination of the pelvic contents per rectum that distinguishes the capable clinician from the mediocre. Time and again in the practice of medicine examination per rectum of either a male or female patient gives the clue that clinches the diagnosis. Furthermore, pelvic examination per vaginam is an essential procedure in the practice of obstetrics and gynecology. Now, with the aid of your specimens you have the opportunity to learn the rudiments of both these fundamental procedures.

EXAMINATION PER RECTUM

Clinically there are several positions the patient may adopt to make it easier for the examiner to perform a rectal examination. The various positions are illustrated in many clinical texts. Frequently the examination is performed with the patient lying on his or her side. Accordingly, place your specimen so that the buttock is toward you; identify the anal canal and rectum. Place the tip of the index finger in the anal orifice. In life, as the finger enters the anal canal, it would be grasped by the sphincter ani. Then, on your specimen, slide the finger onward so that its tip enters the ampulla of the rectum. From there the finger may examine in five main directions, to the right, to the left, anteriorly, posteriorly, and superiorly. Determine what structures are palpable. They are listed as follows:

MALE

Anteriorly:

(1) Posterior surface of the prostate.
(2) Inferior to the prostate, the bulbourethral glands, if they are tender or enlarged.
(3) The seminal vesicles, if they are enlarged and fibrous. Each vesicle is on the superolateral aspect of the prostate.
Superiorly:
The peritoneum.

FEMALE

Anteriorly:

The cervix uteri and the vault of the vagina. In life, a supportive device, a pessary, or a contraceptive device, a diaphragm, located in the vault of the vagina are palpable per rectum.

Laterally:

Although the uterosacral ligaments cannot usually be defined they may be felt. When they are diseased they can be the source of marked tenderness, which may be most deceptive in a differential diagnosis.

Superiorly:

The peritoneum. An ovary may be palpable in the pouch of Douglas. In acute retroflexion of the uterus, the corpus may be easily felt.

BOTH SEXES

Posteriorly:

The anterior surface of the sacrum and coccyx.

To the right and left:

The ischial spines.

OBSTETRICS

Pelvic examination per rectum is an essential procedure in the practice of obstetrics. The obstetrician is well aware that the cervix uteri, in particular the external os, is actually palpable per rectum. Thus the sequence of changes that occur in the os during labor may be determined by regular digital examination per rectum rather than per vaginam. In this way, it is believed, an essential requirement of the conduct of labor is accomplished without the risk of infecting the birth canal.

BIMANUAL EXAMINATION OF THE FEMALE PELVIS

Clinically this form of examination is usually performed with the patient in a modified lithotomy position (Fig. 35-1). Accordingly, place the right half of a hemisection of the female pelvis so that the buttock rests on the table and the hip joint is toward you. Identify the labia, the vestibule of the vagina, the vagina, the fornices, the cervix, and the body and fundus of the uterus. Place the tip of your right index finger in the vagina so that the tip of the finger presses upon the external os uteri. With the left hand steady the fundus of the uterus (in life this hand would palpate the uterus through the anterior abdominal wall). By pressing your two hands toward each other you can determine the size, shape, consistency, and other features of the uterus. In a similar fashion the ovaries may be palpated.

There is much to be learned from your clinical tutors about the technique for this method of examination in the living. Meanwhile you have learned the basic anatomy of the procedure.

Part 4B   The Female Pelvis

by R. D. LAURENSON
and T. R. NELSON

Chapter 34

The Bony Pelvis

For the applied anatomy of the male or female pelvic organs and perineum to be comprehensible, an awareness of the correct orientation of the bony pelvis and its principal landmarks is an absolute necessity. Accordingly, in Figure 34-1 an innominate bone and half a sacrum have been sketched in outline to show the principal bony landmarks of the pelvis correctly oriented one to another. Proceed now to confirm the facts illustrated in Figure 34-1 with the aid of an intact bony pelvis. For an explanation of the adjectives *iliac, ischial,* and *pubic,* refer to Figure 34-2.

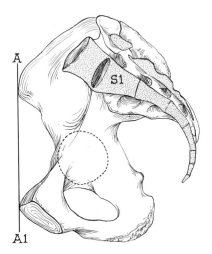

Figure 34-1. Median sagittal section of a female pelvis in the anatomic position. The dotted line indicates the location of the acetabulum. Observe the forward position of S1, the level of the tip of the sacrum and coccyx, and the ischial spine, projecting posteromedially into the midpelvic region. See also Figure 34-3 and text.

(1) The anterior superior iliac spines and symphysis pubis are on the same frontal plane (Fig. 34-1, *A* to *A1*). To demonstrate this fact, place the pelvis against a wall so that those spines and the symphysis make contact. The wall serves well as an actual frontal plane against which the pelvis assumes automatically its correct anatomic position. It is highly unlikely, however, that the pelvis within a living person is ever in the perfect so-called anatomic position, for the pelvis is bound to tilt in response to changes of body position and body posture. Nevertheless, the positions of pelvic bony landmarks remain constant to one another and to the plane of the anterior superior iliac spines and symphysis. Therefore, by taking into account the position of the anterior superior iliac spines and the symphysis pubis, the position of other landmarks in the pelvis can be decided with reasonable accuracy, regardless of the position of the pelvis.

(2) The ischial spine is superior to the ischial tuberosity.

(3) As an exercise to relate (2) to (1), rest the pelvis on a flat horizontal surface with the anterior iliac spines and symphysis pubis uppermost. Now, by changing the plane of those three bony landmarks,

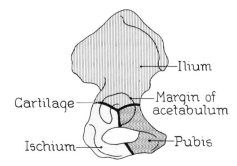

Figure 34-2. The adjectives iliac, ischial, and pubic can be confusing unless one knows their origin. In early life, three parts, separated by a Y-shaped zone of cartilage, can be identified in the innominate bone. They are the ilium, the ischium, and the pubis. The innominate bone shown here, which has an unusual shape, was imported from India.

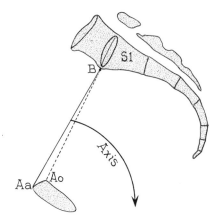

Figure 34-3. B. indicates the sacral promontory. BAo, the obstetric conjugate diameter, is the shortest anteroposterior diameter of the pelvic inlet. This important diameter must not be confused with the anatomic conjugate diameter, BAa, which is of no significance whatsoever to the obstetrician.

observe how the relationship of ischial spine to tuberosity remains constant.

(4) Observe on the pelvis that each ischial spine projects medially rather than posteriorly. The spine has, therefore, a posterolateral surface, a fact difficult to convey by illustration alone.

(5) The sacral promontory (*B*, Fig. 34-3) is on the same horizontal plane as the anterior superior iliac spines. A vertical line dropped from the tip of the promontory intersects a line connecting the symphysis pubis and coccyx (or apex of sacrum) anterior to the midpoint. To many undergraduates it comes as a surprise to realize that the promontory lies so far forward.

(6) In keeping with (5) and because of the pronounced curvature of the sacrum, the first and second anterior sacral foramina face inferiorly rather than anteriorly and the first foramina (and possibly the second) lies anterior to a vertical line through the ischial spine.

If you give careful consideration to the points listed here and get a clear idea of the orientation of the bony pelvis, the anatomic relationships of organs inside the pelvis will be readily understood.

THE PELVIS IN OBSTETRICS

Knowledge of the anatomy of the bony pelvis is of paramount importance to the obstetrician. However, the anatomic facts he selects as being important differ from those included in the total interest of the anatomist. Therefore, as an introduction to obstetrics, the more pertinent facts concerning the pelvic inlet, outlet, and cavity are presented. You will accumulate further relevant anatomic detail as your knowledge of obstetrics grows.

The Pelvic Inlet. Looking with a critical eye at a bony pelvis, you will observe a conspicuous margin, the pelvic inlet, dividing the pelvis into an "open" anterosuperior region and a confined posteroinferior tunnel, the true pelvis. The boundaries, diameters, and orientation of the inlet must be examined closely, for, as the entrance to the bony birth canal, the inlet becomes of critical importance in childbirth.

No doubt in your preliminary gaze upon the pelvis you identified the inlet as extending from the centrally located sacral promontory on to each ala of the sacrum, thence across a sacroiliac joint and along each iliopectineal line on to the superior aspect of each pubic bone beside the centrally located symphysis. If you have done just that, then you have identified the pelvic inlet of classical anatomy rather than the inlet of practical obstetrics. The latter is different, as you will now see. In obstetrics, concerned as it is with the passage of the baby's head through the inlet, attention is focused upon the minimal measurements of the inlet, that is, the real, and not the apparent, inlet. The measurements of the inlet are spoken of as diameters.

Of the various diameters commonly listed, the one to draw your attention to is the one most frequently used, the obstetric conjugate diameter (Fig. 34-3, AoB). *Conjugate* is a mathematical term describing the short axis of an ellipse; if you look again at a female pelvis you will see that the pelvic inlet is nearly a perfect ellipse, with the long axis running from right to left. Accordingly, the short axis or conjugate runs from the sacrum to the symphysis pubis. After studying Figure 34-3, return to a bony pelvis and reinvestigate the posterior sloping surface of each pubic bone. Slide the tip of an index finger up and down upon that surface and you will become aware of an indefinite, but nevertheless palpable, horizontal rise of bone, usually on a level with the obturator canal. This slight rise, corresponding to Ao in Figure 34-3, forms the anterior arc of the real inlet, the brim. In pregnancy and in labor, when the greatest diameter of the head is in the brim the head is said to be engaged. This suggests a close fit, as indeed it is. Trace the brim.

Consider next the angle at which the brim lies. The angle is commonly quoted as 60° to the horizontal, but may be as low as 48° or as high as 85°. What is significant, however, is not so much the size of angle but that there is an angle, or bend, to be negotiated in moving from the vertically disposed lower abdomen into the obliquely disposed true pelvis (see Fig. 15-1).

The Pelvic Outlet. Turn the pelvis upside down and trace the boundaries of the outlet. Posteriorly, begin with the tip of the fifth piece of the sacrum, not the tip of the coccyx, then trace on each side a sacrotuberous ligament between sacrum and tuberosity, next identify the ischial tuberosity, ischiopubic ramus, and finally, anteriorly, the posteroinferior aspect of the symphysis pubis. The outlet is usually described as diamond-shaped, which is a misleading description unless you appreciate that the diamond is bent in the middle to form two triangles, an anal triangle facing posteroinferiorly and a urogenital triangle facing anteroinferiorly. Last, with reference to the outlet, the angle between the ischiopubic rami is called the pubic angle, and the size of this angle gives a fair indication of the size of the pelvic outlet.

The Pelvic Cavity. Between the inlet and the outlet lies the pelvic cavity. Of the several significant facts which could be drawn to your attention, the curve or axis of the cavity (Fig. 34-3) is the one selected here, for the axis is fundamental to all obstetric procedures in the cavity. The axis is best mapped out on a radiograph, but you should also study it in an isolated pelvis. The axis indicates the pathway taken by the baby's head in a normal delivery, and in event of instrumental assistance being required in a difficult delivery, the axis of the pelvis must be kept clearly in mind.

Then, in observing the pelvic cavity, note the dominant position of each ischial spine at the middle of the cavity. Clearly, if the spines are large and project more medially than usual they can readily arrest the onward progress of the baby's head. Accordingly the interspinous diameter is significant.

The Pelvic Joints. An intact bony pelvis examined in the gross anatomy laboratory gives an impression of rigidity that does not really exist in the living and certainly does not occur in pregnant women. The sacroiliac joints, the symphysis pubis, and usually, but not always, the sacrococcygeal articulation, are mobile joints, although their mobility is limited. In the late stages of pregnancy, the pelvic joints become very mobile. This mobility of joints, which enhances the diameter not just of the inlet, but of the cavity and outlet as well, is well known to obstetricians. Thus the anatomy of the pelvic joints deserves your attention.

For review, read an account of the female pelvis as found in any reference book under the heading, Differences Between Male and Female Pelvis.

Exercise: To make more realistic the facts you have just read, pass a rubber ball approximately 9.5 cm. in diameter through the brim, cavity, and outlet. Observe how the ball, representing a baby's head:

(1) Engages at the brim

(2) Advances between the ischial spines

(3) Must pass posteriorly in order to negotiate the pubic angle. Note that the mobility of the sacrococcygeal joint allows the coccyx to be displaced. Thus the apex of the sacrum, which is immobile, becomes the significant posterior landmark of the outlet.

It must be made quite clear that this exercise is an oversimplification of the passage of a baby's head through the pelvis, and that the objective of the exercise is simply to illuminate the principal bony features of the birth canal.

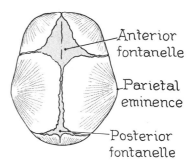

Figure 34-4. Superior view of an infant's skull at birth.

Furthermore, the exercise does not take into account the fact that the baby's skull is incompletely ossified (Fig. 34-4). The existence of membranous areas in the vault of the skull allows the skull to mold to the shape of the birth canal. Even so, there are times when the head is larger than the birth canal, a condition described as cephalopelvic disproportion. Establishment of the relationship of the baby's head to the birth canal is a fundamental step in the conduct of antenatal care and of labor.

Chapter 35

The External Genitalia

INTRODUCTION

The external genitalia occupy the urogenital triangle of the perineum. The perineum is the term applied to the skin and the subcutaneous and deeper structures between the symphysis pubis anteriorly and the coccyx posteriorly, a region bounded on each side by the thigh; it has been calculated that the skin of this confined region represents 1 per cent of the skin of the entire body, a very small percentage, maybe, but one that must be taken into account in the careful assessment of a patient who has been burned extensively.

The perineum is a cleft whose form depends on three factors: first, on whether or not the hip joints are stable, i.e., not dislocated; second, upon the position of lower limbs when the hip joints are stable; third, of less significance but nevertheless a factor, the bulk of the medial thigh muscles. If one or both femoral heads are dislocated from their sockets, then the perineum loses its cleftlike form and "broadening" of the perineum is said to occur, and is noticeable even when the feet are

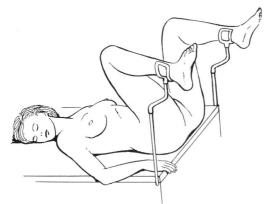

Figure 35-1. Lithotomy position. (From Dorland's Illustrated Medical Dictionary. 24th ed. Philadelphia. W. B. Saunders Co. 1965.)

together. Thus broadening of the perineum is a clue that the hips are dislocated. Last, severe muscle wasting of the adductor muscles, the bulky muscles of the medial thigh, causes an apparent widening of the perineum.

The cleftlike form of the perineum disappears entirely when the patient adopts the lithotomy position (Fig. 35-1). Then the cleft becomes shaped like a diamond. Nearly all operative procedures upon the perineum take place with the patient in the lithotomy position. From what has been said, it is clear that a patient with stiff hip joints may find adopting the lithotomy position impossible.

In the lithotomy position two triangular regions in the perineum may be identified, an anterior region facing inferoanteriorly, called the urogenital triangle, and a posterior region facing inferoposteriorly, called the anal triangle. In both sexes, the feature of the latter triangle is the orifice of the anal canal with, on each side of the orifice, a subcutaneous pad of fat wedged in the ischiorectal fossa.

FEMALE EXTERNAL GENITALIA

The superficial structures occupying the female urogenital triangle are known collectively as the vulva, which includes the labia majora, labia minora, mons pubis, clitoris, and vestibule of the vagina. Pudendum is another name that is sometimes used.

The presenting features of the vulva are the labia majora (singular, labium majus). The two labia merge anteriorly with the mons pubis, a cushion of fat anterior to the symphysis pubis. Posteriorly, the labia diminish in bulk to lose their identity. Within the shelter of the labia majora lie the labia minora (singular, labium minus). Anteriorly, the labia minora provide a frenulum and prepuce for the clitoris. Posteriorly, and this next fact is of obstetric significance, the posterior ends of the labia join to form a ridge called the fourchette, posterior to the vaginal orifice. When a fourchette is present, there lies within its shelter a shallow gutter called the vestibular fossa, sometimes also called the fossa navicularis. The fourchette and vestibular fossa diminish in size and depth, and finally disappear with successive childbirths. Their absence or presence, therefore, is a clue to a woman's parity (parity is a clinical term referring to the number of children a woman has brought forth).

The labia minora bound the vestibule of the vagina. The vestibule is the entire region within the labia minora and, therefore, includes the two orifices, namely the vagina and urethra. In addition, the minute orifices of Skene's glands and Bartholin's glands, bilateral structures, are found within the vestibule. Accordingly, it may be said there are six orifices in all within the vestibule of the vagina.

The position of the urethral orifice and the anatomy of the vaginal orifice will be stressed in the stages of dissection.

ITEM 35-1.   Inspection of the Female Perineum

Hold the specimen by the lower limbs to expose the perineum. Pull the limbs gently apart to expose as much of the perineum as possible, but do not separate the limbs widely or you will tear some tissues of the medial aspect of the thigh. Observe how the perineum may be divided into an anterior urogenital triangle and a posterior anal triangle. Identify the features of the anal triangle: the coccyx, ischial tuberosities, anal orifice, and the subcutaneous bilateral ischiorectal fossa.

Examine the vulva. Identify the mons pubis. Look for the presence or absence of hair, a secondary sex characteristic (in preparation of the cadaver, pubic hair may have been shaved).

Identify the labia majora and separate them and the labia minora to open the vestibule of the vagina (in the laying out of a corpse after death the perineal orifices are plugged, so the anatomy of the orifice may be badly distorted).

Identify the clitoris. Observe that it is bent so that its glans projects posteriorly. It remains in this position even when it is erect, i.e., distended with blood during sexual excitement. Thus, while it is true that the clitoris is the homologue of the penis, it is different in its response to sexual arousal.

In practical obstetrics and gynecology, identifying the urethral orifice is often a challenge to the tyro. Therefore, study your specimen carefully and observe precisely where the orifice lies. The orifice is indeed small and may be obscured by a slight pout of mucous membrane, but it is always anterior and initimately adjacent to the vaginal orifice. Normally, the urethral orifice is 2.5 cm. posterior to the clitoris. Before all obstetric and gynecologic procedures, it is necessary to have the patient's bladder empty; it may be necessary to catheterize the patient and, passing the catheter may well be your responsibility some day. Therefore, make sure you note the position of the external urethral orifice.

Examine the vaginal orifice. Rarely is a hymen present on a cadaver. The shape and size of this fold across the vaginal orifice varies and is usually well illustrated in gynecologic textbooks, to which you should refer. Small fragments of skin, carunculae hymenales, may be present to indicate where the hymen was originally attached. Is a fourchette present?

THE OBSTETRIC PERINEUM

In obstetrics and gynecology, the term perineum is applied more specifically to the skin and subcutaneous structures between the vaginal orifice anteriorly and the anal orifice posteriorly, a limited area of great practical moment. Measure its anteroposterior distance.

You were asked to measure because foreshortening of the perineum is an important condition the examining clinician must look for. If the obstetric perineum has disappeared entirely, in other words there is no skin distance between the vaginal and anal orifices, then it may be deduced that the woman is parous and that her perineum has been badly torn during childbirth. Furthermore, the deeper tissues, supporting her vagina, bladder, and rectum, may also have been badly stretched or torn. If this is so, then support for these organs may be inadequate. Normally the perineum measures approximately 4 cm.

Nerve Supply

When it becomes necessary for the obstetrician to lance the perineum to ease the birth of a child, a procedure called episiotomy, then the nerve supply of the obstetric perineum becomes all-important.

From two pairs of nerves, the bilateral labial and bilateral inferior hemorrhoidal nerves, sensory branches infiltrate the skin of the obstetric perineum. On each side the labial and hemorrhoidal nerves stem from the pudendal nerve posteromedial to the ischial spine. If a liquid anesthetic agent is injected to this region, sufficient agent will be adsorbed by the pudendal nerve to prevent the flow of sensory impulses from the obstetric perineum to the central nervous system to the level of consciousness. This procedure is spoken of clinically as a pudendal nerve block. Clinical observations of the results of pudendal block demonstrate that the anesthesia obtained is unpredictable, presumably because of anatomic variations of the nerve supply of the entire perineum.

Three further aspects refer more to the anatomic perineum, and they are the arterial supply, lymphatic drainage, and venous drainage.

The amount of erectile tissue in the perineum demands a profuse supply of arterial blood. Accordingly, the perineum is a highly vascular region. Injury to the perineum can produce extensive hemorrhage into the tissues and marked bruising.

Lymph from the perineum, including the anal and also the vaginal orifice, drains bilaterally into the superficial inguinal lymph nodes. Accordingly, if those nodes become swollen and tender, indicating an infection somewhere in their field of drainage, your examination must include the perineum as well as the skin of the lower limbs and the anterior abdominal wall.

Last, the venous plexus of the perineum is extensive and significant. Dilatation and even tortuosity of vulvar veins may be disabling as well as dangerous in pregnancy. Furthermore, in the male as well as in the female, the drainage of the anal orifice is mainly into the systemic venous system, thence to the inferior vena cava, and, to a lesser degree, through the superior rectal vein into the portal venous system, thence to the portal vein and liver, Accordingly, this dual arrangement at the anal orifice is referred to as an example of portacaval anastomosis. In the event of occlusion in the portal system, portal blood is diverted through the anastomosis into the systemic veins. A portal occlusion, however, which produces dilated veins at the anal orifice, is usually in the rectum, not in the far reaches of the portal venous system.

MALE EXTERNAL GENITALIA

ITEM 35-2.   Inspection of the Male Genitalia
Proceed according to the first paragraph of Item 35-1.

In the male, in the lithotomy position, the urogenital triangle is only fully exposed when the scrotum and its contents are displaced superiorly on to the pubic region. Deep to the skin of the male urogential triangle lie the three components of the penis, the central and solitary bulb and, on each side, a crus. The bulb and crura are palpable as softish longitudinal masses when the penis is flaccid and are more conspicuous when the penis is turgid. In an embalmed cadaver it is difficult to displace the scrotum.

Examine the scrotum. Observe the midline raphe that can be traced anteriorly from the center of the perineum on to the scrotum, and then on to the ventral surface of the penis. The raphe indicates the line of fusion of the genital swellings, paired embryologic structures that remain apart in the female to become the labia majora.

Note that there are usually two testes, but sometimes only one is in the scrotum. If there is only one testis in the scrotum the other is present elsewhere as an undescended or ectopic testis, or it may have been removed surgically.

Reidentify the spermatic cord, which you exposed when you dissected the inguinal canal. The cord is a subcutaneous structure, and, in the living, is easily palpable.

In a cadaver, examination of the external aspect of the penis is not satisfactory and is best left until you attend a urology clinic. At this present time, however, it is worth emphasizing that examination of the external aspect of the penis is not complete until the prepuce, commonly called the foreskin, is retracted to expose the glans, the expanded end of the penis.

ITEM 35-3. Quite often male cadavers possess a prepuce. In other words, they have not been circumcised. If this is so with your cadaver make a longitudinal slit in the dorsum of the prepuce to mobilize it. Retract the prepuce and observe the frenulum connecting the prepuce to the glans. Examination of the glans is an essential procedure in the management of males with venereal disease. Finally it must be noted that the prepuce is very vascular. Thus hemorrhage is a real hazard in the operation of circumcision.

An Explanation of Terminology

Descriptions of the penis relate to its position when it is erect. Then it projects superiorly and anteriorly from below the symphysis pubis. Accordingly, the penis obtains a dorsal and a ventral surface. The ventral surface is readily distinguishable by the presence of the penile raphe.

The general comments on arterial supply, lymph drainage, and venous drainage of the female perineum apply also to the male.

Chapter 36

Hemisection of the Female Pelvis and Perineum

The first step is to section what is left of the vertebral column. Using an autopsy saw with a broad blade, cut in the median sagittal plane any spinous processes still intact, and then the vertebral bodies to the level of the promontory. Complete the split with the aid of a hand saw. The second step is division of the pelvis in the following order.

ITEM 36-1. Peel peritoneum off the anterior abdominal wall to open the retropubic space. Use a finger to dissect and explore the extent of the space between the bladder and the anterior half of the bony pelvis and related structures.

THE RETROPUBIC SPACE

This space is noteworthy in the female because it allows the gynecologist to reach the bladder and the urethra without entering the peritoneal cavity. He uses the space in the surgical treatment of stress incontinence. Stress is a term freely used and freely interpreted today, but in this condition it specifies the unavoidable expulsion of urine in acts such as coughing, sneezing, and sometimes laughing. This distressing problem is usually the consequence of childbearing; its surgical treatment will be discussed by your clinical teachers of obstetrics and gynecology.

Extravasation of urine into the retropubic space through a rupture of the anterolateral aspects of the bladder occurs in the female, but it is uncommon (see male pelvis, p. 168).

ITEM 36-2. In the midline, incise the mons pubis down to bone. Extend the incision on to the anatomic perineum, proceeding through the clitoris to within 1 cm. of the urethral orifice.

ITEM 36-3. With the aid of a curved instrument, slip a gigli saw (Fig. 56-1) inferior to the symphysis pubis. Saw through the symphysis.

ITEM 36-4. Divide the bladder strictly anteroposteriorly in the midline. To open the bladder of a cadaver, select a point on the superior surface central to the root of the urachus and the two ureterovesical junctions. Stick the closed points of straight scissors millimeter by millimeter through the bladder wall until the cavity of the bladder is reached. Before withdrawing the scissors, open them and keep them open as you withdraw. The cavity becomes more obvious. It is worth emphasizing that the solid chunk of flesh, the usual form of the cadaveric bladder, bears not the slightest resemblance to the delicate texture of the bladder alive.

ITEM 36-5. Identify the urethra. Determine its lumen. Divide it.

ITEM 36-6. Identify the anterior vaginal wall. Divide it in the midline.

ITEM 36-7. Divide the body of the uterus.

ITEM 36-8. Turn now to a division of the sacrum. Run a sharp knife blade through the supraspinous ligament of the lumbar and sacral vertebrae. This procedure allows the saw blade direct contact with bone. Using a strong carpenter's saw, saw through the middle of the vertebrae and sacrum. Take into account the curve of the sacrum. Avoid ripping adjacent soft tissues.

FRACTURES OF THE PELVIS

Now that the symphysis pubis and the sacrum have been split, you have a practical demonstration of the dangers of extensive fractures of the pelvis. The soft tissues are in peril when the pelvis is fractured in two places, especially if the fractures are diametrically opposite each other; the soft tissues cannot withstand the shearing forces that exist at the line of bony separation. What organs may be torn in pelvic fractures and fracture-dislocations involving either the sacroiliac joints or the symphysis pubis? In all fractures of the pelvis, damage to the soft parts must be suspected until the truth is established.

ITEM 36-9.   Return to the perineum. In extending the incision you have already made there, stay strictly in the midline. Proceed to incise the perineum between the vagina and the anal orifice.

ITEM 36-10.   Divide the rectum and anal canal in the midline.

ITEM 36-11.   The final midline cut is essentially through the superior end of the vagina. If this final cut is to one side of the midline it should be possible to expose almost the entire vaginal part of the cervix uteri, leaving the external os intact (Fig. 37-1).

ITEM 36-12.   The pelvis is now in two halves. If not, seek help fron an instructor. At a deep sink, not a washbasin, flush away feces and debris from your specimens.

Chapter 37

The Peritoneum of the Female Pelvis

Review the anatomy of the peritoneum in three locations: (1) lateral, (2) intermediate, and (3) median. Deal with (2) first and examine the broad ligament.

THE BROAD LIGAMENTS

These ligaments are earmarked for comment not to emphasize but to diminish their importance, for it is all too easy to fancy that they support the uterus. That the word ligament is used in a special sense to describe peritoneal folds which may or may not have a supportive role should be clear to a student who has already explored the peritoneal cavity.

In life the broad ligaments are soft, pliant, and easily distorted; inferiorly the two leaves of each ligament are readily separated. Therefore it would be more appropriate and would cause less confusion to describe each ligament simply as a fold of peritoneum between the uterus and the sidewall of the pelvis, a uteropelvic fold, for that is precisely what it is. Furthermore, the broad ligaments are not stationary but adjust themselves to the position of the uterus and the degree of distention of the urinary bladder.

ITEM 37-1. Examine the broad ligament. Note how its form is determined entirely by the shape and position of the uterine tube and related blood vessels. Thus the configuration of the free edge of each broad ligament is determined primarily by the uterine tube and ovarian vessels in much the same way as the free edge of the lesser omentum is determined by underlying structures.

Pull the fundus of the uterus posteriorly and then anteriorly to show that the orientation of the ventral and dorsal surfaces of each ligament is dependent upon whether the uterus is retroverted or anteverted.

ITEM 37-2. Next examine the round ligament and the ligament of the ovary. Both of them are found in the uteropelvic fold (the broad ligament) and are rightly termed ligaments.

You have already identified the round ligament at the deep inguinal ring. Without disturbing peritoneum, trace the round ligament, which lies deep to the ventral leaf of the broad ligament, to its termination at the anterior surface of the cornu of the uterus, close to where the uterine tube joins the uterus. Note that the round ligament is quite a substantial cord composed of muscle fibers, some connective tissue, small vessels, and lymphatics.

ITEM 37-3. Deep to the dorsal leaf of the broad ligament, identify the ligament of the ovary, where it begins on the posterior surface of the cornu of the uterus and trace it to the ovary. This ligament, too, contains muscle fibers and some connective tissue.

Thus in tracing these two ligaments you have in fact established the continuity of a cord of tissue from the labium majus to the ovary, although the continuity is interrupted where the cord fuses with the uterus. The entire cord is the homologue of the gubernaculum testis, believed to be responsible for guiding the testis into the scrotum.

Reconsider the substantial form of the ligament of the ovary, truly a suspensory ligament, in contrast to the so-called suspensory ligament, the infundibulopelvic ligament, which has *no* suspensory role and is merely another peritoneal fold. The ligament of the ovary hitches the ovary to the uterus. Accordingly, one factor governing the position of the ovaries is the position of the uterus.

ITEM 37-4. Now review peritoneum in the lateral location on the sidewall of the pelvis. Identify the ovary, the fimbriae of the uterine tube, and the abdominal ostium, obscured from view by the fimbriae.

ITEM 37-5. Examine the surface of the ovary; it is composed of cuboidal epithelium, in contrast to the squamous epithelium of the peritoneum. Accordingly, there is a debate which can never be resolved, namely, is the ovary intra- or extraperitoneal. Suffice it to say that it is through the ovarian surface you are now examining that an ovum is shed; the forces that guide the ovum through the abdominal ostium into the uterine tube are dimly understood.

Furthermore, because of the continuity of the reproductive tract, it is indeed possible for infection ascending from the vaginal orifice on the perineum eventually to pass through the abdominal ostium to infect the peritoneal cavity.

ITEM 37-6. By maneuvering the uterine tube and the ovarian vessels in their relationship to peritoneum, create a tent of peritoneum between the sidewall of the pelvis and the infundibulum, the lateral part of the uterine tube. To name this elevation the *infundibulopelvic ligament* is to give it undue emphasis as a ligament, but it is, nevertheless, important surgically because it encloses the ovarian vessels and lymphatics.

ITEM 37-7. The importance of the ovarian fossa is also likely to be misconceived. The fossa is that small area of peritoneum anterior to the bifurcation of the common iliac vessels and to which the ovary is related quite often. The fossa is significant not because of its shape, but because of the close proximity posteriorly of the ureter, adherent to and almost embedded in peritoneum. Thus in surgical removal of an adherent ovary from the location just described, the ureter is in peril. Pull the ureter and confirm its relationship to the fossa.

Three particularly significant parts of the peritoneum lie in the midline, the pouch of Douglas, the uterovesical pouch, and the retropubic space.

ITEM 37-8. Observe the relationship of the pouch of Douglas (the rectovaginal recess) (Fig. 37-1) to the vagina, a very special relationship indeed, but do nothing more than observe, because there are particular features of the vagina to be observed at a later stage of dissection.

THE POUCH OF DOUGLAS (FIG. 37-1)

The broad ligaments and the uterus form a septum across the pelvis and thereby create anterior and posterior compartments. On balance, the posterior compartment is more significant, not only because it is surrounded by more organs than the anterior compartment, but also because it extends inferiorly between the rectum and vagina to form the

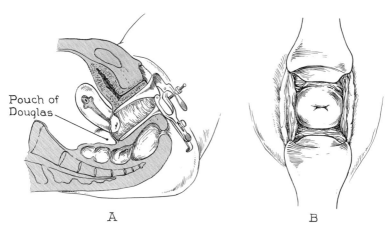

Pouch of
Douglas

A   B

Figure 37-1.   Examination of the vaginal aspect of the cervix uteri. *A* shows a vaginal speculum separating the walls of the vagina. *B* shows a view of the cervix from the vagina with retractors in place.

pouch of Douglas. Observe on your specimen how blood, pus, or contents from viscera of the posterior compartment can gravitate into the pouch.

The pouch is accessible per vaginam as well as per rectum. From what has just been said, it is clear that clinical evidence of fluid in the pouch of Douglas demands a review of widely separate structures, ranging from the rectum and sigmoid to the cecum and appendix, and including the uterine tube and ovary of each side. The pouch of Douglas is indeed the hub of the posterior compartment of the pelvic peritoneum.

ITEM 37-9.   Observe how peritoneum is loosely applied to the superior surface of the bladder and is densely adherent to the body of the uterus. Then observe especially how the peritoneum bridges the space between the two organs and forms the uterovesical pouch. Beneath the pouch loose connective tissue occupies a wedge-shaped interval. Through this interval, after he has incised the uterovesical peritoneum, the obstetrician reaches the lower uterine segment for one method of cesarean section.

ITEM 37-10.   Review the anatomy of the retropubic space (p. 168).

Chapter 38

Rectum and Anal Canal

For practical anatomic reasons, the description of the large bowel was temporarily interrupted at the rectosigmoid junction (p. 118). To refresh your memory, reread the section on the large bowel.

Although the rectum is distinct anatomically from the anal canal and is, therefore, usually described separately, such a clear distinction cannot be made in clinical diagnosis because the applied anatomy of the two structures is so intimately related. Accordingly, the rectum and anal canal are considered together under the headings position, form, peritoneum, mucosa, and musculature. Relations of the rectum and anal canal are dealt with later after they have been exposed. Digital examination per rectum, a basic clinical procedure, will then be reviewed.

ITEM 38-1. Position

Observe the relationship of the rectosigmoid junction to the sacral promontory. Identification of the junction was discussed on p. 114. The flexure of the rectosigmoid junction and the promontory are both significant in sigmoidoscopy (p. 210).

Observe how the rectum, below the rectosigmoid junction, lies clasped to the curve of the sacrum and coccyx. The sweep of the curve continues anteroinferiorly until the rectum reaches the anorectal junction. Pay close attention to the angulation of this junction. From it the anal canal proceeds posteroinferiorly to the anal orifice, the anus, between the ischial tuberosities. Note that it is to the lower sacrum and coccyx that the rectum is related. Thus the rectum lies low in the pelvis. The distance of skin between tip of coccyx and the posterior margin of the anal orifice is usually overlooked. Once observed, however, that distance emphasizes the low and forward position of the anal canal between the ischial tuberosities.

ITEM 38-2. Form

The rectum has a lumen larger than the sigmoid colon and, in addition, a much more obvious dilatation called the ampulla, found just internal to the anorectal junction. The exact position of the ampulla is particularly significant in obstetrics. Review a sagittal section of a normal female pelvis to see how the anterior wall of the ampulla bulges forward (Fig. 37-1) to lie as a superior relation of the obstetric perineum and perineal body. Indeed, it is recognized that the rectum, when empty, is a blind-ended tube from the side of which the anal canal arises. From your specimen you can easily see how, during vaginal delivery, the baby's head pushes the tissues, including the ampulla, toward the perineum. Thus, the anterior wall of the ampulla of the rectum is in peril when an episiotomy (p. 198) is bungled.

The walls of the rectum are in apposition except when feces or gas is present. The anal canal is straight and its walls are in apposition also, except during defecation.

ITEM 38-3. Peritoneum and Rectum

By maneuvering the rectum firmly but with care, observe its relationship to the peritoneum. Observe: first, immediately distal to the rectosigmoid junction, the rectum is covered by peritoneum anteriorly and on each side, but it is not covered by peritoneum posteriorly. Compare the peritoneal covering of the rectum to that of the sigmoid. Second, the intermediate part of the rectum is covered only on its anterior surface by peritoneum. In the male, the peritoneum here passes onto the bladder and creates the rectovesical pouch. In the female, peritoneum passes onto the upper third of the vagina and then superiorly onto the uterus. The pouch so formed is the rectovaginal pouch, the pouch of Douglas (Fig. 37-1). Third, both the ampulla of the rectum and the anal canal are devoid of peritoneum.

ITEM 38-4. Mucosa

In life, the rectal mucosa is red in color, not brown as seen in the embalmed cadaver. Furthermore, embalming stiffens rectal mucosa and, as a result, the anatomy student does not recognize that the mucosa is normally loosely attached. Peel off the mucosa from a small area of rectum — it is about 1 mm. thick — and expose the underlying loosely woven tissue, the submucosa. You may expose a thin, delicate but definite layer of longitudinal muscle fibers termed the lamina muscularis mucosae; translated, this means layer of muscle of the mucosa; the Latin name is usually abbreviated to muscularis mucosae.

Projecting inward from the lateral walls of the rectum are several flangelike folds, placed alternately on the right and left sides of the rectum. In the substance of each fold there is a core of muscle derived from the muscular coat of the bowel. The folds are felt or seen on clinical examination of the rectum, but they are not usually evident in the embalmed cadaver.

To establish the landmarks of the mucosa of the anal canal it is advisable to begin externally with the perianal skin possessing the usual skin appendages, namely hairs, hair follicles, and sebaceous and sweat glands.

Internal to the perianal skin is an easily recognized smooth zone devoid of skin appendages. This zone is the pecten, so-called because of the shape of its superior boundary, the pectinate line (pecten — Latin for comb). The anal valves, soon to be demonstrated more carefully, are attached at the pectinate line. Inferiorly, the junction of the pecten and the perianal skin is referred to as the anal verge. Although the pecten is only a narrow strip, 1 cm. deep, it is a significant landmark in surgical procedures because it is firmly attached to the underlying tissue. Furthermore, its stratified squamous epithelium may give rise to a form of cancer.

ITEM 38-5. The anal valves are not well seen in the cadaver. An anal valve is a very small flap measuring not more than 3 mm. across. To find one fairly easily, identify two anal columns (*Grant's Atlas of Anatomy*, Fig. 203), and slide the tip of a probe between them into an anal sinus; probing toward the anal orifice, and entering an anal crypt you will elevate a very small flap, semilunar in shape, between the bases of the columns—that flap is an anal valve. In many instances, valves are so poorly formed that this exercise is unsuccessful.

ITEM 38-6. In an anal column, blood vessels are present and the veins are of great importance. Therefore, on a well-formed anal column, gently incise the mucosa, separate the edges of the incision, disperse the submucosa, and thus expose a hemorrhoidal vein in the substance of the column.

CLINICAL ANATOMY OF THE RECTAL AND ANAL MUCOSA

In the living, the rectal mucosa may become so loose that it can slide through the anal canal to appear at the anal orifice, a clinical condition described as partial, or mucosal, prolapse of the rectum. (The term complete rectal prolapse is applied when the entire thickness of the rectal wall appears through the anal orifice.) The seriousness of these conditions requires no emphasis.

The passing of a hard mass of feces (the mass is often referred to as a scybalum or as a scybalous mass) can split the mucosa and sometimes tear an anal valve to produce an anal mucosal fissure, a common enough condition, both irritating and painful.

Hemorrhoids

The veins of the anal columns may become dilated and somewhat tortuous. The mechanisms leading to such varicosity are not clear enough to be discussed. One point, however, is beyond argument. Distended veins at the anal orifice may be the outcome of a venous obstruction in the rectal wall. Accordingly, examination of a patient with distended veins at the anus is not complete until the lower bowel has been inspected.

Internal Hemorrhoids. Clinically, distended veins in the anal canal are called internal hemorrhoids, from a Greek word meaning discharging blood. Hemorrhoids are also called piles, from a Latin word meaning ball. When the anal canal is viewed with the patient in the lithotomy position (Fig. 35-1) and internal hemorrhoids of moderate severity are present, they can be distinguished at the 4, 7, and 11 o'clock positions, a disposition that corresponds essentially to the larger primary terminal tributaries of the superior rectal vein. In a more extensive form of hemorrhoids, additional varicosities occur intermediate to the 4, 7, and 11 o'clock positions and are said to correspond to the smaller secondary terminal venous tributaries of the superior rectal vein. Hence, on anatomic grounds, hemorrhoids are described as primary if they occur in primary tributaries of the superior rectal vein; the term secondary is applied to those hemorrhoids occurring in secondary tributaries. Often the distinction is not easy to make. With reference to internal hemorrhoids, there are degrees of severity recognized clinically, a topic to be discussed later by your clinical tutors.

External Hemorrhoids. Hemorrhoids that lie external to the anal canal are, therefore, subcutaneous. In other words, they are covered by skin, whereas internal hemorrhoids are submucosal. When external hemorrhoids are present, as for instance in pregnancy, they are spoken of as perianal varices.

Knowledge of the nerve supply of the anal canal is important in the injection therapy of internal hemorrhoids. External hemorrhoids are never treated by injection, for the following reason. Somatic sensory cutaneous nerves, which respond immediately to painful stimuli such as the prick of a needle, extend into the canal as far as the pectinate line and slightly beyond onto the bases of the anal columns. Thus an injection of a hemorrhoidal vein must be above the pectinate line, where the mucosa is relatively insensitive to lancination.

ITEM 38-7. Musculature of Rectum and Anal Canal

Observe how thin the wall of the rectum is. Measure its thickness. In life it is soft and delicate, almost diaphanous. Delay in the diagnosis of rectal cancer gives the growth not only time to invade the thin wall of the rectum but time also to obliterate the surrounding planes of cleavage upon which successful operative removal of the rectum depends. Here indeed is stark evidence that early diagnosis of rectal cancer is imperative. Fortunately, a rectal cancer is slow to grow.

Within the wall, longitudinal and circular layers of muscle are present. Identify the circular layer, which is the inner layer, and trace it toward the anal canal where the muscle fibers increase in number to form the easily identified internal sphincter. Observe that the lower border of the sphincter is well defined and is level with the anal verge, the lower border of the pecten.

Next trace the longitudinal layer, which is the outer layer of muscle, from the rectum to the anal canal and trace it into the interval between the internal sphincter and the external sphincter.

ITEM 38-8. Identify the external sphincter. Note that the sphincters are named with reference to the lumen of the anal canal and not to the skin surface. Thus, the external sphincter surrounds the internal one. You will observe, no doubt, that the lowermost margin of the external sphincter protrudes beyond the lowermost margin of the internal. However, during relaxation of the anal canal, as for example in defecation or under general anesthesia, the internal sphincter protrudes beyond the external sphincter. The two sphincters have been likened to two tubes, one within the other; as two such tubes can slide up and down in relation to each other so do the two anal sphincters. Thus, a concept of a rigid relationship of internal to external anal sphincter is quite erroneous.

Conjoining the musculature of the anal canal are parts of the levator ani muscles; the levator ani is a bilateral structure slung from the sidewall of the pelvis. If you leave the study of this pair of muscles until the dissection has advanced further (p. 226) you will find their anatomy easy to understand.

Review

Review the anatomy of the anal canal with special emphasis upon the levels of change. All the while, remember that the anal canal is only 4 cm. long, the length of half a finger. Thus your eyes must be sharp and your observations precise.

Read an account of the lymphatic drainage of the rectum and anal canal.

SIGMOIDOSCOPY

The internal surface, namely the mucosa, of the lower sigmoid, the rectum, and anal canal can be seen with the aid of an instrument called a sigmoidoscope. The basic anatomic facts for this important clinical procedure can be seen at a glance. Your specimen shows how first the tip of the instrument must first be advanced in an anterosuperior direction for 4 to 5 cm. to negotiate the anal canal. Then the direction of advance must change to posterosuperior to follow the curve of the sacrum. Observe again that the angle of anorectal junction is nearly 90°. While the tip of the instrument advances through the rectum, the tip must be manipulated past rectal folds. At 10 to 12 cm. from the pectinate line the tip will reach the rectosigmoid junction, where further manipulation will be necessary. To get the scope through the flexure into the sigmoid and beyond for another 10 to 12 cm. the tip must be maneuvered forward and to the left. From the pectinate line, approximately 20 cm. of bowel can be examined. And it is in this length of bowel that the majority of tumors of the large bowel occur.

If you are dissecting a male pelvis proceed to p. 223 to study the lower urinary tract.

Chapter 39

The Vagina

Review the vagina in the following order: the lumen, the urethrovesical angle, the position of the vault, rugae, shape of the vagina in cross section, epithelium, pH of vaginal fluid, fornices, relationships, vascularity, and clinical examination.

If you have left the vagina undisturbed since you made the mid-sagittal section, its walls should be in apposition. Normally the vagina is closed, a fact that is never made clear in illustrations. The lumen of the vagina is potential and is demonstrated only when the vagina is distended (Fig. 37-1). This may be during intercourse, labor, or clinical and surgical procedures: the vagina can retain up to 300 cc. of blood clot. The size of the head of a newborn baby shows how much distention can occur.

The vagina is not straight. Its anterior wall is bent and its long axis is convex forward. Every sagittal section of a female pelvis shows this to some extent, yet it has escaped the eye of many illustrators. Examine your specimen with a critical eye and you will observe that inferiorly the vagina lies parallel to the urethra whereas superiorly it lies parallel to the base of the bladder. In the living, it is while the bladder is continent that the angle at the urethrovesical junction is conspicuous. During the act of micturition the angle is almost completely straightened as the bladder neck descends.

ITEM 39-1. To relate the vagina to the bony pelvis of your specimen place a 12 inch ruler or rod between the superior border of the symphysis pubis and the tip of the coccyx. Note that the vault of the vagina is level with the rod. Reexamine Figure 34-1 to confirm that the ischial spines are at the same level. In fact, the vault of the vagina is midway between the spines. Thus, in life it is possible to palpate each ischial spine from the vagina.

ITEM 39-2.   Separate the walls of the vagina. If the women was of child-bearing age and had not delivered many offspring per vaginam in her lifetime, obvious horizontal folds, called rugae, will be present. If she was well past the menopause, however, and most female cadavers are, rugae will have disappeared and, therefore, the vaginal walls will be smooth as well as thin. If this is so, do not assume that such senile changes are unimportant. The changes that occur in the vagina after the menopause often lead to distressing conditions requiring consultation and therapy. It is worth noting that changes of this nature are commonly classified as postmenopausal or senile.

ITEM 39-3.   Separate the walls of the vagina even more to establish the anterior and posterior extensions present at the lateral edge of the lumen of the vagina. The extensions are best seen on cross section. They will probably not be obvious if your cadaver was multiparous and postmenopausal.

THE CLOSED VAGINA

To emphasize that the vagina is not a straight open tube, a summary of the anatomy of the closed vagina is given: The vestibule is concealed by the labia lying side by side. The H-shaped formation of the vagina and the existence of rugae not only make distention of the vagina easy, but also ensure that at other times the walls are closely apposed. Furthermore, contraction of the muscular pelvic diaphragm increases the convexity of the vagina and thus creates a dynamic barrier. It is relaxation of the pelvic diaphragm that allows the vagina to straighten for penetration as, for example, during intercourse. In that instance, it is clear why this structure was named vagina, which means sheath.

THE VAGINAL EPITHELIUM

It is all too easy to imagine the vaginal epithelium as changeless and to ignore the profound influence hormones have upon the epithelium, not only across the years but also, to some extent, throughout each menstrual cycle. Certainly it is not within the scope of this text to elaborate this comment except to describe the epithelium briefly as follows.

The epithelium is squamous and stratified. Under the influence of estrogen, the epithelium becomes thick and pliant and each cell obtains a high glycogen content. Until puberty, and after the menopause, the epithelium is thin, unyielding, and low in glycogen.

In view of the apparent similarity to skin, it is worth emphasizing here that vaginal epithelium lacks skin appendages; it has no glands.

Under the influence of estrogen, the vaginal epithelial cells themselves secrete a sufficient quantity of fluid rich in glycogen to keep the surface moist.

ᴘH OF THE VAGINA

The pH of the film of fluid that coats the vaginal epithelium is acid, but is regulated by the level of estrogen. Thus the pH is related to the woman's age; more specific factors are, for example, the menstrual cycle, pregnancy, and lactation.

Vaginal acidity is due to the presence of lactic acid. The acid is a breakdown product of the activity of specific bacilli (Döderlein's bacilli) upon the glycogen produced by epithelial cells. The bacilli are an essential link in the regulation of vaginal pH — here, indeed, is an excellent example of symbiosis.

In practice, the pH of the vagina is significant not only for the protection of the vagina against foreign organisms but also in conception. Seminal fluid is normally alkaline and the mucus secreted by the glands of the cervix is also alkaline. During sexual stimulation the cervix increases its rate of secretion, thus raising the pH to an optimal level for the survival of sperm.

ITEM 39-4. The Fornices of the Vagina

Examine the vault of the vagina more carefully and observe how the cervix of the uterus projects into the anterior aspect of the vault (Fig. 37-1). Observe that there is no dramatic change in passing from vagina to cervix, but that the epithelium covering the vaginal surface of the cervix is continuous with and identical to that of the vagina.

The recess between cervix and vagina is termed a fornix, a term that means arch. Observe that the fornix varies in depth and that it is circumferential to the cervix. The fornix is divided, for descriptive purposes only, into posterior, anterior, and lateral fornices. Although these are merely positional terms, their anatomic relationships are highly significant, as you will see.

ITEM 39-5. The Posterior Fornix

What is its most significant immediate posterior relationship? Observe that when the body is recumbent (Fig. 37-1) the posterior fornix is the most dependent part of the vaginal canal and can serve as a receptacle for semen. Semen thus forms a pool into which the cervix dips.

ITEM 39-6. The Anterior Fornix

This fornix is shallow and practically nonexistent. What is the depth of this fornix in your specimen? What is its principal anterior relationship?

ITEM 39-7. The Lateral Fornix

In the later stages of dissection the proximity of both the ureter and the uterine artery to this fornix will become obvious. Meanwhile, press the tip of a finger laterally from the lateral fornix and appreciate the proximity of these important structures.

ITEM 39-8.   Relationships of the Vagina

The relationships of the vagina are few but important. First examine the posterior relationships. From superior to inferior, they are the pouch of Douglas and then the ampulla of the rectum. Between the rectum and the vagina there exists a plane of cleavage of surgical import. Finally, inferiorly, the perineal body is a posterior relation of the vestibule of the vagina.

Anteriorly, note how the urethra is contiguous to the lower third of the anterior vaginal wall. The base of the bladder is related to the middle third with a plane of cleavage between. Superior to the base of the bladder the cervix penetrates the vaginal wall.

The lateral relationships are soon to be uncovered. They are the ureters and uterine arteries as well as the pelvic fascia and levatores ani. In addition, a meshwork of autonomic nerves, an offshoot of the pelvic autonomic supply frequently referred to as Frankenhäuser's plexus, lies in the fascia lateral to the vault of the vagina. Finally, lymph vessels, microscopic and inconspicuous when all is well, travel from the upper part of the vagina to lymph nodes located along the course of both uterine arteries, and thence to adjacent nodes along the internal and external iliac arteries and the obturator artery of both sides.

The vagina is a very vascular organ and there is an extensive anastomosis of the vessels reaching the vagina from above with the vessels arriving from below. The small veins and arteries in the wall of the vagina are not evident in an anatomic specimen, but they do become evident in a clinical emergency when the vagina is bruised or torn. That the vagina is a vascular structure must be emphasized.

The vagina is examined clinically with the aid of a vaginal speculum (Fig. 37-1). From your observations so far and the diagram (Fig. 37-1), you may readily appreciate how simple it is, under the proper circumstances, to examine this part and to carry out such important procedures as cytologic tests for malignancy.

Chapter 40

The Uterus

What the clinical student really needs to know about the uterus can scarcely be acquired from the specimens he is likely to see in the dissecting laboratory. There the chances are great that the female cadavers were long past the menopause at the time of death, whereas the majority of his female patients of the future will be menstruant. Therefore, knowledge of the functional uterus is of prime importance. That this textbook cannot do justice to the function of the uterus is obvious and there has been no attempt to do so. This statement only is made: The student must realize that the size, shape, and consistency of the uterus depend entirely upon age, sexual development, the menstrual cycle, and pregnancy. The position of the uterus depends upon the fullness of the bladder and the position and load of the pelvic colon. Congenital malformations, which are rare, should nevertheless be kept in mind.

The inactive, shrunken, narrow uterus of old age is vastly different from the functioning, plump, pear-shaped uterus of a woman in her prime. The student will learn the more profound physiologic facts about the uterus at the appropriate time. However, since many of his future patients will be beyond the menopause, examination of an atrophic uterus in the gross anatomy laboratory is definitely worthwhile.

ITEM 40-1. Identify the following two major subdivisions of the uterus, corpus uteri and cervix. The uterus of the nulliparous young woman is bent at the junction of the corpus uteri and the cervix so that the ventral surface of the uterus is concave. This angular shape of the uterus is spoken of as anteflexion. Is the uterus of your specimen anteflexed? Anteflexion is not usually present after the first pregnancy.

Anteflexion has to be distinguished from anteversion. The former refers to shape, the latter to position. When the uterus as a whole is directed toward the symphysis pubis the uterus is anteverted; directed toward the sacrum the uterus is retroverted. Is the uterus of your specimen ante- or retroverted?

ITEM 40-2. Examine the cervix. Observe the part external to the vagina (portio supravaginalis) and the part in the vagina (portio vaginalis). The cervix is almost a perfect cylinder in shape, in contrast to the corpus uteri, which has distinct dorsal and ventral surfaces. But the junction of cervix and corpus is not nearly so clearly defined in the uterus of the elderly as it is in the young.

215

THE ISTHMUS UTERI

At the junction of the cervix and corpus uteri there is a special part called the isthmus. The isthmus is not readily visible on gross inspection of the nonpregnant uterus for then the isthmus is scarcely 1 cm. deep. It is generally visible on examination of a longitudinal section of the uterus, between the anatomic internal os and the histologic internal os. There is, however, no sustained agreement upon the exact definition of the isthmus of the nonpregnant uterus. The reason your attention is drawn to the isthmus is as follows:

It is believed that the isthmus is destined to become the lower uterine segment of the pregnant uterus near term. The segment is 5 to 7 cm. deep, on average, and is quite thin. To understand how the cervix thins and how the isthmus expands requires a depth of knowledge of pregnancy. It is sufficient, therefore, for the time being, simply to know the terms isthmus and lower uterine segment. It is through that segment that one method of cesarean birth is performed.

ITEM 40-3. Examine the canal of the cervix and the cavity of the corpus uteri. The cervical canal is normally occupied by mucus secreted by cervical glands. The character and quality of the mucus is determined by the hormones estrogen and progestogen. Under the influence of the former, the mucus is watery, profuse, and crystal clear. With the additional influence of progestogen, the mucus becomes thick, tenacious, and opalescent.

The cavity of the corpus uteri is triangular in shape, and the anterior and posterior walls are apposed. The length of the canal of the cervix and of the cavity of the corpus together measure 6 to 7 cm. in the adult; the cervical canal usually accounts for one-fourth to one-third of this measurement. In childhood, however, the cervical canal is twice as long as the cavity of the corpus.

The average measurement for canal and cavity must be borne in mind in a clinical procedure termed dilation and curettage. The canal is first dilated, then the womb is scraped with a curette (*curette*—scraper, Fr.) to remove the endometrium of the corpus uteri for diagnostic or therapeutic purposes. Measure the length of canal and cavity of your specimen.

ITEM 40-4. Examine the portio vaginalis of the cervix.

EXAMINATION OF THE CERVIX

Doctors assume such immense responsibility in the prevention of cancer of the cervix uteri that this structure requires more than a cursory glance. The vaginal portion of the cervix is accessible per vaginam (Fig. 37-1 *A*) for gross inspection, cytologic examination of its surface cells, and biopsy of its substance. By means of regular inspection of the cervix and periodic cytologic examination using the Papanicolaou technique, malignant change can be detected in the squamous epithelium of the cervix before the malignancy breaks through the basement membrane. Such a degree of early malignancy is termed carcinoma in situ.

To teach you the technique of examining a cervix uteri is a clinician's responsibility. Meanwhile, study carefully where the cervix lies, how it lies in relation to the vagina, and the appearance of the external os. Is the appearance that of the external os of a nulliparous or a multiparous woman? Consult a textbook to learn the difference.

The fundus uteri is a landmark frequently referred to. It is the eminence between the cornua and above the level of uterine tubes.

The supports of the uterus are described on p. 221. The uterine artery is exposed in the dissection outlined on p. 222. Bimanual examination of the uterus is described on p. 190. Read an account of the lymphatic drainage of the uterus.

Chapter 41

The Uterine Tubes

The uterine tubes and the uterus develop from the same embryologic structure, so it is not surprising that they function in similar ways. Indeed, under certain circumstances, nidation (i.e., embedding) of a fertilized ovum occurs in the tube, a condition described as a tubal pregnancy. Unlike the uterus, however, the tube does not have the capacity to carry a pregnancy beyond the early weeks.

The prime function of both the tubes and the uterus is the nourishment of a fertilized ovum, for which they are provided with a highly specialized lining. The lining of the tubes is also designed to allow viable sperm to reach the fimbriated end of the tube, where fertilization of an ovum usually occurs. Why successful fertilization occurs there and not in the uterus puzzles the mind until one recalls that the prime function of the tube is nourishment of a fertilized ovum up to a certain stage of development. In addition to nourishment, however, modern research has revealed that there are factors, as yet unknown, that contribute to the cell division of the fertilized ovum beyond a certain stage. Thus the several days required by a fertilized ovum to move from the fimbriated end of the uterine tube to the uterine cavity are vital.

On the basis of what has just been said, there can be no doubt that both uterine tubes are integral parts of the reproductive tract. Fertilization of an ovum cannot occur when both uterine tubes are blocked, for blockage prevents ascent of the sperm to the fimbriated end of the tube, where optimal conditions for fertilization exist. Furthermore, the further development of a fertilized ovum will cease if the nourishment in the tube is inadequate. It is emphasized that the major causes of infertility in women are related to the uterine tubes.

Ligation of both uterine tubes is one method of birth control. An ovum, shed after ligation, dies in the peritoneal cavity or in the fimbriated end of the tube and is then disposed of by phagocytosis (phagocytosis is the ingestion and digestion of substances by certain cells of the body). Sperm are disposed of in like manner.

There are various methods of testing the patency of the uterine tubes but we need not discuss those further. The student is, of course, at liberty to consult appropriate textbooks in the medical library. At this present time, simply review the anatomy of each uterine tube, and, at the appropriate time, study in detail its histology. Bear in mind that patency of one uterine tube is indispensable to successful reproduction.

In life, peristalsis is a feature of the normal uterine tube; on histologic examination a well-developed muscle wall is seen. At operation, the tube feels like a piece of slender cord, and it is limp. It slips through the gloves of the operator because it is moist with peritoneal fluid. Even the adroit operator can look clumsy if he tries to grasp the uterine tube without the aid of an instrument. When a uterine tube is infected, it may become thick and heavy. Then it prolapses into the pouch of Douglas, because of the natural curve of the tube, to where it meets the ovary on the posterior surface of the broad ligament.

Dissection:

ITEM 41-1. Reconsider the relationship of the tube to the peritoneal cavity and review the anatomy of the broad ligament (p. 202).

ITEM 41-2. Examine the abdominal ostium.

ITEM 41-3. Identify the parts of the tube, namely the infundibulum, the ampulla, and the isthmus, which are in view. There is an interstitial or mural part of the tube, that is lodged in the wall of the uterus and is therefore not seen. The uterine ostium cannot be found easily in an embalmed cadaver.

Chapter 42

The Ovaries

In clinical practice, the feature that distinguishes the ovary from other organs of the body is its ability to produce tumors of incredible diversity and complexity. Certainly many of these tumors are rare. Nevertheless, the occurrence of any one of them reemphasizes the ovaries' remarkable potential for life. For instance, one rare tumor of the ovary resembles the structure of the thyroid gland and, furthermore, the tumor secretes thyroxine. Another tumor contains recognizable elements of various body tissues, including teeth. This type of tumor may be considered an example of disordered parthenogenesis, a zoological term denoting reproduction by the female of a species without fertilization by the male.

To grapple with these and other ovarian disorders, a knowledge of the histology, cytology, pathology, and the function of the ovary is of prime importance, and none of these subjects are within the scope of this text. Accordingly, there is little detail here concerning the ovary, but what is here is significant. In other disciplines the ovary will be discussed in depth.

Dissection:

ITEM 42-1. The relationship of the ovary to the peritoneal cavity is described on p. 83.

At this stage of the dissection, when the abdominal viscera have long since been removed, it is worth recalling that the ovaries have a relationship to the gastrointestinal tract that is of more than anatomic interest. Cancer cells from a primary cancer in the stomach or in the bowel sometimes reach both ovaries, where they initiate a secondary cancer. There is debate about how this happens and what routes the cells take to reach the ovaries from the stomach. The debate need not concern you now. Simply appreciate that the ovaries and the gastrointestinal tract are closely related to each other across the peritoneal cavity, and that they are also linked to each other through the ramifications of the lymphatic system.

ITEM 42-2. The ovaries are firm and palpable on bimanual examination (p. 190), and, for that reason, it is important to know the size of an ovary and its shape. A functioning ovary is usually 3 cm. long, 1.5 cm. wide, and 1 cm. thick, approximately the same measurements as the distal phalanx of a middle finger of average length. The ovary, however, tapers to form tubal and uterine ends and it is, therefore, usually described as almond-shaped.

Measure the size of the ovaries in your cadaver. It is rare to find a cadaver with ovaries of the dimensions given here.

ITEM 42-3. The position of the ovary

To believe that each ovary has an absolutely constant position in the pelvis will lead inevitably to errors in clinical judgment. You must visualize each ovary as a mobile structure suspended by its mesovarium from an equally mobile broad ligament. As a result of its great mobility, the ovary can lie anywhere between the brim of the pelvis and pouch of Douglas. Major factors governing the position of the ovaries are the position of the uterus, nonpregnant and pregnant, and pathologic changes in the pelvis. What is the position of the ovaries in your specimen?

Chapter 43

Dissection of the Female Pelvis — Part One

These are the stages of the dissection:
Part one:
1. Reflection of the peritoneum
2. Identification of the ureter and uterine artery
3. Exposure of the lateral cervical ligament and the uterosacral ligament
4. Identification of the pelvic splanchnic nerves
5. Identification of the ureteric, vesical, and vaginal branches of the uterine artery

Part two (p. 226):
1. Examination of the endopelvic fascia
2. Identification of the levator ani
3. Identification of the branches of the internal iliac artery
4. Identification of the sacral plexus
5. Identification of the pudendal nerve and vessels

ITEM 43-1.   Reflection of the Peritoneum

In reflecting peritoneum on the left side, the presence of the sigmoid colon must be taken into account and reflected medially also.

Furthermore, on the left, you will observe that there is a quantity of fat around the ureter; therefore, the left ureter is not so adherent to the peritoneum as on the right.

With the fundus of the uterus pulled medially to keep the tissue between the sidewall of the pelvis and the viscera under tension, proceed as follows: Cut the round ligament close to the internal inguinal ring and cut the ovarian vessels, which are in the infundibulopelvic ligament. In the following procedure, do not cut blindly. Remain close to the external surface of the peritoneum as you reflect it. Incise the peritoneum parallel to the pelvic brim. Then reflect the peritoneum medially. Continue to do so until the broad ligament is mobilized, and while doing so observe particularly the adherence of the ureter to peritoneum. Release the ureter from the peritoneum.

The next step should be the identification of a significant structure, the lateral cervical ligament. It is not easy, however, for the novice to identify the ligament immediately, for it is not a well-defined ligament with clean-cut edges. It is, rather, a mass of fascia including smooth muscle fibers and supporting blood vessels, lymphatics, and nerves, between the posterolateral aspect of the cervix of the uterus as well as the vault of the vagina and the region of the internal iliac vessels. The lack of anatomic definition of the lateral cervical ligament has resulted in much confusion, mentioned briefly in the following commentary.

THE LATERAL CERVICAL LIGAMENT

This ligament was first emphasized in the literature by a German gynecologist, Mackenrodt, in 1895. Since that time, considerable confusion has developed about the precise nature of the ligament and the several different names applied to it, i.e., lateral cervical ligament, transverse cervical ligament, cardinal ligament, and Mackenrodt's ligament. There are four names, then, for the same structure, and there are other names less well known. If you follow carefully the dissecting instructions given here, there can be no confusion in your mind. You will demonstrate that an aggregation of pelvic fascia extends between the sidewall of the pelvis posterolaterally, and the supravaginal portion of the cervix and the vault of the vagina medially. It is the thickened basal part of this aggregation of fascia that is, essentially, the lateral cervical ligament.

Each lateral cervical ligament becomes particularly obvious when it is pulled tight. Thus the lateral cervical ligaments are seen to advantage, perhaps best of all, at a particular stage during vaginal hysterectomy (removal of the uterus through the vagina), which is commonly illustrated in gynecologic textbooks. Such illustrations show how the cervix is pulled toward the surgeon, the vaginal wall incised, the bladder displaced, and other essential steps taken to expose the lateral cervical ligaments, which are then clamped and cut. Indeed, the uterus cannot be fully mobilized until these paired ligaments and the paired uterosacral ligaments are cut.

Contrary to common belief, the ureter does not enter the surgical cardinal ligament but remains immediately superior to it and lies in the areolar tissue you must remove to expose the ligament. Furthermore, the uterine artery lies superior to the ureter and, therefore, it too is not incorporated in the ligament. Accordingly, during vaginal hysterectomy, these highly significant structures are not in immediate peril when the cardinal ligaments are clamped and cut.

With these facts in mind, proceed to identify the lateral cervical ligament by tracing the ureter, uterine artery, and veins into the vicinity of the ligament.

ITEM 43-2. At the brim of the pelvis, mobilize the ureter and trace it into the pelvis. Observe its relationship to the iliac vessels. The ureter lies superficial to the iliac vessels, then, deep to the uterine vessels. Once the ureter begins its horizontal course anteriorly at the level of the ischial spine, be alert for the uterine veins and artery that will lie superior to and adjacent to the ureter. Then, as the vessels become obvious, proceed cautiously, because you have now reached the locality of the transverse cervical ligament. The veins lie superior to the artery and together they form a sort of superior boundary to the ligament.

ITEM 43-3. To demonstrate the attachments of the lateral cervical ligament, grasp the cervix firmly with toothed forceps from within the vagina and pull the cervix inferiorly. Observe how taut the tissue described as the lateral cervical ligament becomes. Observe its direction toward the internal iliac vessels.

Having demonstrated that this is so, snip away tissue, including veins, to show how the uterine artery proceeds medially across the ureter to reach the side of the uterus. Next, clear away tissue to show how the ureter reaches the bladder. If you have not been too radical in your dissection, the basal part of the lateral cervical ligament, the surgical part, will become more obvious.

To demonstrate the uterosacral ligaments, pull the rectum off the sacrum. While the rectum is pulled anteriorly and medially, pull the cervix anteriorly with toothed forceps. Close to the vault of the vagina, a band of tissue, the uterosacral ligament, will be obvious. Reconstruct the anatomy to show how this band extends posteriorly lying deep to the peritoneal fold that forms the lateral boundary of the pouch of Douglas.

ITEM 43-4. To demonstrate, to some degree, the pelvic splanchnic nerves, pull the bladder and vagina anteriorly and clear away areolar tissue on the lateral aspect of the rectum. Interconnected bundles of nerve fibers, traveling in a posteroanterior direction, usually emerge during removal of this areolar tissue, which lies adjacent to the uterosacral ligament. These bundles are part of the pelvic splanchnic network and they are parasympathetic in function. They may be destroyed during removal of the rectum. It is suspected that their destruction is one factor in the explanation of retention of urine in the bladder after excision of the rectum.

Not now, but at the end of the dissection of the female pelvis, cut the uterosacral ligament and the lateral cervical ligament close to the vault of the vagina in order to demonstrate how mobile the cervix and the vault of the vagina become.

Review

Establish the relationship of the uterine artery to the ureter and also their relationship to the lateral fornix.

ITEM 43-5. If the uterine artery is well injected, you should be able to identify branches to the ureter, urinary bladder (vesical branches), and, certainly, the vagina.

Chapter 44

The Lower Urinary Tract

The lower urinary tract includes the urinary bladder and the male or female urethra. The upper and lower urinary tracts meet at the ureterovesical junctions.

Before we consider the anatomy of the junction, the significance of the ureter below the pelvic brim must be brought forth. This portion of the ureter is referred to as the pelvic ureter. It is 12.5 cm. long, and distinctly curved, the concavity of the curve facing anteromedially. At all times in pelvic surgery the surgeon must be aware of the ureters. Throughout the dissection of the cadaveric pelvis, the student should develop the same awareness.

The ureters are part of the upper urinary tract; the term "upper" is very misleading with reference to the actual position of the lower ends of the ureters in the pelvis.

The Ureterovesical Junctions

"In the distal ureter a mechanism operates to permit an orderly one-way flow of urine from ureter to bladder and to inhibit its return. The nature of this action is ill understood, but our anatomical, pathological and radiological studies indicate that the intrinsic musculature of the ureter rather than extrinsic factors is operative in this mechanism."*

Failure of the mechanism not only allows urine to return to the ureter from the bladder (the clinical term for this return is *reflux*, vesicoureteral reflux) but will also quite often lead to a stasis of urine in the ureter. The failure is usually bilateral, but it can be unilateral. Consequent infection of the upper urinary tract is common, so the anatomy of the junction is of practical significance.

The lowermost end of the ureter is intravesical and can be divided into an intramural segment passing through the bladder wall and a submucosal segment.

The longitudinal muscular coats of the ureter normally persist throughout the intramural and submucosal segments, whereas the circular coat ceases at the bladder wall. Stephens (1963) suggests that it is contraction of the longitudinal fibers that bring the "roof" of the ureteric orifice toward its "floor" to close the orifice after each jet of urine has entered the bladder.

Dissection:

ITEM 44-1. Look into the cavity of the bladder and observe the orifices of the ureters in the bladder. Note their position in relation to the trigone, a smooth triangular area of mucous membrane, the result of the firm attachment of the membrane to the underlying muscle. The two ureteric orifices and the urethral orifice are the apices of the triangle. Is an interureteric ridge or fold to be seen between the ureteric orifices? When present, it indicates the site of a bundle of muscle fibers sweeping from one ureter to the other. The mucous membrane elsewhere in the bladder is loosely adherent to the muscle. In the cadaveric bladder, it is rugose in appearance because the bladder was empty at the time of embalming. In life, when the bladder musculature hypertrophies, thick bands of muscle called trabeculae become prominent. Pockets of mucous membrane into the spaces of this muscular lattice are termed diverticula (singular — diverticulum).

ITEM 44-2. Identify the submucosal segment of each ureter. Examine its orifice. Make a longitudinal incision into the mucosa. Release the segment from its bed of fascia. The intramural segment lies in a muscular tunnel in the bladder wall.

---

*Stephens, F. D.: Congenital Malformations of the Rectum, Anus, and Genito-urinary tracts. Edinburgh, E. and S. Livingstone Ltd., 1963.

The Urinary Bladder

To see what the urinary bladder really looks like, the student is well advised to attend an autopsy or an operation upon pelvic organs. Then he will realize how justifiable it is to describe the bladder as diaphanous and how remotely the embalmed bladder, solid and shrunken, resembles the real thing. Then, too, he will realize why the bladder may be easily torn in a fracture of the pelvis and why steps are taken to protect the bladder during difficult surgical procedures in the pelvis.

Although the cadaveric bladder does give some idea of the position of the bladder and its relationships within the pelvis, the extent to which a full bladder can occupy the pelvic cavity and ascend into the abdominal cavity can scarcely be visualized. Therefore, it should be pointed out that in all clinical procedures in the pelvis, the fullness of the bladder is taken into account and, if need be, the bladder is emptied before the procedure begins.

Sometimes the bladder is deliberately filled with fluid before a surgical procedure. A full bladder elevates peritoneum off the posterior aspect of the lower abdominal wall. Thus the surgeon can reach the retropubic space, the bladder wall, and the prostate without opening the peritoneal cavity.

Read an account of the bladder in the male, in the female, and in the child. The male urethra is described on page 170.

The Female Urethra

The cadaveric urethra is solid and unyielding. It is therefore difficult for you to visualize how this delicately constructed tube can undergo considerable stretching and displacement in labor, yet recover completely, or that it can, indeed, be badly bruised or ruptured in labor. One reason for these effects is the proximity of the urethra to the anterior wall of the vagina. The fascia around the urethra and the fascia around the vagina are fused in the midline.

The female urethra varies in length; it is said to be, on average, 3.6 cm. long; it will dilate to accommodate instruments 1 cm. in diameter. The urethral musculature has been investigated extensively, and its function is debated at length. The location of the urethral orifice on the perineum is described on p. 197.

The Urine

Read the account on p. 174.

Chapter 45

Dissection of the Female Pelvis – Part Two

ITEM 45-1. It is important now to show that the lateral cervical ligament is distinct from endopelvic fascia. This fascia has a parietal and a visceral component. Identify the parietal component first. To do so, slide a finger over the pelvic brim into the pelvic cavity. It is inevitable that you will slide onto a sheet of fascia, easily identified for it is light gray in color and has the appearance and tension of a delicate drumskin. Do not proceed if you are uncertain, because once this sheet of fascia is sundered its anatomy is difficult to reconstruct.

The sheet of fascia identified by your finger is the parietal endopelvic fascia. By blunt dissection, remove all loose tissue until you demonstrate how the parietal part is continuous with the visceral endopelvic fascia. Pull the bladder and vagina medially to demonstrate this fact.

In the parietal endopelvic fascia you will see condensed tissue, white in color, in contrast to the gray of the rest of this fascia. The tissue is in the shape of a letter Y lying on its side. The solitary limb is attached posteriorly to the ischial spine. Anteriorly one stem proceeds to the posteroinferior edge of the pubis while the other ascends to the brim of the pelvis to the anterior boundary of the obturator canal.

This peculiar Y-shaped formation is due to a combination of two tendinous arches, one for the levator ani, the other for the endopelvic fascia. Posteriorly the two arches merge in the solitary limb of the Y, while anteriorly they separate; the arcus tendineous of the levator ani ascends to the obturator canal; the arcus tendineous of the pelvic fascia continues anteriorly to the pubis.

Superior to the arcus tendinous of levator ani, some of the obturator internus muscle is visible through the fascia. Inferior and anterior to the same arcus, the visible muscle fibers are the levator ani.

Levator ani is a bilateral structure. The levatores ani form an almost complete muscular sheet across the cavity of the pelvis, and together they are known as the pelvic diaphragm. The anatomy of each levator ani is difficult to comprehend from descriptions; it is without doubt the one structure that must be seen to be understood.

ITEM 45-2. To see the levator ani, carefully incise the parietal endopelvic fascia parallel to the arcus tendineus of the pelvic fascia. With care, remove as much of the fascia as possible to expose the underlying

226

levator muscle. Observe how bundles of muscle fibers turn medially to the midline, where they would normally meet their fellows from the opposite side. Trace the pubovaginalis fibers from the body of the pubis to a point posterior to the vagina (and thus anterior to the rectum).

Displace the rectum medially and trace the remaining fibers in a dorsal direction to the posterior aspect of the anorectal junction and to the coccyx.

LEVATORES ANI

It must be stressed again that the anatomy of this pair of muscles must be learned from a specimen. The component parts of each muscle are well illustrated in atlases and textbooks, which should be consulted with a specimen in hand. The muscles, known together as the pelvic diaphragm, will be referred to frequently in obstetrics and gynecology, especially, and in pelvic surgery in general.

Two aspects which present difficulty to the student are illustrated in Figure 45-1. Puborectalis is a component of the levator ani that meets its fellow of the opposite side posteriorly to the anorectal junction. The puborectalis sling is believed to be an integral part of the mechanism for the continence of feces.

The second aspect is the ease with which fibers of the levator ani become part of the longitudinal coat of the anal canal. The key fact here is the oblique direction of the anal canal; the arrows in Figure 45-1 show how easily the essentially horizontal fibers of the levatores ani sweep naturally into place in the anal canal. Confusion arises when an illustration of a longitudinal section of the anal canal is interpreted as being in a vertical plane.

ITEM 45-3. To demonstrate the branches of the internal iliac artery, well illustrated in most texts and atlases, identify the common iliac artery and its major branches plus the accompanying veins.

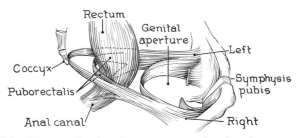

Figure 45-1. Diagram showing the components of each pubococcygeus, which in turn contributes to the formation each levator ani. Observe that the long axis of the anal canal is oblique and note the ease with which some pubococcygeus fibers blend with the longitudinal fibers of the canal. The cut fibers within the genital aperture represent the levator prostatae, or pubovaginalis.

Pursue the internal iliac artery into the pelvis and identify the origins of its many branches. Variations of these origins are very common. In order to save time and avoid prolonged debate, it is best to delay final identification of arteries until the gluteal region is dissected (p. 237). Use illustrations as a guide to the interpretation of your findings in your specimen. If need be, sacrifice without restraint the many veins in this region. Obviously in a surgical procedure veins cannot be treated with such abandon.

The rami of the sacral plexus are in close relationship with several of the branches of the internal iliac artery. *Grant's Atlas of Anatomy*, Figure 213, illustrates the essential facts.

THE PUDENDAL NERVE AND VESSELS

Dissection of these structures has barely begun. They have yet to be identified in the gluteal region, in the ischiorectal fossa, and on the perineum. Nevertheless your attention is drawn to them now, especially to the nerve, which is frequently anesthetized in the region of the ischial spine. Indeed, in pudendal nerve block, the ischial spine is the landmark to be palpated through the lateral fornix of the vagina.

Review the anatomy of this region by identifying the ischial spine and relating it as best you can to the lateral fornix. Do not be misled by the unyielding nature of embalmed tissue; in life the tissues are vastly different.

The continuation of the pudendal vessels and nerve is studied most easily after the gluteal region is dissected and the ischiorectal fossa is cleared of fat.

Proceed to Chapter 33, Pelvic Examination (p. 188).

REFERENCES

Leeson, C. R., and Leeson, T. S.: Histology. Philadelphia, W. B. Saunders Co., 1966.
Prather, G. C.: Injuries of the bladder. *In* M. F. Campbell (ed): Urology, Philadelphia, W. B. Saunders Co., 1963.
Stephens, F. D.: Congenital Malformations of the Rectum, Anus, and Genito-urinary Tracts. Edinburgh, E. & S. Livingstone Ltd., 1963.
Tobin, C. E., and Benjamin, J. A.: Anatomical study and clinical consideration of the fasciae limiting urinary extravasation from the penile urethra. Surgery, Gynecology, and Obstetrics, 79:195, 1944.

PART 5

THE LOWER LIMB, The Organ of Locomotion

by R. D. LAURENSON
and B. J. GREENHILL

Introduction:

The lower limb is also known as the lower extremity. It should be noted, too, that the term lower limb, or lower extremity, includes the thigh, leg, and foot. The leg, then, is only part of the lower limb.

"To make a body of a limb" should be the intent of every student dissecting a limb. In other words, he must view the limb in its entirety, not in a series of parts. Moreover, he must not view the limb as remote from the rest of the human frame for, as George Herbert said:

> Man is all symmetrie,
> Full of proportions, one limb to another,
> And all to all the world besides:
> Each part may call the farthest, brother:
> For head with foot hath privite amitie,
> And both with moons and tides.

> The Church Man

In the following dissection, therefore, emphasis is laid upon a systemic and total approach; the horizons of dissection are: the skin, superficial lymphatics, superficial venous system, deep fascia, gluteal region and ischiorectal fossa, thigh, leg and foot, and, last, joints of the lower limb. In the process of dissection the student's attention will be drawn to the regions of clinical importance.

The student is well advised to study the anatomy of his own limbs, for that is the easiest way to become familiar with living anatomy. For example, the range of movement in a joint and the muscle groups moving the joints are easily established on oneself. In addition many tendons, nerves, and vessels can be seen or felt. This method of learning the anatomy of the lower limb is indeed worthwhile because examination of the lower limb is an essential part of a complete physical examination.

Finally, the junior student about to dissect the lower limb of a rigid corpse must be informed that the prime function of the limb is effortless walking (p. 288). Therefore, at the end of the dissection of the lower limb, walking (known clinically as the gait) is discussed (p. 288).

If you have not yet read the chapter on skin (p. 1) and on fascia (p. 5), you are advised to do so now.

Chapter 46

Skin, Lymphatics, and Veins

Exercise:

Examine the skin of the entire limb. In addition to the general features of skin (Chapter 1), look for evidence of changes in the skin associated with age (p. 3), and also for changes that can occur in certain areas of skin of bedridden patients. Often in the dissecting room there is enough evidence of decubitus ulcers to stress the importance of the care of the skin in the nursing of a helpless patient confined to bed, especially if he has a terminal illness. Decubitus means lying down; decubitus ulcers occur on the heels, hips, and over the sacrum and coccyx.

Look also for scars from a previous injury or surgical procedure.

ITEM 46-1.   To remove the skin from the lower limb, begin at the ankle. Do not skin the foot because the foot of an embalmed cadaver dries out quickly once the skin is removed.

Immediately superior to the medial malleolus make a transverse incision about 2 cm. long and expose the long saphenous vein (Fig. 46-1). It is a common clinical procedure to "cut down" in this manner to expose the long saphenous vein for the administration of blood, plasma

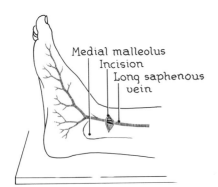

Medial malleolus
Incision
Long saphenous
vein

Figure 46-1. The long saphenous vein, exposed by an incision proximal to the medial malleolus.

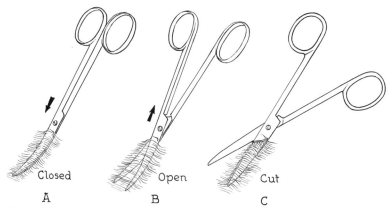

Figure 46-2. The closed-open scissors technique. *A.* Closed scissors are thrust along a plane of cleavage. *B.* The scissors are opened and withdrawn. *C.* The overlying tissue is cut as far as the reach of the scissors.

expanders, and electrolytes. Of course, there is a precise technique for this procedure but, for the moment, you are only concerned with the anatomy.

Then, by means of the closed-open scissors technique (Fig. 46-2) to mobilize skin superficial to the vein, make a longitudinal cut in the skin, superficial to the vein, up to the knee and down onto the anterior aspect of the ankle. Cut the skin at right angles to the long incision to create such flaps as are necessary.

Now that you have identified the depth of the superficial venous plane, strip back the flaps of skin to expose the rest of the superficial veins. Over the calf, ensure that the short saphenous vein remains undisturbed on the leg. In removing skin from the anterior aspect of the patella the prepatellar bursa will be exposed. See Bursa (p. 439).

ITEM 46-2. Look for perforating veins (Fig. 46-3). This is a most important step in the dissection, and the importance of perforators will be explained soon.

ITEM 46-3. Still using the closed-open scissors technique to mobilize skin and superficial fascia before they are cut, expose the long saphenous vein to the groin. The vein and its tributaries are often obscured by fat, especially in the thigh. Most surgeons believe that the superficial fascia of the lower limb can be divided into a superficial fatty layer and a deeper membranous layer. The long and short saphenous veins lie between this deeper layer and the deep fascia, while their tributaries lie in the fatty layer. It is those tributaries, having less support, that become varicose.

Thus you will find that the long saphenous vein is deeper than you expect, for it lies adjacent to the deep fascia. Confirm this point, and confirm the existence of a deeper membranous layer in the superficial

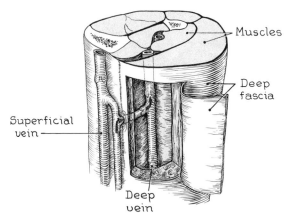

Figure 46-3. A perforating vein, perforating the deep fascia and connecting a superficial vein to a deep vein. The black arrows indicate the direction of normal blood flow.

fascia that must be split in order to release the vein. Skin the entire thigh and observe how the tributaries of the long saphenous vein lie suspended, as it were, in the superficial fatty layer.

Toward its termination, the long saphenous vein passes through a cluster of superficial inguinal lymph nodes. The precise termination of the long saphenous vein will be studied after a brief comment on lymphatic drainage. Meanwhile, remove skin from the entire thigh. Investigate the major tributaries of the long saphenous vein and look for perforators.

THE LYMPHATIC DRAINAGE OF THE LOWER LIMB

The drainage is superficial and deep. Superficial drainage is mainly from skin; deep drainage is from muscle. The two principal groups of lymph nodes, superficial and deep, are located in the groin.

It is difficult, at first, to conceive that lymph from the skin of the toes finally filters through the superficial lymph nodes in the groin, yet that is so. Long and normally inconspicuous lymph vessels accompany the long saphenous vein all the way to the groin. Thus, when the superficial inguinal lymph nodes are tender and swollen, obviously reacting to an infection somewhere in their field of drainage, the skin of the entire limb must be examined. The skin of the entire perineum and of the abdominal wall must also be included in the examination.

The superficial inguinal lymph nodes may be considered in two groups, one parallel to the inguinal ligament and another, a vertical group, adjacent to the termination of the long saphenous vein. Their efferent lymph vessels drain primarily to the external iliac lymph nodes proximal to the inguinal ligament and, to a lesser extent, into the deep inguinal lymph nodes. To reach the latter, the lymph vessels penetrate the fascia covering the saphenous opening (the cribriform fascia).

The deep inguinal nodes are few in number. They lie on the medial aspect of the femoral vein. Their efferents drain into the external iliac nodes.

ITEM 46-4. Examine the superficial fascia of the groin and see if lymph nodes are present. There are usually a few to be found. In life, it is quite common to be able to feel those nodes. Thus you can understand the dilemma of the clinician who, in investigating a patient for a probable lymphatic disorder, finds palpable inguinal lymph nodes; to gain more information it is customary to remove one or two nodes surgically to examine them microscopically. But examination of inguinal lymph nodes in the investigation of a generalized lymphatic disorder is usually unsatisfactory, for those nodes nearly always show extensive chronic inflammatory changes and fibrosis, unlike lymph nodes in the neck and axilla.

TERMINATION OF THE LONG SAPHENOUS VEIN

The long saphenous vein terminates by joining the femoral vein at the saphenous opening, an opening in the deep fascia, and of such surgical importance that its anatomy must be carefully reviewed.

ITEM 46-5. By elevating and gently mobilizing the long saphenous vein near its termination identify its many small tributaries. Three of these tributaries are named; the others—sometimes as many as six—are unnamed but they are nevertheless important in surgical procedures to mobilize and tie off the long saphenous vein.

Continue mobilizing the long saphenous vein to demonstrate how it curves over the edge of the saphenous opening and passes through the cribriform fascia to join the femoral vein. The edge of the opening is usually well portrayed in illustrations, but it is not so clearly demonstrable in a cadaver. One, sometimes two, small arteries about 1 mm. in diameter cross the saphenous opening deep to and at right angles to the long saphenous vein. In a surgical procedure, such vessels must be ligated and then cut, but you are at liberty to destroy them to give a better exposure of the next step. Establish exactly how and where the long saphenous vein joins the femoral vein.

Read an account of the anatomy of the saphenous opening.

THE VENOUS DRAINAGE OF THE LOWER LIMB

Figure 46-3 shows the fundamental facts. Superficial veins are superficial to the deep fascia. Deep veins, situated within the fascio-osseous compartments of the limb, lie in fascia between muscles. Valves are more numerous in the deep than in the superficial veins.

Normally blood flows from the superficial veins to the deep veins. Thus the long saphenous vein joins the femoral vein (and to do so it must pass through deep fascia). The same is true of the short saphenous vein. In addition, smaller veins leaving the tributaries of either the long or short saphenous system penetrate deep fascia to join the deep venous system. These smaller veins are usually referred to clinically as "perforators," but they are also referred to as communicating veins, and sometimes simply as deep connections. The arrows (Fig. 46-3) indicate the direction of blood flow in a normal perforator. Perforators are significant in the etiology, precise diagnosis, and treatment of varicose veins, one of the commonest clinical disabilities. To emphasize the significance of perforating veins one might add: retrograde flow through the perforators, i.e., from the deep veins to the superficial, is an important aspect of the problem of varicose veins.

Furthermore, and this fact is not illustrated in Figure 46-3, the girth of the superficial veins remains essentially the same from their beginning to end. The long saphenous vein is almost the same diameter at the groin as it is at the ankle, even though it has many tributaries. On the other hand, there is a striking increase in the girth of the deep veins. The femoral vein, for example, as it leaves the thigh, has the same diameter as a middle finger—it is a huge vein. One may therefore deduce that the perforating veins play a significant part in the venous drainage of the superficial aspects of the limb.

The venous return from the lower limb of a living person is a physiologic study that can only be touched on lightly here. The venous flow depends heavily upon muscular activity within the fascial compartments. It was pointed out in Chapter 2 that in life the muscles are not shrunken but that they bulge to fill out the fascial compartments. Thus a pressure exists within each compartment, a pressure that varies with muscular contraction. The ever-changing pressure associated with muscular activity promotes venous return.

Clinically, in considering the mechanics of venous return from the lower limb, the calf muscles are referred to as the calf muscle pump. Then the perforators are considered the "input" lines and the deep veins the "output" lines. The cusps of the valves in those lines are so arranged (Fig. 46-3) to maintain an onward flow of blood to and from the pump. The majority of perforators join the deep veins directly, as shown in Figure 46-3, but a variable number join the venous system actually in the substance of the muscles, the gastrocnemius or soleus, whose venous system drains into the deep veins. Thus one may conceive the pump acting in two ways: first, muscular contraction within the limitations of an osseofascial compartment forces blood onward in the deep veins; second, contraction of the muscles empties their venous pool, which refills during relaxation.

In very brief summary, then, it may be said that muscular activity promotes deep venous return and thus promotes also a flow of blood from the superficial to the deep system through the perforating veins.

Finally, for the successful management of all venous problems of the lower limb, the venous system must be seen in its entirety. From each lower limb blood flows into the iliac venous system, thence through the inferior vena cava to the right side of the heart, and then swiftly into the lungs. Now you can appreciate how easily small clots of blood (emboli) can reach the lungs from the lower limbs—and how a massive clot from the deep veins of the lower limb can jam either of the pulmonary arteries or even the pulmonary trunk. Moreover, you can appreciate why disorders of the heart giving rise to an elevation of venous pressure affect the venous return from the lower limbs.

ITEM 46-6. To show the principle of perforating veins, the dissection that follows is adapted from the work of Sarjeant (1964).

Identify the anteromedial surface of the tibia. Identify especially the posteromedial border of that surface. Next identify the tendo Achillis. Then at the junction of the middle and lower thirds of the leg, and about midway between the border of bone and the tendon, incise the investing layer of deep fascia (the surgical incision is different). Your incision creates an anterior and a posterior flap. Peel the anterior flap off the gastrocnemius and the soleus until you demonstrate how the investing layer of deep fascia and the transverse intermuscular septum fuse. Select at least one perforating vein and trace it through the deep fascia, observing its close relationship to the line of fusion, a landmark of great surgical importance, and also observing how the vein terminates. How does it terminate? Peel the posterior flap off the gastrocnemius and you will demonstrate perforators from the short saphenous system entering the muscle.

Clearly a surgeon dealing with varicose veins and their complications must have a sound knowledge of the anatomy you have demonstrated only in principle. But you have demonstrated enough anatomy in principle to be able to understand *Surgical Anatomy in the Treatment of Venous Stasis*, by Sarjeant (1964). It is a masterful account based on an excellent section on the anatomy and function of the veins of the lower extremity.

ITEM 46-7. Valves

Once you have reviewed the anatomy of the superficial veins, make longitudinal slits in some of them to establish the presence or absence of valves. Are there valves present in the long and short saphenous veins? Open one or two perforators and see if any valves are present. Valves in deep veins cannot be exposed yet. The deep veins will be exposed more fully in the course of further dissection.

Chapter 47

The Deep Fascia of the Thigh, Iliotibial Tract, Gluteal Region, and Ischiorectal Fossa

ITEM 47-1. To expose the deep fascia remove the superficial fascia, which may be abundant (see Fat, p. 6). To remove the superficial fascia from an obese cadaver, incise the fascia where it is thickest and expose the deep fascia, gray in color and substantial in texture. Then, from the entire limb, peel off as much of the superficial fascia as you can in one piece. If you proceed with reasonable caution, you will note cutaneous nerves piercing the deep fascia. Even though you do not have time to demonstrate those nerves by dissection, it is useful to know something about their distribution, which is usually adequately illustrated in anatomy texts. If the abdomen has been dissected, it is possible to identify the lateral cutaneous nerve of the thigh, mentioned more often than any other cutaneous nerve of the lower limb, and to trace the nerve beyond the inguinal ligament into the thigh.

ITEM 47-2. The deep fascia around the thigh is termed the fascia lata, the broad fascia. Laterally, observe that a longitudinal strip of fascia lata is thicker than the rest; in a cadaver the strip is whitish in color. This strip, the iliotibial tract (also known as band), is of considerable interest in the functional anatomy of the lower limb. It is an obvious structure whose function is not clearly understood. For discussion of the functional significance of the iliotibial tract read the article by Kaplan (1958). In any event, the tract and the gluteal region must be considered together. Therefore, skin the gluteal region and examine the fascia there. Remove the superficial fascia. Deep fascia is virtually nonexistent upon gluteus maximus, whose coarse muscle bundles lie clearly exposed upon removal of the superficial fascia. Over the anterior aspect of the gluteal region, however, deep fascia is conspicuous where it forms the superior part of the iliotibial tract, which covers the gluteus medius.

THE ILIOTIBIAL TRACT (BAND)

It is all too easy to strip off deep fascia and miss the opportunity to study the iliotibial tract. Make sure, therefore, that you see the tract and its extensive but indirect attachment to the femur, through its connection with the lateral intermuscular septum. In addition the tract is

236

attached to the pelvis superiorly and to the tibia inferiorly; three quarters of the gluteus maximus and all of the tensor fasciae latae are inserted into the tract. The superior and inferior attachments are readily recognized. The anterior and posterior margins of the tract blend imperceptibly with the rest of the deep fascia. In the living, however, the margins of the tract, especially inferiorly, are readily recognized as follows:

Exercise: Stand with the knee slightly bent and raise the heel off the ground. Then, on the lateral aspect of the thigh, above the knee palpate a vertical band, about 5 cm. broad, the iliotibial tract.

ITEM 47-3. This dissection to demonstrate the two muscles inserting into the tract and the further attachments of the tract is based on demonstrations by Kaplan (1958). Proceed as follows: Identify the greater trochanter deep to the iliotibial tract. Over the greater trochanter make a longitudinal incision into the tract. Extend the incision superiorly toward the iliac crest and inferiorly to a point about a handsbreadth above the knee. In passing, identify the bursa between the tract and the trochanter. Like all bursae, this one may become distended with sufficient fluid to make an obvious swelling that fluctuates.

ITEM 47-4. At approximately the midpoint of the tract, make a horizontal incision into both the anterior and posterior portions of the tract. It is now much easier to manipulate the normally tense iliotibial tract and so to study it further.

Peel the lower posterior quadrant of the tract posteriorly to expose more and more of the vastus lateralis. By remaining on the internal surface of the iliotibial tract and by displacing the vastus lateralis anteromedially, the continuity of the iliotibial tract and the lateral intermuscular septum will become obvious. The lateral intermuscular septum projects much further posteriorly than its name implies (Fig. 48-1). If, however, you remain on the internal aspect of the tract you cannot fail to reach the anterolateral surface of the septum. By blunt dissection with the fingers superiorly and inferiorly, reveal as much of the septum as you can. Where is it thickest?

Review the inferior attachments of the tract, into the quadriceps expansion, and into the tendon of biceps as well as into the tibia.

ITEM 47-5. Peel the upper anterior quadrant of the cut iliotibial band anteriorly to expose the tensor fasciae latae. It may be necessary to incise the fascia to expose the tensor; do so neatly.

The next region to be dissected is the gluteal region. Before proceeding there, review the anatomy of the iliotibial tract.

GLUTEAL REGION

ITEM 47-6. Identify the cephalic (anterosuperior) border of the gluteus maximus. Accurate identification is of prime importance for success in the next dissection. Using Figure 47-1 as a guide, make an incision parallel to the cephalic (anterosuperior) border of maximus into the gluteal fascia that overlays gluteus medius. Slip the fingers of one hand deep to maximus. If you have incised the deep fascia correctly, your fingers will slide easily into a plane of cleavage deep to maximus. Seek guidance if you are not sure. Then proceed to mobilize the cephalic (anterosuperior) border of maximus by extending this latest incision to join the longitudinal incision made previously into the iliotibial tract.

ITEM 47-7. Next cut the femoral attachment of maximus. Finally identify the caudal (inferior) border of gluteus maximus, and in line with that border make a horizontal cut through the deep fascia. Continue the cut along the inferior border of the muscle (but in doing so watch out for the posterior cutaneous nerve of thigh that lies subjacent to the deep fascia and at right angles to the border of the muscle).

In mobilizing the gluteus maximus in this fashion, you have in fact created the "gluteal lid" as described by Henry (1957). Lift the lid and tilt it back to expose the structures deep to gluteus maximus. In a cadaver, the muscle may not lift and bend too easily; firm pressure may be required. Tie the muscle back with a loop of string.

Several muscles, nerves, and vessels can now be seen or found. The muscles from anterior to posteroinferior are the gluteus medius, piriformis, obturator internus (whose tendon is concealed to some extent by the gemelli), and quadratus femoris. The gluteus minimus lies deep to the gluteus medius. The tendon of the obturator externus lies at the same depth as the gluteus minimus; the entire obturator externus is seen most easily when the hip joint is dissected as described later (p. 273). The gluteus medius and minimus are hip abductors, and the piriformis, obturator internus, quadratus femoris, and obturator externus are the so-called short external rotators of the hip.

The most obvious structure now in view is the sciatic nerve, descending vertically into the thigh midway between the greater trochanter and the ischial tuberosity. Slip an index finger around the nerve, and, by

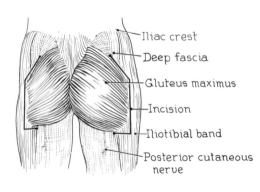

Iliac crest

Deep fascia

Gluteus maximus

Incision

Iliotibial band

Posterior cutaneous nerve

Figure 47-1. The incisions to create the gluteal lid. Observe carefully which side of the body you are dissecting so that you employ the appropriate incision.

blunt dissection with the fingers, mobilize the nerve superiorly and inferiorly as far as you can.
ITEM 47-8. The key anatomic structure, however, is the piriformis. Identify the piriformis and establish its relationship to the superior and inferior gluteal vessels and nerves and, especially, to the sciatic nerve. Establish the continuity of these distal parts with their proximal parts within the pelvis. Having identified the sciatic nerve and piriformis, identify the other muscles found in this region. Begin anteriorly with the gluteus medius and, with the fingers, mobilize its posterior border. For orientation purposes it is important to observe how the gluteus medius is only partially covered by the maximus. Identify the posterior border of the medius and relate it to the cephalic border of the maximus. Slip a finger deep to the gluteus medius and open the plane of cleavage between the medius and the underlying gluteus minimus.

Review

Identify the following muscles in order: the gluteus medius, the piriformis, the tendon and the gemelli of the obturator internus, and the quadratus femoris.

Of all the structures deep to the gluteus maximus, the sciatic nerve is by far the most important to the practicing physician.

INTRAMUSCULAR INJECTIONS INTO THE BUTTOCK

In the everyday practice of medicine, this region has special importance as the commonest site for intramuscular injections. Simple observation of the extensive venous and arterial plexuses on the deep surface of the gluteus maximus and of the close proximity of the sciatic nerve indicates why care must be exercised in giving an intramuscular injection in this region, especially in a thin person with poorly developed muscles.

Exercise: Place an index finger on the sciatic nerve where it emerges from the shelter of the piriformis. Keep the finger in place and restore the gluteus maximus to its anatomic position. Now establish where you would inject a substance into gluteus maximus so as not to damage the sciatic nerve. If your dissection has been well done it should be obvious that the so-called upper-outer quadrant of the gluteal region is a relatively safe site for an intramuscular injection.

THE ACTION OF THE GLUTEUS MEDIUS AND MINIMUS

Examine the region of the hip joint of a skeleton and establish, with the aid of an illustration, the proximal and distal attachments of those

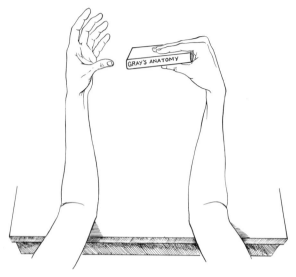

Figure 47-2.   A demonstration of how the muscles of one hand must tighten to hold a book horizontal when the other hand is taken away. If the left hand is taken away the muscles of the right hand tighten to keep the book horizontal. Thus the right gluteus medius and minimus steady the pelvis when the left foot is off the ground.

two muscles. Their function is of paramount importance in normal hip function; their care dominates rehabilitation after surgery.

Not only do they abduct the hip joint, they also stabilize the pelvis when the opposite foot is raised off the ground. To demonstrate their function, proceed as follows: with elbows on a desk hold a book, as in Figure 47-2. Then let go one hand. Immediately the muscles of the other forearm and hand spring into action to hold the book horizontal. In like manner, when you raise your right foot off the ground the left gluteus medius and minimus spring into action to stabilize the pelvis.

It must be made clear, however, that two essential factors govern the success of stabilizing the pelvis in the manner just described; the muscles must be normal; the bony skeleton must be normal. The effect of muscular paralysis is readily understood. On the other hand, the muscles may be normal but unable to function to perfection because the skeletal lever system is unstable, for example, because the neck of the femur is fractured.

THE PUDENDAL NERVE AND VESSELS

ITEM 47-9.   Pull gluteus maximus vigorously toward its sacral attachment, cutting the inferior gluteal vessels if need be, to expose the posterolateral aspect of the ischial spine between piriformis and the obturator internus. The dissection usually fails because the student is not bold enough in his approach. Expose also the sacrospinous ligament posteromedial to the ischial spine. As you proceed, you will expose the pudendal nerve and vessels. Establish their continuity with their proximal parts within the pelvis. Where precisely does the pudendal nerve lie in relation to the ischial spine and the sacrospinous ligament?

Since the distal parts of the pudendal vessels and nerve lie masked by fascia on the lateral wall of the ischiorectal fossa, exploration of that fossa is now appropriate.

THE ISCHIORECTAL FOSSA

Immediately anterior to the caudal border of the gluteus maximus there is a mass of fat that can be more fully exposed if the gluteus maximus is retracted as much as possible toward the sacrum. Some of the fibers of maximus arise from the sacrotuberous ligament; it may be necessary to scrape the maximus off the ligament to get a full exposure of the region you are now entering.

Fat occupies the ischiorectal fossa, and is bounded posteriorly by the gluteus maximus and the sacrotuberous ligament, laterally by fascia on the internal surface of obturator internus and the ischial tuberosity, medially by the anal canal (note—anal canal, not rectum), and superomedially by the inferior aspect of levator ani. The anterior boundary is ill-defined; from the ischiorectal fossa, by blunt dissection, one can tunnel anteriorly immediately inferior to the levator ani. The most important boundary, however, from the point of view of the practicing physician, is skin. Pus in considerable amount may collect in the fossa as a result of a bacterial infection. An ischiorectal abscess is opened and drained by means of an incision into the skin which forms, really, the inferior boundary of the fossa.

ITEM 47-10. In cleaning out fat from the ischiorectal fossa, you will encounter the inferior hemorrhoidal vessels and nerve crossing the fossa from the fascia upon obturator internus to reach the anal canal. Stick a finger into the fossa and hook out the fat. Use the inferior hemorrhoidal structures to guide you to the lateral wall of the fossa. Get as much fat as possible out of the fossa before returning to the gluteal region to trace the pudendal vessels and nerve from there into the fossa. They enter a fascial tunnel called the pudendal canal. From the canal, branches of the vessels and nerve are distributed to the perineal structures. Branches proceed as far as the dorsal surface of the penis. You may dissect the branches further if you wish.

Chapter 48

The Thigh

Introduction

The following text must be read before the dissection proceeds. The key to an understanding of the thigh is a knowledge of the location and nomenclature of the three muscle groups (Fig. 48-1). Clinicians name the three groups the extensors, flexors, and adductors on the basis of their principal function; the first two groups act powerfully on the knee joint; the third group acts equally powerfully on the hip. Anatomists, however, prefer to name the three groups anterior, posterior, and medial femoral, so that smaller muscles of lesser functional significance may be included. In summary, then, clinicians name these groups on the basis of function while anatomists name them on the basis of location.

In the course of your dissection you will see that some of the muscles cross two joints. These muscles are referred to clinically as two-joint muscles, and that action is of considerable significance in the coordination of the movements of the joints of the lower limb. The action of a two-joint muscle is not as simple as it appears to be on first consideration, so a discussion of the action on an elementary basis would no doubt mislead the student. Accordingly, the function of two joint muscles is not discussed further, but this should not prevent the student from identifying the muscles that span two joints.

The anterior group of thigh muscles includes the quadriceps muscle mass. This group acts primarily on the knee, but one of the quadriceps, namely the rectus femoris, is a two-joint muscle, for it is attached proximal to the hip joint; thus the rectus femoris may act as a hip flexor as well as a knee extensor. The sartorius, the additional member of the anterior group, is another example of a two-joint muscle.

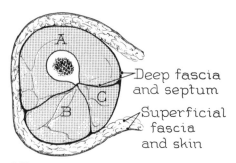

Figure 48-1. Cross section of thigh. A is the extensor (anterior) compartment, B the flexor (posterior) compartment, and C the adductor (medial) compartment. The septum between compartments B and C scarcely exists.

The posterior group is the flexor group. The three muscles are called the hamstring muscles because of their tendons, but they are called, more commonly, simply the hamstrings. They act powerfully as flexors of the knee and they also assist extension of the hip.

The medial group is the adductor group. The gracilis, however, unlike its companions in this group, is attached to the tibia, i.e., distal to the knee joint. Presumably, then, it may act on the knee joint, possibly as a flexor, as well as giving noble support to the powerful pull of the main adductor mass.

The sartorius overlaps, almost all the way, the junctional zone between the anterior and medial group. It is a long straplike muscle that has its proximal attachment proximal to the hip joint and its distal attachment distal to the knee joint. Between these attachments it lies like a snake across the anterior and medial aspects of the thigh.

Observe on Figure 48-1 the breadth of the anterior group, from the well-defined lateral intermuscular septum, posterolateral in relation to the femoral shaft, to the ill-defined medial intermuscular septum between the sartorius and adductor longus. The mass of muscle posteromedial to the two septa and the femoral shaft includes both the posterior and medial group. Their separation into two groups is unreal, for the septum that supposedly separates them scarcely exists.

ITEM 48-1. Locate the three main muscle groups of the thigh as follows. Grasp each group and establish its extent. It is much easier to manipulate the muscle groups in the living. Then, with care so as not to lacerate underlying structures, remove as much deep fascia as possible to establish more clearly the muscle groups and their relationship to the intermuscular septa (Fig. 48-1)

NERVES ENTERING THE THIGH

Three major nerves enter the thigh to proceed to each group of muscles. The femoral nerve enters the thigh lateral to the femoral artery and supplies the anterior group (extensor group); the obturator nerve enters the thigh through the obturator canal and supplies the medial (adductor) group; the sciatic nerve enters the gluteal region in relationship to the piriformis. This nerve supplies not only the posterior femoral group of muscles (the flexor group) but also the muscle groups of the leg, i.e., below the knee.

ITEM 48-2. Identify the femoral nerve in the interval between the psoas and iliacus and trace the nerve to the inguinal ligament.

ITEM 48-3. Identify the obturator nerve at the brim of the pelvis and trace the nerve to the obturator canal.

ITEM 48-4. Identify the sciatic nerve, first, on the anterior surface of the piriformis in the pelvis, and, second, in the gluteal region.

MAJOR ARTERIES ENTERING THE THIGH AND GLUTEAL REGION*

ITEM 48-5. Identify, first, the common iliac artery and trace it to its bifurcation into the external and internal iliac arteries. Trace the external iliac artery to where it disappears into the thigh, posterior to the inguinal ligament. At this point it is renamed the common femoral artery (in the vascular surgeon's terminology). Anywhere up to a distance of 10 cm. beyond the ligament the common femoral artery bifurcates into the superficial femoral and deep femoral arteries. Identify that bifurcation. Further exploration of these major vessels must await dissection of the thigh. But learn now that in the living, blood in the common femoral artery is destined to nourish almost the entire lower limb and the peripherai parts of the gluteal region.

ITEM 48-6. Identify the obturator artery at the brim of the pelvis. Establish where it arises from the internal iliac artery. Trace it to the obturator canal through which it disappears to nourish the proximal part of the adductor region.

ITEM 48-7. Review the gluteal arteries, superior and inferior. Establish their origin from the internal iliac artery, their course through the greater sciatic foramen, and their distribution to the gluteal muscles.

MAJOR VEINS LEAVING THE THIGH AND GLUTEAL REGION

ITEM 48-8. Identify the femoral vein lying medial to the femoral artery. Trace the vein distally to the point where it is joined by the deep femoral vein. Observe the size of these veins and their tributaries. They

---

*The terminology preferred by vascular surgeons in describing the femoral artery is used here (Fig. 48-2).

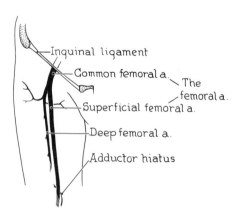

Inquinal ligament

Common femoral a.

The femoral a.

Superficial femoral a.

Deep femoral a.

Adductor hiatus

Figure 48-2. For descriptive purposes, vascular surgeons divide the femoral artery into the common femoral artery and the superficial femoral artery.

convey most of the blood from the lower limb. Establish the continuity of the venous pathway between the limb and the inferior vena cava.

ITEM 48-9. Identify the obturator vein emerging from the obturator canal and trace it to its junction with the internal iliac vein.

ITEM 48-10. Identify the gluteal veins (they may have been cut already) and appreciate their continuity from the gluteal region to the internal iliac vein.

Now that you are aware of the muscle groups of the thigh and have recognized the major nerves and vessels entering or leaving the limb, proceed to study in detail the organization of the nerve supply to the lower limb.

Chapter 49

The Nerve Supply to the Lower Limb

To prevent the student of gross anatomy from jumping to the conclusion that the nerve supply of the lower limb begins and ends in the lumbosacral plexus, a concept that will be developed in much greater detail in neuroanatomy is described briefly now.

The predominant control of voluntary activities of the upper and lower limbs of the same side of the body is from the motor cortex of the opposite cerebral hemisphere. Similarly, the sensory representation of the limbs is contained predominantly in the opposite cerebral hemisphere. However, present knowledge of the functional activity of the central nervous system shows clearly that to consider the motor control and sensory representation of any limb to be confined entirely to the opposite cerebral hemisphere is far too simple a concept. Much integrated activity of widely separated parts of the entire central nervous system is involved in both voluntary and reflex movement. Also, sensory input affects more than those areas in which conscious impressions are generated. Any single sensory stimulus evokes widespread activity in many parts of the central nervous system. These facts, as well as the concept of contralateral motor control or of contralateral sensory representation, must be borne in mind in the interpretation of the signs and symptoms of injury or disease of the central nervous system.

Now that you have been reminded of the part the central nervous system plays in the function of the limbs, proceed to examine the peripheral nervous system in the lower limb. Begin with the cord and its ventral and dorsal roots.

ITEM 49-1. After the vertebral column was sectioned (p. 156), perhaps a portion of the conus medullaris of the spinal cord was left. If not, at least the dorsal and ventral roots that form the cauda equina should still be present. Observe the lengths of these roots and how they make a vertical descent in the subarachnoid space.

ITEM 49-2. Observe that the ventral root, which is motor, and the dorsal root, which is sensory, leave the subarachnoid space in separate sleeves of the arachnoid and dura mater. That the sleeves remain separate as far as the posterior root ganglion is not obvious, but it can be demonstrated once the intervertebral foramen is opened (Fig. 83-2).

ITEM 49-3. Pull the dura medially to see the dural sheath that encloses the dorsal and ventral roots. The sheath is surrounded by fat and veins of the extradural space. Clinicians refer to the sheath and its contents as the "nerve root." See how the lowermost nerve roots are essentially vertical to begin with, then each root curves inferior to the pedicle of the vertebra above. The relationship of the proximal part of the nerve roots L5 and S1 is important, and is examined next.

ITEM 49-4. Identify the cut surface of the disc between L4 and 5. Observe its relationship to the fifth lumbar nerve root.

A protrusion of the disc between L4 and 5 vertebrae impinging on the L5 root produces signs and symptoms in the motor and sensory distribution of that root. The classic findings in an L4 and 5 disc protrusion are weakness in dorsiflexion of the toes and numbness of the skin of the anterolateral aspect of the leg and of the dorsum of the foot, regions remote from the actual protrusion. Similar signs and symptoms occur elsewhere, according to the nerve root involved. Such clinical details are introduced here merely to indicate the breadth of vision that is necessary in the successful diagnosis of the cause of a peripheral disorder. It is apparent that knowledge of the root value of motor and sensory nerves is necessary in the accurate diagnosis of nerve root disorders.

ITEM 49-5. In the next step, the student must use his initiative to gain as wide exposure as possible with minimal destruction. Using bone forceps and an autopsy saw to remove bone, trace the fifth lumbar root into the intervertebral foramen. Observe its curve inferior to the pedicle above.

The posterior root ganglion is soon exposed. It is an obvious swelling and serves as an ideal landmark. Beyond the ganglion identify the fifth lumbar spinal nerve and its division into an anterior and posterior ramus. Note the following facts:

(1) The posterior root ganglion is located in the intervertebral foramen. This is true of all posterior root ganglia except in the sacral region, where the ganglia are located in the sacral canal.

(2) The actual spinal nerve is short (Fig. 83-2), for it quickly divides into an anterior and posterior ramus. This is true of all spinal nerves. Each spinal nerve is only slightly longer than an intervertebral foramen.

ITEM 49-6. The anterior rami of spinal nerves L1, 2, 3, and 4 enter the psoas muscle, where they form the lumbar plexus from which two major nerves of the thigh arise. They are the femoral and obturator nerves. Identify the femoral nerve in the interval between the iliacus and psoas. Trace it proximally to where it emerges from the psoas, then distally to where it disappears deep to the inguinal ligament. Then identify the obturator nerve within the pelvis on the medial side of the psoas. Trace it proximally and then distally to where it leaves the pelvis through the obturator canal.

ITEM 49-7. A part of the anterior ramus of L4 and all of the anterior ramus of L5 form the lumbosacral trunk (both parts are lumbar in origin, yet their union is described as lumbo*sacral*). The lumbosacral trunk crosses the ala of the sacrum, then the anterior aspect of the sacroiliac joint. Identify the trunk and trace it to where it joins with anterior rami of nerves S1, 2, and 3 to form the sciatic nerve.

ITEM 49-8. The sciatic nerve has already been exposed in the gluteal region. From that region, establish its continuity with the sacral plexus within the pelvis.

THE ANATOMY OF THE STRAIGHT LEG RAISING TEST

The investing sheaths of the sciatic nerve, like the sheaths of all nerves, are continuous with the coverings of the central nervous system. Thus the epineurium of the sciatic nerve is continuous with the dura mater. It follows that if the epineurium is pulled upon, some degree of tension will be transmitted to the dura mater and to the nerve roots.

Therefore, clinically, one method of exerting tension on the nerve roots and the dura mater is to exert a pull upon the sciatic nerve by means of the straight leg raising test. The nerve is a close posterior relation of the hip joint and the two branches of the nerve are close posterior relations of the knee joint. Furthermore, the sciatic nerve is 2 cm. broad and its supporting sheaths are strong. Thus when the hip is flexed while the knee is extended, as in the straight leg raising test, tension is transmitted back to the L4, L5, S1, S2, and S3 nerve roots and to the dura mater. In performing the test, the clinician may elicit pain not only from the nerve roots and the dura mater, but also from other structures. Therefore, clinical experience is necessary for the interpretation of the results of the test, but the anatomy of the test can be readily demonstrated now.

ITEM 49-9. To demonstrate the anatomy of the test, grasp the sciatic nerve firmly and pull it distally while you observe the effect upon the nerve roots and the dura mater. The tissues of an embalmed cadaver are often difficult to manipulate, but you should be able to see some tension develop in the dura mater close to where the L5 root was exposed.

ITEM 49-10. Review the main distribution of each of the three nerves entering the thigh. The femoral nerve supplies the anterior (extensor) group of thigh muscles. The obturator nerve supplies the medial (adductor) group. The sciatic nerve supplies the posterior (flexor) group, then supplies all the muscle groups below the knee.

Chapter 50

Exploration of the Muscle Compartments of the Thigh

Each muscle is connected to at least one nerve, artery, and vein, collectively known as a neurovascular bundle. Individual neurovascular bundles will not be earmarked for identification. In general as each muscle is identified its neurovascular bundle will become obvious.

The quickest way to dissect the muscles of the limbs is with the fingers (Fig. 50-1). In this way, the muscle can be elevated and mobilized to its proximal and distal attachments without damaging the neurovascular bundles.

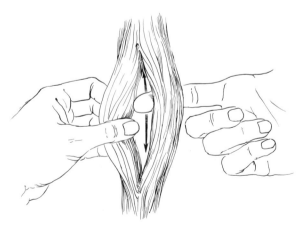

Figure 50-1. The muscles of the limbs are easily separated by dissecting with the fingers, a technique referred to as blunt dissection.

It is a practical necessity for the student to know how to test the action not only of a muscle group, but also of many significant individual muscles. The method is illustrated in Figure 53-1, where the patient is keeping his foot in a position of dorsiflexion while the clinician pulls in the opposite direction. All muscle groups or individual muscles, including the thigh muscles, are tested in this way, and the required position of the patient and the most suitable grip for the clinician are fully illustrated in Aids to the Investigation of Peripheral Nerve Injuries, M. R. C. War Memorandum No. 7, from which Figure 53-1 has been adapted.

DISSECTION OF THE MUSCLES OF THE ANTERIOR FEMORAL COMPARTMENT

ITEM 50-1.   The Sartorius
About midthigh, mobilize the muscle until you can get a finger deep to it. Then cut the muscle across. Snipping and breaking fascia with blunt dissection using the fingers, strip the proximal half of the muscle proximally to the anterior superior iliac spine to which sartorius is attached. Then mobilize the lower half of the muscle. Elevate and put tension on the muscle to demonstrate its attachment to deep fascia and the quadriceps expansion as well as to the tibia. To demonstrate the tibial attachment particularly well, the muscle must be deliberately mobilized until its attachment to bone is clearly seen. Do so.

The full extent of the superficial femoral artery and vein can now be appreciated although a sheet of fascia obscures them from view. However, rather than dissect them free at this time, wait until the popliteal fossa is dissected. Then the continuity of the vascular system of the thigh is easier to comprehend.

ITEM 50-2.   The four muscles of the quadriceps are attached distally to the patella. They are also attached to the tibia by means of the patellar retinacula and the ligamentum patellae, which are dealt with when the knee joint is dissected. Identify, first, the rectus femoris proceeding from the anterior inferior iliac spine to its attachment into the quadriceps tendon, proximal to the patella. Observe the bipennate form of the rectus femoris and compare it with the straplike form of sartorius.

On each side of the rectus femoris, observe the vasti. Vastus lateralis is an extensive muscle extending as high as the greater trochanter; it is also a bulky muscle with a copious blood supply; in life considerable hemorrhage may occur into the muscle as a result of a severe blow to the lateral aspect of the thigh. The vastus medialis is not as bulky as the vastus lateralis, but it is nevertheless a big muscle; its strength is of supreme importance in the stability of the knee joint, particularly in athletes.

Deep to the three muscles just listed lies the vastus intermedius. To expose the vastus intermedius adequately, proceed as follows:

ITEM 50-3. Identify the line of separation between the vastus lateralis and the rectus femoris. Split the muscles apart and, in doing so, observe the neurovascular bundle entering the vastus after crossing the superior part of the vastus intermedius. Then observe the fibers of intermedius running parallel to the shaft of the femur.

Review

In the course of the dissection just completed, the neurovascular bundles to each muscle would have been encountered. To review the anterior femoral region, trace the femoral nerve into the region and establish that this nerve supplies the muscles of the region, namely, the quadriceps and sartorius.

SURGICAL APPROACH TO THE FEMORAL SHAFT

In the treatment of fractures of the femoral shaft, for example, it may be necessary to expose the shaft surgically. The usual approach, which you have already demonstrated to some extent, is on the plane of the lateral intermuscular septum, posterior to the vastus lateralis muscle. Explore this plane further until you reach the femoral shaft. You may be able to identify the perforating arteries approaching this region from a posteromedial direction and coming through the lateral intermuscular septum. At operation, those arteries are more easily identified; they must be ligated before the femoral shaft can be successfully exposed.

THE MUSCLES OF THE MEDIAL FEMORAL (ADDUCTOR) COMPARTMENT

The muscles of this compartment are recognized in three layers. The most anterior layer consists of the pectineus and adductor longus; the adductor brevis forms the second layer, and the adductor magnus the third. The gracilis is superimposed upon the medial aspect of the three adductors just named.

ITEM 50-4. Mobilize the gracilis first. Slip a finger around the muscle at midthigh. Once the midriff of the muscle is free, mobilize the entire muscle by blunt dissection with the fingers. It may be an advantage to divide the muscle at its midpoint, just as you did with the sartorius, and then peel the proximal and distal parts right to their attachment. In particular, observe the relationship of the tibial attachment of the gracilis to that of the sartorius, and of the semitendinosus, soon to be mobilized.

ITEM 50-5. Identify the stout white tendon of adductor longus attached to the body of the pubis at a position inferomedial to the pubic tubercle. In life, when the legs are spread apart the tendon is readily palpable. It is crossed by the spermatic cord.

Slip a finger around the tendon. Then by blunt dissection with the fingers, mobilize the entire muscle. The plane of separation between the adductor longus and pectineus will become obvious. At this time, the obturator nerve and vessels are seen emerging from the obturator canal.

ITEM 50-6. Next, slip the tip of a finger posterior to pectineus and mobilize it. Be careful: in a cadaver this muscle ruptures and fragments very easily. If it is difficult to determine the superior border of pectineus, trace the medial circumflex femoral artery posteriorly—the artery passes superior to the pectineus.

ITEM 50-7. Close to the pubic bone, cut the tendon of the adductor longus and reflect the muscle with reasonable care toward the femoral shaft to expose the adductor brevis.

ITEM 50-8. Posterior to the brevis lies the massive adductor magnus. Textbook descriptions of this muscle are not easy to follow, but is attachments are easy enough to understand on a specimen.

Identify, first, the tendon of the adductor magnus. The tendon forms the medial boundary of the region through which the superficial femoral vessels are seen to disappear. Trace the tendon distally to where it attaches to the adductor tubercle. Then trace the part of the muscle attached to the tendon proximally to the ischial tuberosity, where the most posterior fibers of the adductor magnus are attached. It is now possible, by blunt dissection toward the femoral shaft, to demonstrate the rest of the adductor magnus. Observe, for interest only, that the pelvic attachment of the adductor magnus is essentially anteroposterior in direction, whereas the femoral attachment is vertical. Such a change of direction explains the unusual and interesting shape of the muscle.

Review

To review the adductor compartment, trace the obturator nerve into the region and establish that the nerve supplies the gracilis, adductor longus and adductor brevis, and most of the adductor magnus. The part of the adductor magnus that is attached to the ischial tuberosity along with the hamstrings is supplied by the sciatic nerve.

THE MUSCLES OF THE POSTERIOR FEMORAL (FLEXOR) COMPARTMENT AND THE SCIATIC NERVE

This compartment was partially exposed during dissection of the gluteal region. To demonstrate the tendons of these muscles posterior to the knee joint, it is necessary to remove deep fascia that is quite dense and holds the tendons toward the midline of the limb. This regional zone of fascia is named the popliteal fascia and forms the roof of the popliteal fossa.

Complete the dissection as follows:

ITEM 50-9.   Identify the tendon of the semitendinosus, lying posterior to the tendon of gracilis. Mobilize the entire muscle and its tendon. Check its tibial attachment in relationship to the gracilis and sartorius.

ITEM 50-10.   Deep to the belly of the semitendinosus, the belly of the semimembranosus and its membranous attachment to the ischial tuberosity are easily recognized. Its distal attachment to the tibia is overlapped by the gastrocnemius, one of the calf muscles, and must be left obscured from view, meantime. Figure 269, (*Grant's Atlas of Anatomy*), in which the gastrocnemius is cut away, shows how the distal tendon of semimembranosus reinforces the capsule of the knee joint.

ITEM 50-11.   Now identify the long head of the biceps femoris, a bulky muscle deep to which the sciatic nerve disappears. By finger dissection mobilize the muscle proximally to the ischial tuberosity. Then, distally, identify the short head arising from the femoral shaft and, next, the tendon of the entire muscle proceeding to the head of the fibula. Leave the fibular attachment until you dissect the knee joint.

ITEM 50-12.   Establish now where the division of the sciatic nerve occurs on your specimen. The nerve divides into medial popliteal and lateral popliteal parts. In the anatomic nomenclature (1966), however, these two parts are renamed the tibial nerve and common peroneal nerve. Many clinicans still use the former terminology. Accordingly, the new names are used here and the old names are included in parentheses.

The division may occur anywhere between the pelvis and the popliteal fossa. Identify the common peroneal (lateral popliteal) nerve and trace it distally to the posterior aspect of the head of the fibula. Its further course will be studied in the leg.

Now trace the tibial (medial popliteal) nerve into the popliteal fossa, where it gives off several distinct branches that form a superficial barrier to entry into the popliteal fossa. Besides, there is usually a considerable pad of fat in the fossa. Do not delay over the branches of the tibial (medial popliteal) nerve at this time. Later, when the gastrocnemius is split, the branches are more readily seen.

REGIONS OF THE THIGH

Review the three compartments and their muscles. Reconstruct the following regions, the femoral triangle, the subsartorial canal, and the popliteal fossa.

The femoral triangle is bounded superiorly by the inguinal liga-ment, laterally by the sartorius, and medially by the medial border of the adductor longus. The iliopsoas, pectineus, and adductor longus lie in the floor.

The subsartorial canal is bounded posteriorly by the adductor longus and magnus, anterolaterally by the vastus medialis, and antero-medially by the sartorius.

The popliteal fossa in bounded superiorly by the biceps femoris laterally, and the semimembranosus and semitendinosus medially; in-feriorly by the two heads of the gastrocnemius. The femoral shaft and the posterior aspect of the knee joint form the floor of the fossa.

The adductor hiatus connects the subsartorial canal to the popliteal fossa.

These three regions, where the major blood vessels may be quite easily exposed, are key regions in vascular surgery. What are the prin-cipal nerves and vessels of each region?

Chapter 51

Review of the Major Blood Vessels of the Thigh

You are reminded that the femoral arteries are named here ac-cording to the terminology of the vascular surgeon. If necessary, refer to Figure 48-2. Throughout the three principal regions of the thigh, the major vein and major artery have a varying relationship to each other. If you read individual accounts of each region you will be confounded. Therefore, beforehand, study Figure 51-1 and then study a specimen; you may find that your specimen does not match the Figure, so use the Figure only as a guide.

ITEM 51-1. Mobilize the vessels from the inguinal region to the popliteal fossa.

ITEM 51-2. At the apex of the femoral triangle, where the common femoral artery bifurcates into the superficial and deep femoral arteries, a significant grouping of arteries and veins occurs. In the fork created by the bifurcation of the common femoral artery, the superficial femoral vein and the deep femoral vein join. The two veins lie within the fork so that an artery-vein-vein-artery relationship exists. The vessels lie one behind the other, and all four may be transfixed by a knife. An

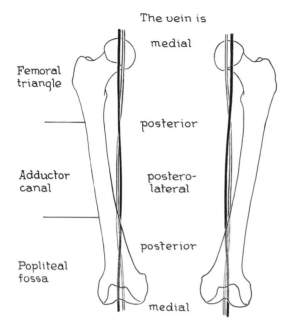

Figure 51-1. With the aid of a composite diagram, it is easy to understand the changing relationships of the major vein of the thigh to the major artery.

accident of this kind is common enough among butchers; thus the apex of the femoral triangle came to be known as butcher's point.

HUNTER'S CANAL

An observation by John Hunter, a surgeon and anatomist of the eighteenth century, has illuminated for all time the anatomy of the mid-thigh. John Hunter, realizing that the popliteal artery was simply the continuation of the superficial femoral artery, observed that the latter is more accessible than the former. Thereafter, when he had to ligate the popliteal artery in the treatment of popliteal aneurysm Hunter ligated the vessel in the subsartorial canal, i.e., before the vessel passes through the adductor hiatus and not after. Thus the subsartorial canal became known as Hunter's Canal. With this historic fact in mind, reexamine the course of the superficial femoral artery deep to the sartorius, thence through the adductor hiatus, to be renamed the popliteal artery.

ITEM 51-3. In the vicinity of the bifurcation of the common femoral artery, identify the medial and lateral circumflex femoral arteries. Where do they arise?

ITEM 51-4. The adductor longus has already been peeled laterally to expose the adductor brevis. Peel the adductor longus further toward the femoral shaft to expose the deep femoral artery and to observe how the artery tapers to its end near the adductor hiatus. Look for at least one perforating artery (three are described), leaving the deep femoral artery to encircle the femoral shaft. The perforating arteries pass through tendinous arches in the femoral attachment of the other adductors, hence the description perforating. They supply most of the blood to the posterior femoral compartment.

In mobilizing the popliteal artery you will expose genicular arteries that encircle the skeleton in the neighborhood of the knee joint. Do not delay over the genicular arteries, even though they are of some importance in the arterial anastomoses of the limb.

AN ARTERIAL ANASTOMOSIS

Trace the descending branch of the lateral circumflex femoral artery into vastus lateralis. Distally, this vessel anastomoses with the lateral superior genicular artery, but you may not see this in your specimen. This alternate channel, although small, can transmit blood to distal parts in event of chronic occlusion of the superficial femoral artery.

It is evident that the occlusion must be distal to the origin of the lateral circumflex femoral artery and proximal to the origin of the lateral superior genicular artery for this anastomosis to be effective. What other possible anastomoses are present in the thigh and gluteal region?

ARTERIAL DISTRIBUTION

Now is the time to establish with you a concept of the extent of the distribution of an artery. Too much emphasis is often placed upon the position and relationships of an artery, while too little emphasis is placed upon all the tissues the artery supplies—and there are many such tissues. It may be stated quite simply that all tissues of the body require the nourishment of arterial blood. The amount of nourishment depends, above all, upon their metabolic rate, which in turn depends upon their function. Thus an artery, especially in a limb, may be expected to supply skin, fat, muscle, tendon, bone and joint, and nerve as well as microscopic branches to nourish its very own walls. Branches to all these different tissues may be found in the course of the dissection of a limb. Branches to bone and bone marrow are referred to as nutrient arteries. To see an artery to a nerve, look closely at the sciatic nerve for the arteria comitans nervi ischiadici; all nerves have similar arteries. Finally it is not generally recognized that tendons, thick and solid though they are, require a modicum of blood for survival; deprive a tendon of its blood supply and it will degenerate. Without doubt, knowledge of these facts will increase your awareness of the endless distribution of the arterial system.

THE STRUCTURE OF AN ARTERY

Make a longitudinal slit in the superficial femoral artery at a point proximal to the adductor hiatus. Extend the slit proximally toward the groin and clean out all debris within the artery so that you have a perfect view of the tunica intima that lines the lumen of the vessel. Its normal structure and function and its diseases are under intensive investigation today because of the high incidence of occlusive arterial disease.

Next examine the longitudinal section of the arterial wall; external to the tunica intima lies the tunica media and then the tunica adventitia. That the tunica media is composed of muscle and elastic fibers is best determined with a microscope.

An extract from the writings of John Hunter shows that the microscope is not always essential for good observation. In John Hunter's time microscopes were rare. Nonetheless, he wrote as follows:

From the account we have given of those substances which compose an artery, we may perceive it has two powers, the one elastic and the other muscular. We see also that the larger arteries are principally endowed with the elastic power, and the smaller with the muscular, the elastic is always diminishing in the smaller, and the muscular increasing...

Quaint in style, John Hunter's treatise on arteries, based on what he saw when he cut the arteries of an animal, still alive, or of a human, recently dead, is enjoyable and instructive reading (Clinical Orthopaedics, No. 28).

Chapter 52

The Deep Fascia, Retinacula, and Synovial Sheaths of the Leg

Figure 52-1, a cross section of leg, shows how the deep fascia is attached to the anterior and posteromedial borders of the tibia and forms an external investment to the leg. From the investing layer, several septa create compartments bounded by fascia and bone. In the forthcoming stages of dissection you will explore the contents of each compartment.

In the leg the compartment mentioned most often clinically is the

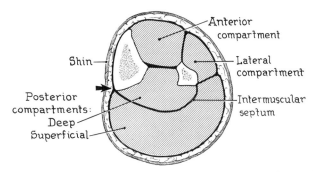

Figure 52-1.   Cross section of the leg. The black arrow indicates the junction at which several perforating veins are usually located.

anterior tibial compartment, for the following reason: In the living the deep fascia is tense, not slack; the muscles are full, not shrunken. Sometimes, as in the management of swelling of the muscles of the forearm (p. 441), it is necessary to incise the deep fascia of the anterior tibial compartment (fasciotomy) to safeguard the underlying muscles from the effects of increased pressure. If fasciotomy is not done the pressure may increase to a degree that the muscles perish. To understand how serious this is the student should consult an orthopedic textbook for an account of the anterior tibial syndrome.

RETINACULUM

The various retinacula, described in the region of the ankle joint, are portrayed in vivid lines in anatomic illustrations, yet they can scarcely be seen on a cadaver. A retinaculum is a thickening of deep fascia deep to which minor septa create compartments for tendons. Thus it would seem the purpose of a retinaculum is to prevent excessive displacement of tendons. There is an extensor retinaculum superior to the anterior aspect of the ankle joint and another inferior; presumably they help to prevent bowstringing of the extensor tendons across the anterior aspect of the ankle joint. A flexor retinaculum prevents the flexor tendons from slipping anteriorly over the medial malleolus. A peroneal retinaculum prevents the peroneal tendons from slipping anteriorly over the lateral malleolus. In a cadaver retinacula are not easily identified on examination of the external aspect of the deep fascia. Their existence can be appreciated when they are cut during the opening of the fascio-osseous compartments. Then the retinacular compartments will be revealed.

ITEM   52-1.   Moisten the deep fascia around the ankle joint, and then, with the fingers, smooth the fascia on the anterior, lateral, and medial aspects of the ankle joint. Generally this maneuver demonstrates the whiteness of the retinacula, but do not be disappointed if the retinacula are not demonstrable.

SYNOVIAL SHEATHS

There are many synovial sheaths around the ankle. Although a synovial sheath is quite long, usually, the principle of the sheath can be demonstrated best with the aid of a ballon (Fig. 52-2). Press a pencil into a partially inflated balloon until the balloon completely envelops the pencil (Fig. 52-2B). The pencil represents a tendon, the balloon a synovial sheath. Figure 52-2C demonstrates how the tendon obtains a visceral and a parietal layer of synovial sheath; the potential cavity between them is distended with air, for normally visceral and parietal layers are adjacent, separated only by a thin film of fluid. Figure 52-2C also demonstrates the mesotendon whereby minute blood vessels reach the tendon without penetrating the synovial sheath. Figure 52-2D reveals how the synovial sheath is closed at each end, an arrangement that can be easily understood by referring to Figure 52-2B.

Distention of synovial sheaths may be achieved by the injection of air, liquid, or latex. Clinically, distention of a synovial sheath with fluid is not uncommon; synovitis is frequently associated with an unusual amount of wrist or ankle work, e.g., snow shoveling or hiking, but it sometimes occurs because of a bacterial infection.

To demonstrate each synovial sheath around the ankle (or wrist) in the gross anatomy laboratory is time-consuming and not too successful. Fortunately, anatomic illustrations of them are plentiful and clearly illustrate their shape and extent. You should be able to visualize the precise location of the synovial sheaths on your own ankle or wrist. Then as your experience grows you will be able to recognize clinically that a sausage-shaped swelling set longitudinally across a joint is more than likely a distended synovial sheath. Clinicians will advise you of the additional pointers to clinch the diagnosis.

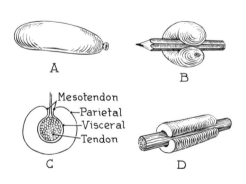

A

B

Mesotendon
Parietal
Visceral
Tendon

C   D

Figure 52-2. The basic principle of a synovial sheath. See text.

Chapter 53

The Leg

Introduction

The following text must be read before the dissection proceeds. As in the thigh, in the leg the key to understanding the layout is a knowledge of the location and nomenclature of the muscle groups. In the leg, fascial septa create four compartments, namely the anterior, lateral, superficial posterior, and deep posterior. Figure 52-1 shows their locations.

The muscles of the anterior compartment are the tibialis anterior (Fig. 53-1), extensor hallucis longus, and extensor digitorum longus (and sometimes a small muscle called peroneus tertius). These muscles are powerful extensors of the ankle joint and of the toes; more commonly they are described as dorsiflexors. Dorsiflexion, which is an alternate name for extension, is the upward movement of the foot that occurs with every footstep as the leg is swung forward and the heel strikes the ground. The power of the dorsiflexors is clearly seen when a person stands on his heels.

The superficial group of posterior leg muscles includes the gastrocnemius and soleus, which are inserted into the tendo Achillis; they are frequently referred to as the calf muscles. The deep group of posterior leg muscles includes the tibialis posterior, flexor hallucis longus, and flexor digitorum longus. In general, all these muscles in action flex the ankle — in other words they act to point the toes to the ground; they are plantar flexors, plantar flexion being the term opposite to dorsiflexion.

The lateral group of muscles includes the peroneus longus and

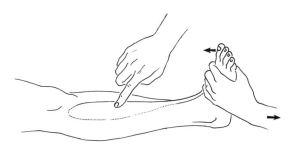

Figure 53-1. A quick method of testing muscle power. The patient is bending his foot up while the doctor resists the movement. Normally the muscle belly and tendon of tibialis anterior become very prominent, as they are here. In assessing the power of any muscle, the influence of gravity upon the moving part must be taken into account.

259

brevis. They evert the foot so that the sole of the foot faces laterally, a movement termed eversion. Thus this muscle group is frequently referred to as the evertors.

The opposite movement to eversion is inversion. During inversion, the foot is twisted so that the sole faces medially; when both feet are inverted the soles face each other. Inversion or eversion occur to a lesser but nonetheless significant degree when, with each step, the foot twists slightly to accommodate to the terrain. The invertor muscle group, however, is not isolated in a discreet compartment but includes the tibialis anterior of the anterior compartment and the tibialis posterior of the deep posterior compartment.

Exercise

On your own leg, at some convenient time, palpate the malleoli, the anterior border and the broad subcutaneous anteromedial surface of the tibia; all of them are subcutaneous. Dorsiflex the foot and feel the anterior tibial muscles. Raise the heels off the ground and feel the muscles of the superficial posterior compartment. Evert the foot and feel the muscles of the lateral compartment. Finally invert the foot, first in the dorsiflexed position and second in the plantar flexed position, and palpate the tendons of tibialis anterior (anterior compartment muscle) and tibialis posterior (deep posterior compartment muscle).

ITEM 53-1. Make a longitudinal incision into the fascia of the anterior and lateral compartments. Reflect the fascia and identify the septa and the muscle group in each compartment.

The deep fascia of the posterior compartment has already been incised when the perforating veins were explored. Complete the removal of the fascia from the muscles of the superficial posterior compartment. Leave the intermediate septum between the superficial and deep posterior compartments undisturbed.

NERVES ENTERING THE LEG

Two major nerves enter the leg to supply the muscles of the four compartments. The common peroneal (lateral popliteal) nerve supplies both the lateral compartment and the anterior compartment. To do so it divides into the superficial peroneal (musculo cutaneous) nerve and the deep peroneal (anterior tibial) nerve.

The tibial (medial popliteal) nerve supplies both the superficial and deep posterior compartments, and eventually the sole of the foot.

ITEM 53-2. Return to the division of the sciatic nerve and identify the common peroneal (lateral popliteal) nerve. Trace the nerve distally posterior to the head of the fibula. Just beyond the neck of the fibula the nerve divides into the superficial peroneal (musculocutaneous) nerve supplying the muscles of the peroneal compartment and the deep peroneal (anterior tibial) nerve supplying the muscles of the anterior tibial compartment. The division occurs in the superior portion of the peroneus longus and will not be seen until fascia and muscle are torn asunder. The division is exposed later in the dissection.

The tibial (medial popliteal) nerve travels through the popliteal fossa from where it innervates the superficial group of the posterior leg muscles. Trace the nerve through the popliteal fossa and observe its branches. Its course through the deep compartments, where it supplies the muscles, will come to light later, as well as its ultimate division into the medial and lateral plantar nerves that innervate the muscles of the sole of the foot.

THE MAJOR ARTERY ENTERING THE LEG

The popliteal artery, which is the continuation of the femoral artery, passes through the popliteal fossa to enter the leg. Soon thereafter the main arterial stem gives off the anterior tibial artery, then the posterior tibial artery, and finally continues to its termination as the peroneal artery. Each of these arteries nourishes the muscles in its respective compartment, but it should be noted that the gastrocnemius and soleus are nourished by vessels arising directly from the popliteal artery. The posterior tibial artery proceeds to the sole of the foot. The anterior tibial artery proceeds to the dorsum of the foot.

THE MAJOR VEIN LEAVING THE LEG

The arteries throughout the leg are accompanied by veins, the venae comitantes, usually two in number and intimately related to the arteries. Ultimately, these accompanying veins join in the popliteal fossa to form the one massive popliteal vein, which continues on as the femoral vein.

Now that you are aware of the muscle groups of the leg and have recognized the major nerves and vessels entering or leaving the leg you are ready to explore the muscle compartments.

Chapter 54

Exploration of the Muscle
Compartments of the Leg

The muscle compartments of the leg are: (1) the superficial posterior compartment, (2) the medial side of the leg and the deep posterior
compartment, (3) the peroneal compartment, and (4) the anterior tibial
compartment.

THE SUPERFICIAL POSTERIOR COMPARTMENT

ITEM 54-1.   By blunt dissection mobilize the two heads of the gastrocnemius. Separate them from the underlying soleus. Then establish
how the gastrocnemius and soleus merge to form the robust tendo
Achillis. Clear away all fat and fascia on the anterior aspect of the tendo
Achillis in order to expose the transverse intermuscular septum. Split
the gastrocnemius vertically in its middle to obtain a clearer view of the
neurovascular structures emerging from or entering the popliteal fossa.
These structures will become much more obvious in the next step of the
dissection.

THE MEDIAL SIDE OF THE LEG AND THE DEEP POSTERIOR
COMPARTMENT

With the exception of the peroneus longus, all the structures destined to pass into the sole of the foot do so on the medial side of the
ankle, where they lie posterior to the medial malleolus. The order of
structures at that location are the tendon of the tibialis posterior, the
tendon of flexor digitorum longus, the posterior tibial artery and its
accompanying veins, the tibial nerve, and the flexor hallucis longus,
named from medial to lateral within the flexor retinaculum.

A concentration of structures such as this and the ease with which
the calf and the sole of the foot can be opened and explored allow an
excellent opportunity to demonstrate the continuity of these structures
from the level of the knee to the toes. Below the knee those structures
lie, first, deep to the soleus, second, deep to the transverse septum of
fascia, third, deep to the flexor retinaculum, and fourth, deep to the

abductor hallucis, the muscle that lies along the medial side of the foot. The following steps, then, are the order of dissection.

ITEM 54-2. Identify the soleus "bridge" (A. K. Henry, 1957) between the fibula and the tibia. The popliteal artery and the tibial nerve disappear deep to soleus. They pass beneath the soleus bridge. Carefully, so as not to damage underlying structures, detach the soleus from the tibia and expose the underlying vessels and nerve. Pull the soleus posteriorly to expose the transverse intermuscular septum covering the flexor digitorum longus and the flexor hallucis longus, and between them the tibialis posterior; the tibial nerve and the posterior tibial vessels are also in view.

ITEM 54-3. Split the transverse intermuscular septum in the line of the vessels. Reflect the septum, identify the muscles, and trace the muscles to their tendons, which are located on the posteromedial aspect of the medial malleolus. In doing so do not lacerate the vessels and nerve.

ITEM 54-4. The trifurcation of the popliteal artery is an important landmark in vascular surgery; it is important to see its anatomy as it really is and not as it is portrayed in illustrations. It is convenient to study it now.

The main arterial stem gives off, first, the anterior tibial artery, which arises almost at right angles to proceed anteriorly from the anterior aspect of the stem. Mobilize the anterior tibial artery and, by using the closed-open scissors technique (Fig. 46-2), expose it as far as you can on its way anteriorly between the tibia and fibula to reach the anterior tibial compartment. Beyond the point of departure of the anterior tibial artery, the main arterial stem continues on to become the peroneal artery. On the way the posterior tibial artery arises from the medial aspect of the arterial stem. Confirm this, and realize that although the peroneal artery seems to be the major vessel because of its size and direction, it is indeed the posterior tibial artery that becomes the major vessel ultimately to supply the sole of the foot. The peroneal artery, then, usually tapers to an end in the vicinity of the ankle.

To do an intelligent dissection at this next stage, it is necessary to have a basic outline of the layers of the foot in mind. Therefore, while it would seem logical to open the flexor retinaculum next, it is best to proceed to the medial border of the foot. Read the following introduction first.

INTRODUCTION TO THE FOOT

The bones of the foot form a longitudinal arch into which the soft tissues of the sole are molded, a fact that is quite obvious when you examine the imprint of a wet foot on a dry floor. To see easily the bones

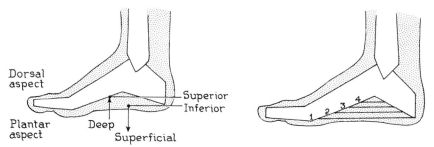

Figure 54-1.   In the sole of the foot, *superior* is equivalent to *deep* and *inferior* to *superficial* when the sole is dissected from the plantar aspect.

Figure 54-2.   The muscles of the foot are divided into four groups for descriptive purposes. The groups are numbered 1, 2, 3, and 4, from superficial (i.e., inferior) to deep (i.e., superior). In his dissection, the student will find that layers 3 and 4 are much further anterior than they are in this diagram.

that form the arch, examine the foot of a skeleton and identify the bones, beginning posteriorly with the calcaneum; next is the talus (taking part in the ankle joint), then the navicular, the three cuneiforms, and the three medial metatarsal bones; laterally the arch is completed by the cuboid and the lateral two metatarsal bones. The talus is the most superior bone of the arch; thus one can imagine the calcaneum as forming the posterior pillar of the arch and the remaining bones the anterior pillar. At a convenient time, examine your own foot and, by referring to a text on surface anatomy, identify the significant bony landmarks. Also, observe a footprint and note the areas where contact is made; the actual weight-bearing areas, however, are much smaller than a footprint indicates; most of the weight is distributed onto the anterior and posterior pillars.

In approaching the dissection of the sole of a foot, the terms superior and inferior must be clearly understood. As Figure 54-1 reveals, deep structures are superior to superficial structures. In other words, skin is the most inferior and also the most superficial part of the sole of the foot. These facts are important because the small muscles of the foot are described in four layers. It follows, then, that layer 1 is the most inferior or the most superficial, as is shown in Figure 54-2.

TWO TENDONS THAT CROSS EACH OTHER

A key landmark in the anatomy of the sole of the foot is the crossing of the tendon of the flexor digitorum longus inferior to the flexor hallucis longus. Figure 54-3 shows how the crossing comes about. The flexor digitorum longus arises from the medial side in the leg, but it is inserted into the lateral digits, whereas the flexor hallucis longus arises

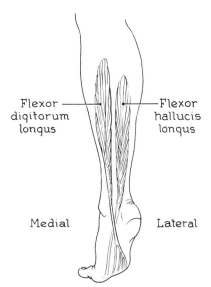

Figure 54-3.   The tendons of the flexor digitorum longus and flexor hallucis longus cross in the sole of the foot. The crossover is a major landmark of the second layer in the sole.

from the lateral side in the leg and is inserted into the big toe. The crossover occurs shortly after the tendons enter the sole of the foot.

Layer 2 is the key layer and consists of the crossover of the two tendons, the flexor hallucis longus and flexor digitorum longus; associated with them are two sets of small muscles.

Layer 1, superficial (inferior) to layer 2, and layer 3, deep (superior) to layer 2, each consist of three small muscles. Layer 4 is adjacent to the skeleton.

Figure 54-4 shows two small muscles, the abductor hallucis and flexor brevis hallucis, and indicates that one belongs to layer 1 and the other belongs to layer 3 — yes, layer 3. Why? Your dissection will shortly reveal that the flexor hallucis brevis lies superior to the tendon of the flexor hallucis longus, which belongs to layer 2. Thus, the flexor hallucis

Figure 54-4.   Medial aspect of the foot. Structures entering the sole of the foot pass deep to the abductor hallucis.

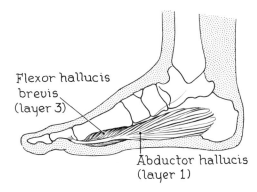

brevis is allocated to layer 3, although it "pouts" medially to lie in a subcutaneous and obvious position. Review the above points carefully, and then proceed with the dissection and see for yourself.

Remove the skin from the dorsum and sole of the foot. Removal of the skin from the toes of a cadaver is time-consuming. Skin the big toe only.

THE WEIGHT-BEARING AREAS OF THE FOOT

The two weight-bearing areas are the heel and the heads of the metatarsal bones. The superficial fascia covering these areas is usually overlooked by the junior student in the urgency of a cadaveric dissection. Yet the fascia is recognized as important by orthopedic surgeons because of its cushion-like action, especially when the full weight of the body is borne by one limb. Examine the fascia: observe that it is like sponge rubber with fat instead of air in the spaces; recognize that the function of the superficial fascia is to cushion the tread.

ITEM 54-5. Remove the superficial fascia, but be careful not to lacerate the deep fascia, represented by the plantar aponeurosis, and the adjacent small muscles of the sole of the foot.

ITEM 54-6. Establish the attachment of abductor hallucis to the flexor retinaculum and to the calcaneum. Then trace the straplike tendon of the abductor hallucis anteriorly, where it lies superficial to the flexor hallucis brevis (Fig. 54-4). Mobilize the tendon, and in doing so establish the plane of cleavage between the flexor hallucis brevis and the abductor hallucis muscles. Separation may require a little skillful dissection, but proceed cautiously until the flexor can be retracted superiorly and the abductor inferiorly to expose the two long flexor tendons (Fig. 54-3). Wiggling the big toe and the digits will reveal their position. By cutting what A. K. Henry* describes as the master knot you will expose the tendons fully. Once you have exposed the crossing of the tendons, do not explore the foot further, for your exploration can be more successful after the next stage of dissection.

Return now to the flexor retinaculum and slit it to expose the bifurcation of the posterior tibial artery and nerve deep to the retinaculum and the retinacular attachment of the abductor hallucis.

In the cadaver it is often necessary to detach the abductor hallucis completely in order to get an adequate exposure of the structures in the sole of the foot. Do so if necessary.

ITEM 54-7. Trace the medial plantar vessels and nerve anteriorly. They lie between layers 1 and 2 and terminate in muscular and cutaneous branches to the sole and to the big toe and its neighboring digit.

---

*Extensile Exposure. Edinburgh, E. & S. Livingstone Ltd., 1957.

ITEM 54-8.   The lateral plantar artery and nerve pass to the lateral aspect of the foot between layers 1 and 2. To demonstrate their course, slip unopened curved scissors along the direction of the vessels and nerve. Opening and closing the scissors, insinuate them as far laterally as you can. Then, leaving the scissors in position to protect the vessels and nerve, cut the plantar aponeurosis and flexor digitorum brevis and whatever fascia is necessary to reveal the vessels and nerve. Peel the distal part of the aponeurosis and the flexor digitorum brevis toward the toes to improve your exposure. In doing so you will see, in full view, the quadratus plantae muscle joining the tendon of the flexor digitorum longus, and, between the tendons of that flexor, the lumbricales. Furthermore, you will see how the flexor hallucis longus tendon rests on the undersurface of the flexor hallucis brevis.

ITEM 54-9.   Review the second layer of the sole of the foot by identifying the tendons of the flexor hallucis longus, the flexor digitorum longus, and the small muscles, the quadratus plantae (also called flexor accessorius) and the lumbricales.

ITEM 54-10.   Confirm the muscles of the first layer, three in number, namely the abductor hallucis, flexor digitorum brevis, and abductor digiti minimi. Then confirm that the lateral plantar vessels and nerve proceed laterally between layers 1 and 2.

ITEM 54-11.   Deep to, i.e., superior to, layer 2 is the third layer of muscles. Do not delay on their precise attachments, but identify the flexor hallucis brevis and note its relationship to the tendon of the flexor hallucis longus; identify also the adductor hallucis and the flexor digiti minimi brevis.

ITEM 54-12.   Layer 4 of the muscles of the foot consists of the interossei. In your present dissection, some of them lie inferior to the metatarsal bones and are partially exposed, lying between the flexor digiti minimi brevis laterally and the adductor hallucis. The term interossei (between bones), therefore, is misleading, but in the main the interossei do lie between the metatarsal bones. Do not delay on the interossei of the foot. A study of the interossei is best left until you dissect the hand, for the interossei of the hand and foot are similar but not exactly alike.

ITEM 54-13.   Also included in the fourth layer is the tendon of the peroneus longus and the tibialis posterior. The tendon of the peroneus longus will be traced once the peroneal compartment has been explored.

EXPLORATION OF THE MUSCLES OF THE PERONEAL COMPARTMENT

Identify the muscle belly and tendon of both the peroneus brevis and longus. The tendon of the peroneus brevis lies nearer to the lateral malleolus and terminates on the lateral side of the foot, distal to the calcaneocuboid joint. Trace the tendon to its termination. The tendon of the peroneus longus enters a groove on the inferior surface of the cuboid and crosses the sole of the foot. Trace the tendon of the peroneus longus across the sole of the foot. Cut the fascia and ligaments as needed. A sesamoid bone or a fibrocartilaginous thickening occurs in the tendon of peroneus longus, where it is related to the lateral aspect of the cuboid.

SESAMOID BONES

In the interpretation of radiographs, particularly of the foot, it is necessary to be aware of the existence of sesamoid bones. Sesamoid means "like a sesame seed." Sesamoid bones are radiopaque, small in size, and, on a radiograph, are seen to lie a few millimeters from an adjacent definitive bone. Accordingly, on a radiograph taken after an accident, a sesamoid bone may be mistaken by the novice for a fragment of bone.

Sesamoid bones occur in the foot (and in the hand), usually in pairs, and they lie adjacent to the metatarso (metacarpo) phalangeal joints and sometimes to the interphalangeal joints. Although their function is obscure, their existence must be kept in mind in the interpretation of radiographs of the foot and hand.

EXPLORATION OF THE MUSCLES OF THE ANTERIOR TIBIAL COMPARTMENT

ITEM 54-14. Before you disturb the muscles, observe that the muscle bellies of the tibialis anterior (which lies next to the tibia) and of the extensor digitorum longus (which obscures the fibula from view) are adjacent. Superior to the ankle joint, however, the tendon of the extensor hallucis longus is interposed between the tendons of those two other muscles. Thus, the belly of the extensor hallucis longus is obscured from view by the bellies of those two other muscles. These facts are of importance when you seek the vessels and nerve of the anterior compartment.

ITEM 54-15. To mobilize tibialis anterior muscle belly, remain close to the surface of the muscle until you establish the plane of cleavage between it and the extensor hallucis longus.

ITEM 54-16. Mobilize all the muscles of the anterior compartment and their tendons. Observe how the tibialis anterior is attached to the medial side of the foot distal to the talonavicular joint. Observe also that the tendon of the tibialis posterior, lying posterior to the medial mal-

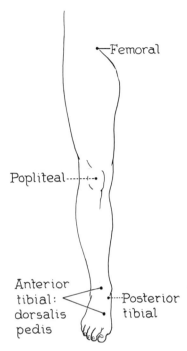

Figure 54-5. Pulse points. An essential step in the physical examination of each lower limb is to confirm the presence or absence of arterial pulsation.

leolus, has an almost parallel course and an almost similar attachment. These two muscles, one of the anterior compartment, one of the posterior compartment, are the principal muscles of the invertor group.

ITEM 54-17. Use the tendons to guide you to the correct plane of cleavage, and separate the tibialis anterior and the extensor hallucis longus to expose the anterior tibial artery entering the anterior compartment from a posterior direction. Establish its continuity with its parent stem in the posterior compartment. Observe its accompanying veins.

Trace the anterior tibial artery on to the dorsum of the foot where the artery is renamed the dorsalis pedis artery and confirm that the dorsalis pedis artery lies in the interval between the big toe and the second toe. It is an essential part of the clinical examination of the cardiovascular system to confirm the pulsations of this artery and of the posterior tibial artery, where it lies posterior to the medial malleolus (Fig. 54-5).

THE COMMON PERONEAL NERVE

Clinical experience dictates that the importance of the relationship of the common peroneal (lateral popliteal) nerve to the neck of the fibula cannot be overstressed. The nerve is vulnerable to pressure at this location, and must be safeguarded in the application of plaster casts to this region of the limb. The precise technique for safeguarding the nerve will be taught by your clinical tutors. Meantime, return to the nerve and study its anatomy.

ITEM 54-18. Trace the common peroneal (lateral popliteal) nerve from the shelter of the biceps tendon across the head of the fibula. Then, using the closed-open scissors technique, open up the pathway of the nerve through the peroneus longus. Slit the peroneus longus. Clear away all tissue until you establish the division of the nerve into its superficial peroneal (musculocutaneous) and deep peroneal (anterior tibial) parts. Then establish which muscles are supplied by each part.

Realize that if the common peroneal (lateral popliteal) nerve is damaged then the muscles of both the anterior crural and lateral crural compartments will be paralyzed. As a result, the main disability is the lack of dorsiflexion of the foot, which is spoken of clinically as dropped foot. Commentary upon this crippling condition is included in the discussion of gait.

Chapter 55

What to Look for or Consider in Dissecting a Synovial Joint

In dissecting a joint, there are certain structures that are immediately obvious and other structures that can only be displayed by meticulous dissection or by microscopic examination.

The first obvious structure is the capsule, which in this context refers to the fibrous sleeve that envelopes a joint. The shape of the sleeve depends on the shape of the joint. To give an example, the shape of the capsule of the hip joint (Fig. 55-1) has been likened to a windsock seen at an airport. One margin of the capsule of the hip joint is attached around the acetabulum, the other around the neck of the femur. Although the capsules of the knee and ankle joints have the same principle in design and attachment, they are not the same shape. It is important to realize that in some joints the anatomic capsule is hidden from view by ligaments that reinforce the external surface of the capsule.

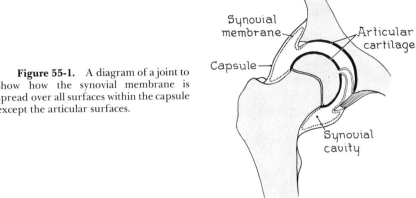

Figure 55-1. A diagram of a joint to show how the synovial membrane is spread over all surfaces within the capsule except the articular surfaces.

The presence of a joint capsule means that a bone has intracapsular and extracapsular parts and, on this basis, fractures may be classified as intra- or extracapsular. Moreover, intracapsular bone may be articular and, therefore, covered by articular cartilage, or nonarticular, covered by periosteum; intracapsular fractures that break the articular surface can have particularly serious consequences.

The internal aspect of the capsule is lined by a synovial membrane, but the membrane is not confined to the capsule. Indeed, it is spread over all surfaces within the capsule except the actual articular surfaces. That synovial membrane disappears at the edge of the articular cartilage is worth emphasizing (Fig. 55-1). Thus, a synovial cavity is lined partly by synovial membrane and partly by articular cartilage. It follows that a synovial cavity and a serous cavity are different. In what way?

The synovial membrane is easily recognized once the joint cavity is opened. The membrane has a smooth surface that gleams with a coating of synovial fluid, slimy to touch, like the white of an egg. Although under normal conditions there is scarcely more than 1.0 ml. of synovial fluid in any human joint, you must appreciate that, today, the bio-chemistry of synovial fluid is studied in detail because of its tremendous significance in the mechanics of a normal joint and in articular disease.

Adult articular cartilage is interesting in that it is devoid of nerves, blood vessels, and lymphatics. Nevertheless, articular cartilage does not lack a source of nourishment. There is evidence that synovial fluid provides most of the nourishment required.

Furthermore, on microscopic examination, articular cartilage is seen to lack mitotic cells which are so characteristic of growth, maintenance, and repair. Thus it is not surprising that articular cartilage is slow to heal. Occasionally, evidence that articular cartilage does not regenerate quickly is found in the gross anatomy laboratory. Accordingly, it is recommended that in due time you examine carefully the articular cartilage of each joint and look for erosions, small irregular depressions on otherwise smooth articular surfaces. The cause of erosions is obscure.

Finally, in some joints there are intraarticular structures that are obvious once a joint is opened.

The structures that are difficult to reveal except by special techniques are nerves, blood vessels, and lymphatics. The nerves are sensory. One group of sensory nerves conveys impulses to the central nervous system so that at the level of consciousness one may be aware of the exact position of a joint or of movement in a joint. Such impulses, which arise in joints and also in muscles, tendons, and bones, are termed proprioceptive. When nerve fibers conveying proprioceptive impulses are destroyed the awareness of the exact position or movement of a joint is lost. A second group of nerves, profuse in number, is believed to be concerned with pain, and their presence no doubt explains why, for example, pain is experienced in a joint when its capsule or ligaments are torn or stretched excessively.

The close interrelationship of sensory supply to a joint and the motor supply to muscles controlling the joint was realized by John Hilton in 1863. He realized that the nerve supply to a joint was not obtained at random but as follows:

> The same trunks of nerves whose branches supply the groups of muscles moving a joint also furnish a distribution of nerves to the skin over the insertions of the same muscles, and—what at the moment more especially merits our attention—the interior of the joint receives its nerves from the same source.

Since John Hilton wrote those words in his book, *Rest and Pain*, little has changed, except that it is now known that synovial membrane is relatively insensitive to painful stimuli, whereas the capsule and ligaments are highly sensitive. Even so, that quotation, known as Hilton's Law, is still valid.

That small arteries are plentiful in the capsule and ligaments of a joint and that arteries are copious in the synovial membrane are well known facts. The role of capsular vessels, however, is obscure, even though it is clear that they are in large measure the source of blood to intracapsular bone. On the other hand, the copious blood supply to synovial membrane is to be expected, for the prime purpose of the membrane is the production and absorption of synovial fluid. The arteries are accompanied by veins that drain an extensive capillary plexus, mainly in the synovial membrane but also in the capsule. Lymphatic vessels from a synovial joint are profuse and eventually drain to regional nodes.

In conclusion of this brief summary of some of the main features to be sought in dissecting a joint, it is recommended to the student who wishes to study synovial joints in depth that he read *Synovial Joints, Their Structure and Mechanics* by Barnett, Davies, and MacConaill (1961).

Dissection of Joints

Although dissection of joints is a destructive procedure because all tissues related to each joint must be removed to expose the capsule and ligaments, it can be a most instructive procedure to the student who identifies significant structures and gives them some consideration before removing them. Also, it is a good idea to dissect the joints of one limb only, leaving the other limb for review. Detailed instructions for the removal of all soft tissue will not always be given. The student must use his initiative to see that an adequate exposure of the joint is obtained.

Chapter 56

Dissection of the Hip Joint

The hip joint is completely surrounded by muscles, some of them quite small. Accordingly, exposure of the hip joint is difficult; because of this, orthopedic surgeons have devised various surgical approaches to the hip, which also take into account the presence of the sciatic nerve posteriorly and the femoral nerve and vessels anteriorly. These approaches are not described here, however, for they are fully described in standard orthopedic texts, which should be consulted for further detail. Here, only a step by step anatomic dissection of the soft tissues around the hip joint is described.

Today it is quite common to substitute a prosthesis for a head of femur or an acetabulum, or both, when they are distorted by disease. Accordingly, in the course of your dissection give some consideration to all that is involved in prosthetic surgery of the hip.

ITEM 56-1. Taking into account the presence of the femoral nerve and vessels, begin to expose the hip joint anteriorly by dividing the psoas and iliacus within the pelvis. Then peel the distal part of the muscle inferiorly. Often, deep to the muscle, between it and the hip joint, there is a bursa that sometimes communicates with the synovial cavity. This may be so in your specimen. Peel the muscle distally to its attachment to the lesser trochanter.

Close to their pelvic attachments cut the sartorius, rectus femoris, and tensor fasciae latae. Make sure that the anterior aspect of the hip joint capsule is fully exposed. Usually one gets a good demonstration of the iliofemoral ligament at this stage of the dissection.

ITEM 56-2. Take note of the medial circumflex femoral artery. Trace it superior to the pectineus and the adductor group. This artery ultimately supplies the head of the femur.

ITEM 56-3. Close to the pelvis, cut the adductors: the pectineus, (the adductor longus has already been cut), adductor brevis, gracilis, and adductor magnus. To find the upper border of the adductor magnus easily, demonstrate the obturator externus by blunt dissection. The obturator externus lies on an essentially horizontal plane and the upper border of the adductor magnus can be quickly separated from it by blunt dissection. Make sure that the adductor magnus is cut right through. The hamstrings now lie exposed.

ITEM 56-4. Displace the sciatic nerve and cut the hamstrings close to the ischial tuberosity.

ITEM 56-5. To displace the hip abductors return to the region of the greater trochanter. By blunt dissection slip scissors or a probe inferior to the tendon of the obturator internus (and the gemelli), piriformis, and gluteus minimus. In other words, make a track for a gigli saw along the medial side of the greater trochanter (Fig. 56-1). With the saw, cut off the greater trochanter. Peel the trochanter and attached muscles proximally to expose the capsule of the hip joint. Sometimes the gluteus minimus is missed in this procedure; if so, cut it close to its attachment to the trochanter and peel it proximally.

ITEM 56-6. Cut the quadratus femoris close to the ischial tuberosity.

ITEM 56-7. To see the obturator externus to advantage, saw the femur across immediately distal to the lesser trochanter and divide all soft tissue of the thigh. The hip joint can now be examined with ease, and it is especially easy to trace the obturator externus muscle to its tendon. Observe the relationship of the tendon to the neck of the femur, and then cut the tendon.

ITEM 56-8. Maneuver the proximal segment of the femur and examine the movements of the hip joint. Examine especially the effect of movement on the iliofemoral ligament. What movement tenses the ligament most?

ITEM 56-9. Posteriorly, make an incision into the capsule, then cut it. Observe the thickness of the capsule anteriorly and the strong reinforcement from the iliofemoral ligament.

Greater trochanter

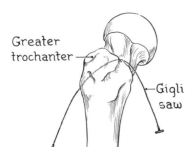

Gigli saw

Figure 56-1. View of the upper end of the femur with a gigli saw on the medial side of the greater trochanter.

ITEM 56-10. Gradually, as the capsule is cut, the head of the femur will become more obvious until you can dislocate it from its socket and reveal the ligamentum teres.

ITEM 56-11. Examine the acetabulum. Determine the principal weight-bearing area of the acetabulum. In what direction does the acetabulum face?

THE WEIGHT ON THE FEMORAL HEAD

With the head of the femur in the acetabulum, measure the horizontal distance from the center of the head to the symphysis pubis and to the tip of the trochanter (Fig. 56-2). In standing with one foot off the ground, the weight-bearing femoral head is a pivot and the lines PC and PB represent levers. The distance PC is approximately twice PB. Using the measurements PB and PC, and knowing the body weight, one can calculate the kilograms pressure imposed upon the femoral head. Methods of calculating the pressure vary and results differ, but it is clear that when one foot is off the ground the pressure exerted on the supporting femoral head may be as much as four to seven times the superimposed weight. When PB is decreased or PC increased the pressure exerted on the femoral head is increased.

ITEM 56-12. Identify the acetabular labrum, spoken of clinically as the limbus, which means margin. Observe how the synovial membrane lines the external surface of the limbus and how the capsule of the hip joint is attached to the base of the limbus, so creating a synovial pocket.

ITEM 56-13. Examine the neck of the femur and identify the synovial retinacula thereon. Deep to these retinacula lie the terminal

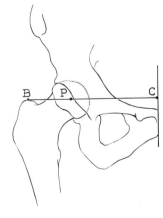

Figure 56-2. The measurements BP and PC are used to calculate the kilograms of pressure imposed on the femoral head. See text.

branches of the medial circumflex artery, en route to nourish the femoral head.

ITEM 56-14. Measure the angle of the femoral neck to the shaft. What is the normal angle? Examine an intact femur and note that the femoral head points anteriorly as well as medially in relation to a line transverse through the femoral condyles. This forward twist of the femoral shaft is spoken of as an anteversion. Measure the angle of anteversion. What is the normal angle? Both anteversion and the angle of the neck are important factors in the biomechanics of the hip joint.

THE BLOOD SUPPLY OF THE FEMORAL HEAD

The articular cartilage upon the head of the femur extends beyond the epiphyseal plate toward the shaft, so part of the metaphysis is included in the anatomic femoral head (Fig. 56-3). Accordingly, Trueta (1957) has classified the arterial supply of the femoral head into a metaphyseal and an epiphyseal group.

The metaphyseal arteries are in two groups, superior and inferior, and they are branches of the medial circumflex femoral artery. The epiphyseal arteries are also in two groups, medial, from the obturator artery, and lateral, from the medial circumflex femoral artery. Obviously, the medial circumflex femoral artery is an important source of blood to the femoral head. Moreover, Howe, Lacey, and Schwartz (1950) demonstrated that the lateral circumflex femoral artery supplies the neck and greater trochanter and contributes little to the vascularity of the actual femoral head.

That the blood supply of the femoral head varies with age has been clearly shown by Trueta (1957), whose paper should be consulted for further detail. It is sufficient to point out here that the possible effect upon the blood supply of the upper femoral epiphysis is seriously considered in nearly every clinical procedure involving the hip joint, no matter what the age of the patient, for the epiphysis is important both in the support of the body weight and in movements of the hip joint.

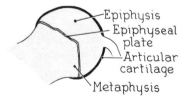

Figure 56-3. Diagram to show the relationship of the metaphysis to the epiphysis of the femoral head. Trueta (1957) classified the arteries supplying the femoral head as epiphyseal and metaphyseal.

Chapter 57

Dissection of the Knee Joint

It is unfortunate that the knee joint was ever described as a hinge joint, because the description has created the common impression that the tibia moves on the femur much the same way as a door swings on its hinges. This is not so. The door has fixed axis, the knee does not. In movement of the knee joint there is certainly an obvious hingelike component, but there are also less obvious gliding and rotatory components, so there is a constant shift of the axis of movement. In other words, the axis of movement present when the knee is almost straight differs from the one present when the knee is almost fully bent. The factors responsible for this shifting axis of movement are highly complex and can only be touched upon in the present context.

Furthermore, to describe the knee joint as a hinge joint gives an impression of stability that is wrong. The impression may be corrected immediately by examining the insecure articulation of the femur with the tibia of a skeleton. Clearly, on the basis of its skeletal structure, the knee cannot be considered a stable joint. Viewing the position of the joint between two long levers in a weight-bearing limb, one can readily appreciate the force the femur or the tibia can exert on the joint, especially in any athletic activity, in which the impetus of the body is added to the weight of the body itself. What stability there is, therefore, is due entirely to the surrounding stress-resisting structures, namely the knee joint ligaments and muscles.

In all studies of the function of the knee joint, it is recognized that a dissection of the knee joint is prerequisite to a study of function. Unfortunately, it is sometimes not easy to make a satisfactory dissection of some of the important ligaments of the knee in an embalmed cadaver. Embalming alters natural colors, causes fascial layers to stick together, and solidifies tissue that is readily dispersed in the living. Yet, in an embalmed cadaver, the main form of the ligaments can be seen. Accordingly, proceed to dissect the ligaments of the knee as follows, and, in doing so, be alert for evidence of injury or disease.

The Medial Aspect

ITEM 57-1. Reflection of Deep Fascia
The deep fascia on the medial side of the knee has already been disturbed by reflecting the sartorius, gracilis, and semitendinosus to

277

their attachments to the tibia. The conjuction of those attachments is referred to clinically as the pes anserina. Manipulate the pes anserina to demonstrate how it conjoins with the deep fascia. Then peel the pes anserina and adjacent deep fascia anteriorly towards the patella and the ligamentum patellae to reveal the underlying medial patellar retinaculum, known also as the quadriceps expansion. The retinaculum is an expansion from the medial vastus muscle to the tibia.

ITEM 57-2. The Medial Patellar Retinaculum and the Medial Ligament

Together they form a plane of aponeurotic tissue deep to the one formed by the deep fascia and the pes anserina. Having pulled the pes anserina well forward and the deep fascia well back, bend and straighten the knee joint to demonstrate how the retinaculum and the medial ligament conjoin. Sometimes, in a cadaver, the retinaculum adheres to the tibial condyle and so spoils the demonstration.

ITEM 57-3. The Medial Ligament

The superficial part of this ligament is separated from the pes anserina by a bursa.

Observe that the superifical part of the ligament is triangular, with its very long base anterior. The apex blends, posteriorly, with the capsule, just superior to where the semimembranosus tendon runs deep to the ligament. By bending and straightening the knee, demonstrate how the capsule fits like a hood over the medial femoral condyle. Note that the posterior part of the ligament becomes slack on flexion, whereas the vertical conspicuous anterior fibers remain taut. Demonstrate that the posterior part and the capsule become taut on full extension.

Cut the medial ligament at its inferior end and peel it superiorly to expose the deep fibers of the ligament spanning the interval between the femoral and tibial condyles. These deeper fibers are attached to the meniscus, which is a knee joint cartilage, still to be seen.

The Lateral Aspect

ITEM 57-4. The deep fascia on the lateral aspect is essentially the inferior part of the iliotibial band. Pull the band in various directions to demonstrate how the deep fascia blends with the lateral patellar retinaculum. Did you observe that the deep fascia on the lateral aspect blends with the patellar retinaculum, whereas on the medial aspect they form two distinct layers?

Move the patella and the lateral vastus from side to side and up and down to demonstrate how the lateral patellar retinaculum descends to its tibial attachment.

ITEM 57-5. The Lateral Ligament

Cut the biceps femoris muscle just superior to the knee joint and peel its tendon inferiorly toward the head of the fibula. Deep to (i.e., medial to) the tendon the cordlike lateral ligament will be easily exposed by scratching away extraneous tissue. Slip the tip of curved, blunt-ended scissors deep to the ligament to demonstrate how it stands aloof from the capsule of the knee joint. Bend and straighten the knee to demonstrate to some extent that the ligament is taut only in full extension.

The Anterior Aspect

ITEM 57-6. The quadriceps tendon, suprapatellar bursa, patellar retinacula, and ligamentum patellae are to be examined now.

Immediately superior to the patella, make a vertical incision, 10 cm. long, into the quadriceps tendon. Cut down to bone. Retract the edges of your incision and insert a fingertip into the suprapatellar bursa. Explore its superior limit. Then slide the finger inferiorly posterior to the patella to prove the continuity of the suprapatellar bursa and the cavity of the knee joint.

To demonstrate the ligamentum patellae, bend the knee and observe the stout band extending from the inferior apical end of the patella to the tibial tuberosity.

The next step is to cut the retinacula to open the joint so, first of all, revise the attachments of the retinacula.

ITEM 57-7. Opening the Knee Joint

On each side of the patella, make an incision to create a flap containing the patella. At this time the extent of the attachment of each vastus into the patella may be compared. Observe, in particular, that the muscular fibers of vastus medialis are attached to half the medial border of the patella. It is held that reduction in the length of this attachment is a significant factor in idiopathic lateral dislocation of the patella. Turn the flap down to expose the internal aspect of the patella. Examine that aspect and observe how it fits into the groove between the two femoral condyles. When the posterior surface of the patella is poorly defined the patella may be displaced easily from the femoral groove.

ITEM 57-8. Within the Knee Joint

Gently bend the knee. Usually one can demonstrate a central synovial strand that extends inferiorly from the intercondylar notch. In its descent the strand widens to form the alar folds that merge imperceptibly with infrapatellar fat pad. If a synovial strand is present, detach it and expose the anterior cruciate ligament. In a cadaver the strand is usually broken when the knee is forcibly flexed.

The Posterior Aspect

ITEM 57-9. To expose the capsule you must remove, but first identify, all the superficial structures at the back of the knee. Then pull on semimembranosus and observe the effect on the joint capsule. Next, on the tibia, identify the popliteus muscle and trace its fibers superiorly and laterally to its tendon, which disappears deep to the lateral ligament. Often a large part of popliteus is attached to the lateral meniscus, a knee joint cartilage to be fully exposed later. The tendon of the popliteus penetrates the capsule and is then attached to the lateral femoral condyle.

To demonstrate anatomically how the popliteus is concerned with rotation at the knee joint, rotate the femur one way and the tibia the opposite way and observe how the popliteus becomes taut or buckles. In life, the popliteus rotates the tibia medially upon the femur. The muscle also retracts the lateral meniscus during knee movements.

Now, to expose the posterior cruciate ligament, by blunt dissection break into the capsule. Almost immediately you will expose the posterior cruciate ligament. It *is* posterior and it ascends almost vertically from the tibia to the intercondylar surface of the medial femoral condyle. If you dissect with care you will demonstrate how two slips from the lateral meniscus join the posterior cruciate ligament. These anterior and posterior meniscofemoral ligaments are significant in guiding the lateral meniscus during the movement.

ITEM 57-10. The cruciate ligaments, however, are best exposed by splitting apart the femoral condyles (Fig. 57-1). It is recommended, therefore, that at alternate tables the condyles be split apart as in Fig. 57-1. Reexamine the cruciate ligaments, now that they are fully exposed. You can now appreciate how the two cruciate ligaments form a sort of septum that partially divides the knee joint into two parts. In other words, the knee joint is not truly a single joint.

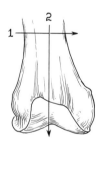
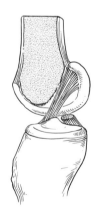

Figure 57-1. 1. The saw cut to mobilize the lower end of the femur. 2. The saw cut to separate the condyles and expose the cruciate ligaments. (In this specimen the posterior cruciate ligament has been cut and the medial condyle of the femur removed.)

STABILITY OF THE KNEE JOINT

For its stability, the knee joint depends upon the following (*not* listed in order of merit): the medial and lateral ligaments, the cruciate ligaments, the capsule, reinforced by expansions from adjacent tendons or muscle aponeuroses, and the activity of the surrounding muscles. A simple demonstration of one of those factors is as follows. Lift the right foot off the ground. Palpate the left quadriceps while you bend and stretch the left knee. What are your findings?

The next order of dissection is a demonstration of the stability provided by one of the ligaments of the knee.

ITEM 57-11. At those tables where the femur has not been split, demonstrate the importance of the anterior cruciate ligament as follows: Cut all soft tissues around the perimeter of the joint so that the cruciates alone hold the femur and tibia together. Next, with the knee joint in full extension, try to open the lateral aspect of the joint (Fig. 57-2), then the medial side. Repeat the test with the knee flexed to 45°. Finally, repeat the tests after dividing the anterior cruciate. What are your findings?

The test you have just performed in the laboratory is one of several clinical tests to review the integrity of the knee joint ligaments. The test is introduced here to demonstrate to you the principle of testing knee joint ligaments, namely by assessing the stability of the joint in a certain position while a certain stress is being applied. Because of the interrelationship of the cruciate ligaments and the medial and lateral ligaments with each other and with the capsule and retinacula during movements of the knee, the results of testing knee joint ligaments must be interpreted with care.

ITEM 57-12. To separate the femur from the tibia (do so on those

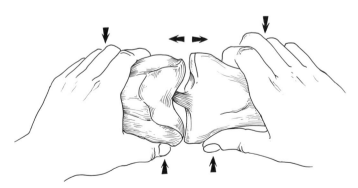

Figure 57-2. A demonstration of the principle utilized in testing the integrity of the knee joint ligaments. The arrows indicate the direction in which the thumbs and fingers press in order to open the lateral aspect of the joint.

specimens in which the anterior cruciate ligament is already cut) cut the posterior cruciate ligament. Examine the joint surfaces and the menisci.

Observe that the long axis of the lateral femoral condyle is essentially anteroposterior, whereas the axis of the medial condyle runs obliquely medial to lateral. Observe also that three articular areas separated by indistinct grooves may be identified: a circular convex area on the base of the lateral condyle, an oval convex area on the base of the medial condyle, and an intermediate concave area. Each convex area extends posteriorly on the posterior surface of a condyle.

Observe that the concave articular surfaces on the superior surface of the tibia have shapes similar in outline to the femoral condyles—the lateral tibial surface is circular, the medial one, oval. However, it is important to realize that the femoral and tibial articular surfaces are congruous only when the knee is extended. In the various degrees of flexion, the opposing joint surfaces are incongruous, as one would expect in a joint in which there is a constant shift of the axis of movement.

ITEM 57-13.   The attachments of the menisci are of some importance. The medial meniscus is firmly attached to the deep part of the medial ligament and loosely attached by coronary ligaments to the tibial plateau. Its horns are firmly attached to the tibia, but not to the cruciate ligaments. On the other hand, the lateral meniscus is attached not only to the tibia but also to both cruciate ligaments, as well as to the femur, by the meniscofemoral ligaments. In addition to the coronary ligaments, present between the lateral meniscus and the tibial plateau, the lateral meniscus receives muscle fibers from the popliteus.

The attachments of the lateral meniscus suggest it might be less mobile than the medial meniscus. On the contrary, it is well recognized that it is the medial meniscus that is less mobile.

MOVEMENT OF THE KNEE JOINT

Helfet (1959) provides a neat summary of the movement of the knee joint. "As the tibia glides on the femur from the fully flexed to the fully extended position it descends and then ascends the curve of the medial femoral condyle and at the same time slowly rotates outwards. These movements are reversed as the tibia passes back to the fully flexed position." Helfet then provides a simple demonstration to show that rotation does take place. "The tibial tubercle of the flexed knee is in line with the medial half of the patella. When the knee is extended, the tubercle rotates outward toward the outer half of the patella." Prove this point on your own knee.

All that need be said now concerns the ligaments. In full extension of a normal knee joint, all the ligaments are taut and no movement can be demonstrated between the femur and tibia. In flexion of the knee, however, the lateral ligament relaxes while the other ligaments remain taut. In flexion some degree of movement between femur and tibia can be elicited. Finally, with one or more of the ligaments torn, the degree of movement between femur and tibia when the knee joint is flexed is greatly increased. But, as has been stressed previously, evidence of instability of the knee joint must be assessed with care in order to pinpoint precisely the torn ligament or ligaments.

Chapter 58

Dissection of the Ankle Joint and the Joints of the Foot

The ankle joint is a hinge joint, and, in examining the joint, you should look for the features that lend stability to the hinge.

ITEM 58-1. In removing soft tissues from around the ankle joint observe particularly the major vessels and nerves. They are vulnerable in fracture-dislocations of the ankle. Examine your specimen and observe how the tibia and fibula are held together inferiorly by strong fibrous tissue. This very strong fibrous tissue is the interosseous tibiofibular ligament, and it is the most important factor in keeping the tibia and fibula firmly together to create a mortice for the talus.

ITEM 58-2. Manipulate the ankle joint and observe how thin the capsule is anteriorly and how strong the medial and lateral ligaments are; deltoid ligament is another name for the medial ligament. To demonstrate the mechanism of sprain, a common mishap to the ligaments of the ankle joint, plantar flex and invert the foot forcibly so as to tense the anterior talofibular ligament, part of the lateral ligament (Fig. 58-1). Then tilt the calcaneum (not easy to do on a cadaver) so as to tense the calcaneofibular ligament, which is the intermediate strut of the lateral ligament. The calcaneofibular ligament is especially vulnerable during forced inversion because the ligament spans two joints, the ankle joint and the subtalar joint (Fig. 58-1). Cut the capsule anteriorly and observe that the proximal part of the neck of the talus is intracapsular. Then cut the deltoid ligament close to the medial malleolus. Observe the instability of the ankle joint once this ligament, one of the collateral ligaments, is divided.

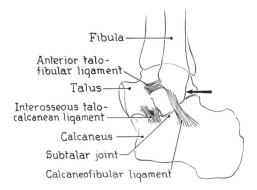

Fibula

Anterior talo-fibular ligament

Talus

Interosseous talo-calcanean ligament

Calcaneus

Subtalar joint

Calcaneofibular ligament

Figure 58-1. The lateral ligaments of the left ankle joint. The calcaneofibular ligament spans both the ankle and the subtalar joint. The black arrow indicates where the student must look to find the posterior talofibular ligament.

ITEM 58-3. To examine the joint posteriorly, proceed as follows: Approach the capsule from a posterior direction and break it with closed, blunt-ended scissors. Be vigorous because the capsule is tough. By blunt dissection using transverse strokes of the scissors, disperse the capsule until two transverse bands come into view (Fig. 58-1). The superior band is the transverse tibiofibular ligament; observe how this ligament also articulates with the talus and serves to deepen the joint cavity. The inferior band is the posterior talofibular ligament, a part of the lateral ligament that often eludes the student because he doesn't appreciate that the posterior talofibular ligament lies transversely across the posterolateral aspect of the ankle joint. Cut the posterior talofibular ligament, then the calcaneofibular ligament, and, finally, the anterior talofibular ligament. The entire foot can now be removed from the limb.

ITEM 58-4. Examine the superior surface of the talus and note that it is broader anteriorly than posteriorly. Restore the ankle joint and, by moving the foot into dorsiflexion and plantar flexion, observe how the socket grips the talus more firmly in dorsiflexion than in plantar flexion.

ITEM 58-5. Next, observe that the medial malleolus is 2 cm. shorter than the lateral malleolus and, accordingly, that the size of the medial and lateral articular facets upon the talus are unequal. The medial facet on the talus is much smaller; the rest of the medial surface of the talus gives attachment to the deep fibers of the deltoid ligament. Obviously the entire deltoid ligament is substantial. Observe how the lateral malleolus lies more posterior than the medial malleolus; at this time you should take note of how the head of the fibula lies posterior to the lateral condyle of the tibia; thus you can see that the fibula really lies more posterior in relation to the tibia than is normally appreciated.

The muscular, and bony factors promoting stability of the ankle joint become really significant in fracture-dislocations of the joint, and they will be discussed again by your clinical tutors in orthopedics.

JOINTS OF THE FOOT

There are numerous joints in the foot, all of them synovial, which may be grouped as tarsal, metatarsal, and phalangeal. Each joint has a fibrous capsule reinforced by ligaments, which may be grouped according to their anatomic position, e.g., plantar, dorsal, collateral, and interosseous. Many of the ligaments receive individual names based on the bones they are attached to, but, in practice, it is recognized that there is little to be gained by such a painstaking exercise. In the dissecting procedure that follows, the student should concentrate on the shape and extent of the articular surfaces and relate his findings to the range of movement that can occur in the joints of a normal foot. It is recommended that you examine the articulations on the foot of a skeleton so that you are always correctly oriented during the dissection.

THE TALAR ARTICULATIONS

You have already seen how the talus articulates with the tibia and fibula. The next stage is to examine how the talus articulates inferiorly with the calcaneum and anteriorly with the navicular bone.

Although the talus is named as the first bone of the foot and lies superior to all the other bones, it is, in fact, the central bone from the functional point of view and, in that respect, it occupies a commanding position in the foot. Talking in general terms, one may say that all the other bones of the foot rotate around the talus, which is held fast in the grip of the tibia and the fibula. That fact is demonstrable to some extent on a foot disarticulated from a cadaver, but, best of all, on your own foot. Hold the calcaneum firmly in one hand, then move the talus. Even in a cadaver there is considerable mobility between the undersurface of the talus and the calcaneum. At the same time, you will also observe that there is mobility between the anterior end of the talus and the rest of the foot. Now look at your own foot. Twist it in and out. The range of the movements you have just demonstrated in the cadaver is greater in the living body. Once the talar articulations have been dissected these movements will be discussed in greater detail.

ITEM 58-6.   The Talocalcaneonavicular Joint

The body, neck, and head of the talus are readily recognized. Examine the direction of the neck with a critical eye and you will observe that the long axis of the neck is deviated approximately 15° medially and 40° inferiorly. Hence the articular surface of the head faces medially and inferiorly as well as anteriorly. Such a fine point of detail must be taken into account in orthopedic procedures on this region of the foot. The point is raised here merely to give a simple example of the many scientific facts that complicate surgical procedures on the foot.

The surface of the head is almost entirely articular, and articulates anteriorly with a reciprocal facet on the posterior surface of the navicular bone. In addition, the medial surface of the head articulates with the "spring" ligament slung between the sustentaculum tali and the navicular bone. Also, the inferior surface of the head articulates with a facet (sometimes divided into two) upon the superior surface of the body of the calcaneus and its medial platform-like projection, the sustentaculum tali.

ITEM 58-7.   Trace the tendon of the tibialis posterior into the foot and observe how it lies adjacent to and sends a slip to the plantar calcaneonavicular ("spring") ligament.

Identify the joint cavity between the head of the talus and the navicular bone. Incise the capsule and cut it so as to open the talocalcaneonavicular joint widely *without* cutting the spring ligament. Make sure that you cut the capsule as far laterally as you can. Examine the direction of the neck of the talus and compare it with the neck of other specimens of the talus. Examine the articular surfaces. If the joint does not disarticulate easily, it will do so once the calcaneocuboid joint is opened. That is what you do next.

The Calcaneocuboid Joint

The anterior end of the calcaneus articulates with the posterior surface of the cuboid. Laterally, the tuberosity of the cuboid projects to provide a polished surface upon which the tendon of the peroneus longus glides.

ITEM 58-8.   Trace the tendon of the peroneus longus toward the lateral aspect of the foot and identify its sesamoid bone and where the sesamoid bone rests. Identify the cavity of the calcaneocuboid joint by twisting the foot, and incise its capsule widely, so that you may examine its articular surfaces. Make sure that you cut the capsule of the calcaneocuboid joint as far medially as you can.

The calcaneocuboid joint and the talocalcaneonavicular joint are often referred to as the transverse tarsal or midtarsal joint. Bend the foot to open the two joints widely and examine their articular surfaces.

The Subtalar Joint

Upon the superior surface of the calcaneus there are two articular areas. The anterior facet takes part in the talocalcaneonavicular joint. (It is sometimes divided into two; if so, the facets are described as anterior and middle.) The posterior area, which is dome shaped, articulates with a reciprocal facet on the inferior surface of the talus to form the anatomic subtalar joint.

Examine the subtalar region of the tarsus of a skeleton and you will see the sinus tarsi, a tunnel you can spy through. It runs obliquely from the anterolateral aspect of the talocalcaneal junction to the posteromedial aspect. In an intact specimen, the sinus tarsi is occupied by a powerful interosseous ligament that serves to divide the talocalcaneonavicular joint from the subtalar joint.

ITEM 58-9. With a knife sharp to the point, cut the capsule of the subtalar joint, then the talocalcaneointerosseous ligament. The talus is now free. After reading the following commentary, replace the talus and demonstrate that it is indeed the central bone of the foot from a functional point of view.

SUPINATION AND PRONATION

All movements of the foot are a combination of many movements at many joints. A significant combination links inversion and adduction to produce the movement of supination. Pronation, the opposite of supination, is a combination of eversion and abduction.

It is not possible to adduct and abduct the forefoot without inversion or eversion. To prove this point, at some convenient time grasp the heel of one foot firmly so that it cannot move, then try abducting and adducting the forefoot. Neither movement is possible without releasing the heel. Accordingly, the terms supination and pronation have, to a large extent, become synonymous with inversion and eversion respectively. Even so, one should remember that inversion and eversion are predominantly subtalar movements, whereas adduction and abduction occur primarily in the transverse (midtarsal) joint. Furthermore, one should remember that in both subtalar movement and midtarsal movement the talus plays a dominant role.

The muscles responsbile for supination are the tibialis anterior and posterior; the calf muscles, especially the soleus, assist in inversion when the foot is plantar flexed. The muscles responsible for pronation are the peroneus longus and brevis, assisted by the extensor longus digitorum.

TRIPLE ARTHRODESIS

Although triple arthrodesis, a term to be explained in a moment, is a highly specialized orthopedic surgical procedure, it is introduced to you to illuminate the great significance of the tarsus in the functional anatomy of the foot. When the muscles of the leg are paralyzed beyond all hope of recovery, the stability of the subtalar, calcaneocuboid, and the talocalcaneonavicular joints is lost, and the patient endures considerable handicap, not just in walking, but even in standing. In order, therefore, to restore stability to the tarsus, the articular surfaces of the three joints named are shorn off; the opposing raw bony surfaces left are allowed to "weld" together; thus three bones become one and a degree of stability is restored. It is a fortunate reflection of the great scientific discoveries of our time, however, that the development of poliomyelitis vaccine has largely eliminated the need for reconstructive procedures such as triple arthrodesis.

THE METATARSOPHALANGEAL JOINT OF THE BIG TOE

No review of the anatomy of the joints of the foot is complete without reference to the big toe joint. A limp is inevitable if the big toe joint is painful, and there are two very very common conditions affecting this joint, namely hallux rigidus and hallux valgus, both producing stiffness and pain. These two conditions and their treatment are adequately described in clinical texts and need not be described here. Enough has been said to show that the metatarsophalangeal joint of the big toe warrants your careful examination.

ITEM 58-10.   In dissecting the big toe joint, look for evidence of hallux rigidus and hallux valgus. First cut the capsule. Then examine the articular surfaces and movements. Confirm the close relationship of the long flexor and the long extensor tendon to the joint. In any operative procedure on the joint, those tendons must be safeguarded. Identify the abductor and adductor hallucis muscles and note the attachment of their tendons to the proximal phalanx of the big toe. Finally, expose the sesamoid bones located in the tendons of flexor hallucis brevis.

Chapter 59

The Gait

To believe that the practice of medicine is restricted to the care of patients confined to bed is a common error. Medical practice, in fact, deals with a very high percentage of ambulatory patients of all age groups, from the very young to the very old and, in many of those patients, the problem is exclusively in the locomotor system. Furthermore, the same type of problem exists in many patients confined to bed. Thus the diagnosis of a locomotor disorder is a common request in the practice of medicine.

In the diagnosis of a locomotor disorder it is always necessary to observe how a patient walks. For you to understand why a patient cannot walk, or can walk but with an abnormal gait, you must have a comprehensive knowledge of all that is involved in normal walking.

Before an analysis of normal walking is presented, however, it is necessary to correct a preconceived notion that some students may have, namely that normal walking involves continuous muscular activity. Electromyographic studies have shown that in normal walking muscular activity is intermittent. The generally accepted explanation of this is that gravity must be taken into account. Indeed, Hall (1965) likened the lower limb to a pendulum. Thus the electromyograph records muscular activity only when a muscle initiates a movement or controls the inertia of the limb. In the following analysis no attempt is made to state precisely when muscular activity or the influence of gravity is maximal. Such an attempt would no doubt complicate the analysis of gait at a time when the general aim is to present principles with minimal detail.

Analysis of the normal gait is complicated by the number of joints moving at the same time. The analysis of the movements of the lower limbs, however, is less difficult if the gait is considered in two phases, "stance" and "swing." Figure 59-1 illustrates those phases in one step. In 59-1A, the left limb is in the stance phase, while the right limb is beginning to push off into the swing phase. The rest of this description concerns the right limb only. The push-off involves primarily plantar flexion of the ankle and slight extension of the knee. In 59-1B, the swing phase is underway. Observe the flexion of the hip and knee and the dorsiflexion of the ankle. In 59-1C the swing phase is complete. The knee may remain slightly flexed or become fully extended, depending on the length of the step. The ankle is dorsiflexed. Soon the heel will strike the ground and the rest of the foot will bear more and more weight as the right limb moves into a stance phase.

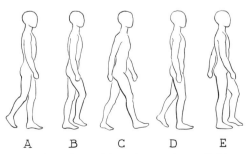

A   B   C   D   E

Figure 59-1.   These illustrations of the gait are to be studied in conjunction with the text.

In 59-1*D* the stance phase of the right limb is obvious. The knee is very slightly flexed. Then, in 59-1*E*, as the stance phase ends, the knee straightens for the push-off into the next swing phase. It should be added that during the peak of the stance phase the foot may be inverted or everted, depending upon the type of surface the foot happens to rest upon.

What has been said so far concerns the obvious elements of walking. Two less obvious but nevertheless highly important elements involve the hip joints, namely hip joint rotation and stabilization of the pelvis through the action of the hip joint abductors.

To demonstrate rotation of the hip joints, stand with the right foot well in front of the left, as if you had been stopped dead in your tracks. Observe that the pelvis is rotated so that its anterior aspect is directed anteriorly and to the left. Now bring the left foot forward beside the right and observe that the pelvis faces directly anteriorly. Finally advance the left foot forward well in front of the right. Observe the pelvis is now facing anteriorly and to the right. Figure 59-2 demonstrates that medial rotation occurs in one hip while lateral rotation occurs in the other. Medial rotation occurs in the hip joint of the limb in the stance phase, while lateral rotation occurs in the hip joint of the limb in the swing phase. As a result of these rotations of the hip joints, the feet continue to point more or less forward throughout the phases of walking. Accordingly, hip joint rotation is one of the significant, yet unapparent, components of normal gait.

Stabilization of the pelvis refers to the fact that throughout the stance phase the pelvis is maintained more or less in a horizontal position by the ipsilateral hip abductors. A demonstration of how the gluteus

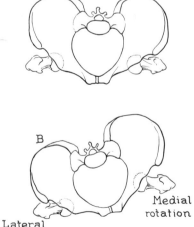

A

B

Lateral
rotation

Medial
rotation

Figure 59-2. Superior view of the pelvis to illustrate how the hip joints rotate in walking. *A.* The feet are together. *B.* The right foot is forward.

medius and minimus act to maintain the pelvis in a horizontal plane was described on p. 239. In summary, then, it may be said that when the right lower limb is in its swing phase, the left gluteus medius and minimus act to stabilize the horizontal position of the pelvis.

Review

Review the main elements involved in normal walking. Then consider what would happen to the gait in the following examples.

(1) The left leg is 7 cm. shorter than the right
(2) The right gluteus medius and minimus are paralyzed
(3) The left hip joint is dislocated
(4) The left quadriceps is paralyzed
(5) The right common peroneal nerve is severed
(6) The left foot is irreversibly plantar flexed
(7) The right tendo Achillis is divided

There are many more factors other than those listed here that can produce an abnormality of the gait. Your clinical tutors will advise you how to classify all the factors responsible for abnormalities of gait. Meantime, concentrate on a consideration of the normal gait. The clearer your understanding of the normal gait, the easier your interpretation of the abnormal gait.

REFERENCES

Barnett, C. H., Davies, D. V., and MacConaill, M. A.: Synovial Joints, Their Structure and Mechanics. London, Longmans Green & Co. Ltd, 1961.
Hall, M. C.: The Locomotor System; Functional Anatomy. Springfield, Ill., Charles C Thomas, 1965.
Helfet, A. J.: The Management of Internal Derangements of the Knee. Philadelphia, J. B. Lippincott Co., 1959.
Henry, A. K.: Extensile Exposure. Edinburgh, E. & S. Livingstone Ltd., 1957.
Howe, W. W., Lacey, T., and Schwartz, R. P.: A study of the gross anatomy of arteries supplying the proximal portion of the femur and acetabulum. Journal of Bone and Joint Surgery, 32A:856, 1950.
Kaplan, E. B.: The iliotibial tract. Journal of Bone and Joint Surgery, 39A:1436, 1958.
Sargeant, T. R.: Surgical anatomy in the treatment of venous stasis. The Surgical Clinics of North America, Vol. 44, No. 5: 1383, 1964.
Trueta, J.: The normal vascular anatomy of the human femoral head during growth. Journal of Bone and Joint Surgery, 39B:358, 1957.

PART 6

HEAD AND NECK

Chapter 60

The Face

Much that goes on in the depths of the body is revealed on the surface of the face. An experienced clinician observes the face of his patient with a kind but searching gaze while he listens to the medical history. The range of his observations quickly convinces the novice that clinical observation is an art to be acquired only by diligent practice and long experience. When Dr. Schumann of Katherine Anne Porter's *Ship of Fools* smiled and said, "Father Garza does not know one face from another. He sees only souls," he indicated the difference between an experienced clinician and his fellow men. To create that difference, let the student of medicine begin now to observe the human face. The following facts will set him on his way.

The human face is much more extensive than is generally thought. To trace the boundary of the face, begin at the tip of the chin and trace a line along the lower border to the angle of the jaw, where the line changes direction abruptly to ascend anterior to the tragus of the auricle and reach the summit of the skull. A similar line on the opposite side completes the boundary of the face. In brief, the face extends from auricle to auricle and from the summit of the skull to the chin (Fig. 60-1). Some instructors may not agree with the superior boundary of the face as defined here, but the definition is deliberate, designed to include the hairline and forehead, which are significant in a clinical examination of the face.

A horizontal line through the palpebral fissures divides the face almost exactly into halves (Fig. 60-1). It may surprise you that so much of the face lies above this line. However, once this division is recognized and is applied in drawing for example, it is indeed surprising how lifelike even a badly drawn face looks, and how, on clinical examination of the face, physical signs previously unseen become immediately obvious.

That a vertical line through the nose and the tip of the chin also divides the face into halves is obvious, but what is not obvious is that rarely if ever is one half the mirror image of the other.

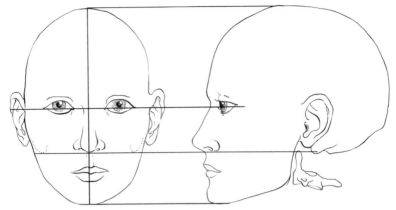

Figure 60-1. For an explanation of these lines see text, p. 293. The tip of the odontoid process of vertebra C2 is level with a line through the tips of the mastoid processes. The odontoid process is on the same level as the philtrum of the upper lip.

ITEM 60-1. On your specimen, scratch in the vertical and horizontal lines to create four quadrants. These quadrants are described clinically as the right and left upper and lower quadrants. In a physical examination of the face the features of each quadrant must be inspected and the findings compared to those of the opposite side. Examine each quadrant.

ITEM 60-2. Observe the following regions of the face: the hairline, the forehead, the two orbital apertures and eyebrows, the parotid regions and cheeks, the nose and nostrils, the oral aperture and lips, and the lower jaw and chin.

ITEM 60-3. Useful clues to the medical history of the cadaver may be obtained by looking for abnormal findings such as scars. Today it is also essential to look for evidence of prosthetic surgery. In clinical practice, when a part of the body has been replaced by a prosthesis it must be established why the original part was removed. Today the eyeball, the cheekbone, the jaw, and even the auricles may be replaced with such artistry that the replacement remains undetected except by a shrewd observer.

The Skin of the Face

The chapter on skin (p. 1) should be read before removing skin from the face. In addition to what is said in that chapter, the following short, unqualified examples of skin changes are presented to encourage the student to take every opportunity to look more closely at the living face, especially at the nature of the skin and its appendages, for it takes but a moment of time to skin the face of a cadaver.

The condition of the epidermis and dermis of the skin of the face indicates the external environment to which the individual has been exposed. The skin of the face also reflects, so very often, the internal state of the individual; for example, blistering of the epidermis is a common manifestation of allergy to a particular kind of food.

Thickening of the subcutaneous tissues and dryness of the skin are characteristic of myxedema, an adult variety of hypothyroidism. In its earliest stages, myxedema may remain undetected but as the hypothyroidism deepens, the facial tissues coarsen and a facies, characteristic of myxedema, develops. Also noted in myxedema are brittleness of the hair and loss of hair from the hairline and from the eyebrows.

Sebaceous glands are particularly numerous on the face and, in a variety of conditions, they may secrete excessive amounts of sebum.

Sweat glands of the face respond rapidly to the emotions as well as to the environment, as every student, and oral examiner, knows.

There is no doubt that methodical inspection of the structural elements of the skin of the face becomes more and more rewarding as one's clinical experience grows.

Nerve Supply of the Skin of the Face

The skin of the face is supplied by the sensory root of the trigeminal nerve, the fifth cranial nerve, also labeled nerve V. Once the skull is opened, nerve V located (p. 371), and its three divisions seen, it is very easy to understand the basis of diagrams such as Figure 60-2, in which the skin of the face is divided into three areas, each supplied by a di-

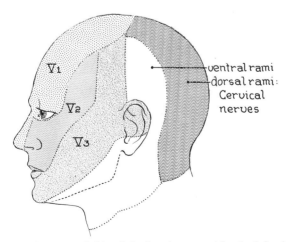

Figure 60-2. The areas of skin of the face innervated by the left trigeminal nerve. Observe that the cornea of the eyeball and the ridge of the nose are both innervated by V_1, the ophthalmic division of the trigeminal nerve.

vision of nerve V. The divisions are the ophthalmic nerve, the maxillary nerve, and the mandibular nerve, sometimes referred to as V^1, V^2, and V^3, respectively. Each division of the trigeminal nerve has several branches that are distributed throughout the area innervated by the division.

Observe in Figure 60-2 that V^2, the intermediate division, supplies an area of skin that includes the lower lid, part of the nose, and part of the cheek above the level of the corner of the mouth. The posterior boundary of the area is an imaginary line that begins at the corner of the mouth and runs superiorly parallel to the nose to meet a similar line from the lateral canthus, i.e., the junction of the eyelids. The area of skin superior and anterior to V^2 is supplied by V^1, and the area inferior and posterior by V^3, except for a small area of skin over the angle of the jaw. The explanation of why V^1 is distributed to the ridge of the nose is available in any textbook of embryology.

In clinical practice, knowledge of the nerve supply of the skin of the face is necessary for the accurate diagnosis of pain, particularly referred pain. An example of referred pain is the pain felt in the ear when the cause is located in a tooth in the lower jaw.

Exercise

With a sharp point scratch on the face of your cadaver the boundaries of the divisions of nerve V (trigeminal) as illustrated in Figure 60-2.

The terminal branches of the trigeminal nerve that are commonly referred to are the supraorbital nerve, V^1; the infraorbital nerve, V^2; and the mental nerve, V^3. These nerves are exposed later in the dissection. Meanwhile, identify, first on a skull, then on your own face, and then on the cadaver, the following landmarks: the supraorbital notch, the infraorbital foramen, and the mental foramen.

The Arteries of the Face

Although there are many arterial branches nourishing the face, they are all either primary or secondary branches of the right and left external carotid arteries, with the exception of the small branches to the upper and lower eyelids, to the skin on the ridge of the nose, and to a central strip of the skin on the forehead. Those exceptional branches spring from the ophthalmic arteries, which are branches of the internal carotid arteries. The branches, whatever their source, anastomose freely with each other and across the midline. Because of the profuse arterial distribution, cuts of the face bleed freely, and because of the free anasto-

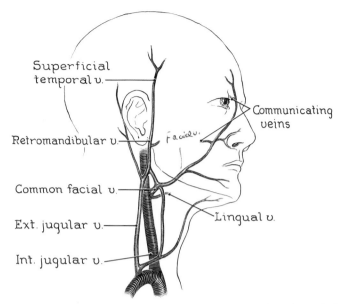

Figure 60-3. The retromandibular vein forms a venous plane through the parotid gland. At the inferior end of the gland the vein divides to join the common facial vein and the external jugular vein.

moses, bleeding may not be readily controlled unless compression is applied to more than one part. The principal arteries on the face are obvious once the skin of the face is removed and they should be identified then.

Venous Drainage of the Face*

Venous blood from the face flows into the right and left facial and retromandibular veins. The right facial vein is illustrated but not labeled in Figure 60-3. If the student finds that the veins on his specimen do not conform to the pattern illustrated, he should not waste time struggling to match specimen to illustration. Instead he should concentrate on the specimen and use the illustration merely as a guide. The veins of the face are classified as superficial veins, and, therefore, they must at some time penetrate deep fascia to join the deep venous system (p. 7). The deep fascia of the neck is introduced on p. 377.

Before the advent of antibiotics, serious bacterial infections of the face were sometimes accompanied by a dangerous complication within

*For dissection see p. 301.

the cranium. Such a complication is extremely rare today, however, in those regions of the world where antibiotics are readily available. Nevertheless, an experienced clinician, anywhere in the world, treats a serious infection of the face as a potentially dangerous event.

The complication occurs because the veins of the face communicate with a pair of venous sinuses at the base of the skull. Each of those venous sinuses is about the size of the tip of a little finger, yet each is named cavernous (Fig. 64-2). The superior communicating vein (Fig. 60-3) enters the orbit to join the ophthalmic veins that drain into the cavernous sinus (Fig. 64-2). The inferior communicating vein (Fig. 60-3) communicates with the pterygoid plexus, which then communicates by a very small emissary vein with the cavernous sinus. Briefly, the complication is clotting of blood in the cavernous venous sinus, a condition described clinically as cavernous sinus thrombosis, and characterized by engorgement of the veins of the orbit as well as by edema of the orbital contents.

The lymphatic drainage of the skin of the face is commented upon later (p. 382).

REMOVAL OF SKIN*

Removal of only skin from the face is extraordinarily difficult because the underlying muscles of facial expression are attached to the dermis; muscle fibers even enter the dermal papillae that protrude into the epidermis. Moreover, there is little or no superficial fascia to be recognized in the face of an elderly cadaver, although small collections of fat are found, depending on the age and the state of nutrition. There is no definite layer of deep fascia. Thus, the proximity of the muscles of the face to the skin means that the muscles will inevitably be lacerated as the skin is removed. It took a competent anatomist untold hours of patient toil to prepare a museum specimen of the muscles of the face. Proceed, therefore, as swiftly and effectively as time permits.

ITEM 60-4. To establish the correct plane of cleavage, it is recommended that you begin at the clavicles, where it is easy to identify the platysma muscle by peeling back the skin. Do not advance until you are sure the platysma is correctly identified. Then, keeping the blade of the knife toward the skin, reflect skin from the entire anterior aspect of the neck and from over the lower jaw. As you proceed make a midline cut in the skin extending from the suprasternal notch to the tip of the jaw, and so create two flaps.

ITEM 60-5. Continue to reflect the skin off the platysma over the lower part of the face. Then, remaining at the same depth, skin the rest of the face. To skin the forehead may be difficult, if not impossible, so

---

*See also Item 74-1.

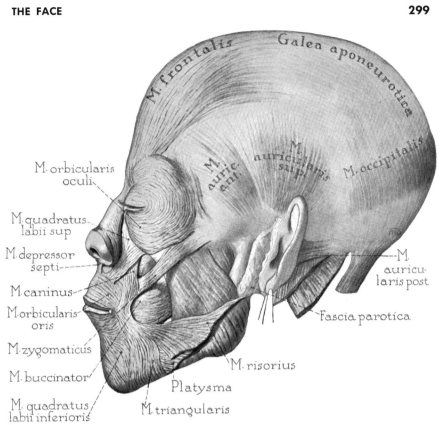

Figure 60-4. Muscles of facial expression; lateral view. The platysma muscle has been transected at the angle of the mandible, together with the adjacent risorius. (From B. J. Anson: An Atlas of Human Anatomy. 2nd ed. Philadelphia, W. B. Saunders Co., 1963.)

do not delay. Remove enough skin to see some of the orbicularis oculi and frontalis muscles. Then leave the rest until the scalp is removed. Do not delay on the nose. Figure 60-4 and 60-5 show where the muscle fibers of the face are concentrated to form recognizable muscles.

THE MUSCLES OF FACIAL EXPRESSION

By definition, the term muscles of facial expression includes only those muscles supplied by the facial nerve, and they are to be distinguished from the muscles of mastication supplied by the motor root of the trigeminal nerve. The muscles of facial expression move the skin of the face, whereas the muscles of mastication control the temporomandibular joints, hinging the jaw to the skull.

Characteristic features of the muscles of facial expression are their

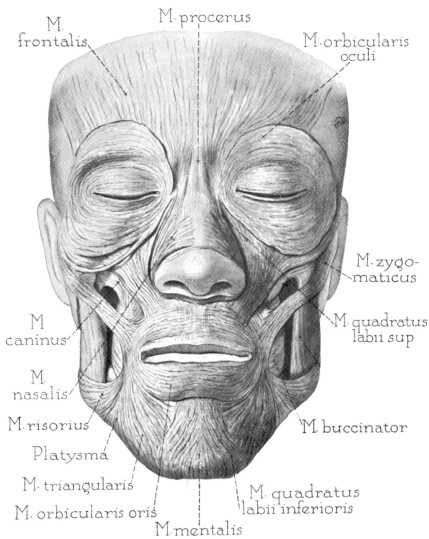

Figure 60-5.   Muscles of facial expression; anterior view. (From B. J. Anson: An Atlas of Human Anatomy. 2nd ed., Philadelphia, W. B. Saunders Co., 1963.)

limited attachment to bone and their extensive attachment to the dermis. In addition to the unusual distribution of muscle fibers to the skin of the face, the small number of muscle fibers controlled by each motor unit must be taken into account. The ratio of muscle fibers to motor unit is probably between 3:1 and 5:1. Such a ratio provides for extremely fine control over the movements of a muscle. Accordingly it is possible to twitch precise parts of the skin of the face, and one can understand why the skin of the face sags and becomes inert when the facial nerve is cut.

Clinically certain muscles of the face are commonly mentioned: frontalis, orbicularis oculi, orbicularis oris and buccinator, and platysma (Figs. 60-4 and 60-5). The muscles of the nostrils are rarely named but their action is observed when the nostrils move in labored respiration. The orbicularis oculi, in particular its palpebral parts, keeps the eyelids apposed to the eyeball. When this muscle is paralyzed the lower lid falls away from the eyeball and the conjunctiva is exposed to dust and daylight; furthermore the ability to blink is lost.

When the orbicularis oris and buccinator are paralyzed, the cheek droops and the angle of the mouth sags so that saliva trickles out onto the skin of the face. Apart from the disfigurement, both the inevitable inflammation of the conjunctiva and the excoriation of the skin at the angle of the mouth are most distressing. Facial nerve paralysis, therefore, is indeed a serious malady. These are the bare facts, but they have been vividly woven into a clinical presentation by Sir Charles Bell, whose descriptions of facial palsy written in the eighteenth century are now classic. (They are reprinted in *Sir Charles Bell*, by Gordon-Taylor and Walls, 1958.)

In the days of Sir Charles Bell, muscles of the nostrils were necessary to take a good sniff of snuff. Accordingly Sir Charles reported: "Our friend here finds it a mere waste of snuff to put it into this nostril: he tells you it does not go high enough." Furthermore, when the patient was asked to laugh, Sir Charles reported: "He exhibited a very singular distortion of countenance; at each cachination his left cheek was puffed out, flapping like a loose sail; and the forehead and eyelids of this side remain perfectly still; whilst upon the right side the whole mouth was drawn upwards, the cheeks were strangely wrinkled, and the eyelids puckered."

There are four simple tests of the muscles of the face: first, raising the eyebrows, second, closing the eyes tight, third, showing the teeth, as in smiling, or pursing the lips, as in whistling, and fourth, pulling down the corners of the mouth so as to raise the skin of the neck. If these four procedures can be carried out successfully then the muscles of the face, the right and left facial nerves, and their connections deep within the central nervous system must be intact and normal. It is clear that the entire test need take only a matter of seconds.

Exercise

Perform on yourself and your partner the four simple tests just described.

ITEM 60-6. Now that the muscles of facial expression are exposed, identify the principal arteries and veins on each side of the face (see *Grant's Atlas of Anatomy*, Figures 466 and 467).

Make a vertical cut into the middle of the upper and lower lips and identify the superior and inferior labial arteries. How would you control the severe bleeding that usually results from a split lip?

ITEM 60-7. To expose quickly the supraorbital nerve, the infraorbital nerve, and the mental nerve proceed thus. On a skull confirm the following landmarks, the supraorbital notch, the infraorbital foramen, and the mental foramen. Over each landmark make a vertical incision down to bone. Separate the soft tissues and expose the nerves.

After examination of the principal muscles of facial expression it would be logical to seek the facial nerve, but the nerve proceeds through the substance of the parotid gland, a salivary gland that also deserves careful study. Therefore study the gland before exposing the facial nerve.

THE PAROTID GLANDS

There are three pairs of salivary glands—the submandibular, sublingual (p. 418), and parotid. They are usually classified as the major salivary glands to distinguish them from the many minute glands studded throughout the oral cavity. The salivary glands secrete 1000 to 1500 ml. of saliva in 24 hours, which is an indication not just of their biochemical activity but also of the considerable part they play in the function of the digestive system and in the fluid balance of the body.

It is of considerable importance to gain the correct first impression of the position of the parotid gland. The gland has an extensive flat lateral surface that is separated from the skin only by dense fascia, but the gland also has an extensive uneven medial surface that is separated only by various longitudinal structures from the pharynx and soft palate. In other words, the parotid gland extends more deeply into the side of the neck than is immediately apparent. To emphasize the point it is worth adding that a tumor of the parotid gland sometimes presents as a mass that can be seen on examination of the soft palate. Unfortunately in an embalmed cadaver it is impossible to demonstrate at this stage the close proximity of the pharynx to the parotid region.

In the course of the dissection of the parotid region you will see how the parotid gland forms a cleft anteriorly for the ramus of the mandible and a lesser cleft posteriorly for the mastoid process and the anterior border of the sternomastoid. These are the main landmarks essential to begin dissection and they should be identified first on a skull. Once the student is more familiar with the region he may wish to read a more detailed account, such as *The Parotid Mold or Bed* by Grant and Basmajian (1966).

ITEM 60-8. Identify the fascia over the masseter and trace the fascia posteriorly where it thickens to form the parotid fascia. The fascia is described as splitting to enclose the parotid gland, but it is not usually possible to show this in a cadaver. Together the two fascia are named the parotideomasseteric fascia. The dense, unyielding nature of the parotid fascia is the reason why acute swelling of the gland, as in mumps, is so painful.

Identify the anterior border of the gland and the parotid duct. Mobilize the duct and trace it to where it disappears through the buccinator to open into the vestibule of the mouth. Exploration of the opening of the duct in the mouth must be delayed until a more convenient time in the dissecting program. It should be stressed now, however, that clinical examination of the parotid gland is not complete until the orifice of the duct inside the mouth has been examined (Fig. 60-6).

ITEM 60-9. Splitting the Parotid Gland

First of all the superficial temporal artery must be found. It is readily seen in life and easily found in a cadaver. The artery pierces the superior boundary of the parotid fascia close to the auricle; then subcutaneously it winds across the temporal region. If you have not already done so, remove skin as far as the auricle to find the superficial temporal artery as it emerges from the parotid fascia. Immediately behind the artery lies the auriculotemporal nerve and the superficial temporal vein. The nerve is slender and not easily found, and sometimes the vein is not filled.

It is, however, necessary to find the vein; within the parotid gland the facial nerve is an immediate lateral relation of the vein (in the gland the vein is renamed the retromandibular vein). At the inferior end of the gland it is also helpful to reflect the platysma sufficiently to find the external jugular vein. It is a continuation of the retromandibular vein.

Next grasp the superficial temporal vein and incise the parotid fascia where the vein emerges. Push the tip of a pair of curved scissors into the substance of the gland. Open the scissors and begin to split the gland. Using the closed-open scissors technique (Fig. 46-2) advance along the pathway of the retromandibular vein until the gland is com-

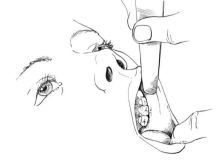

Figure 60-6. Method of examining the opening of the left parotid duct. The opening is found in the vestibule of the mouth on a level with the second upper molar tooth.

pletely split. Then look closely on the lateral surface of the retromandibular vein and find the facial nerve, which is usually plastered onto the vein. Find the stem of the nerve; then trace its branches anteriorly through the parotid gland. Parotid tissue superficial to the nerve should be removed entirely. Of the several branches of the facial nerve the one not to be ignored is the cervical branch, which goes to the platysma. This branch is a structure to be safeguarded by the surgeon when he makes incisions near the angle of the jaw.

Points To Be Observed Once the Parotid Gland is Split

(1) Irregular septa within the gland divide it into lobes and lobules of salivary tissue. The numerous septa fuse with the investing parotid fascia. Thus the general impression of the gland is that it is tough and stringy.

(2) The gland may be divided artificially into superficial and deep parts between which the facial nerve and the retromandibular vein lie. The plane of cleavage through which the division may be made is termed the fasciovenous plane (Patey and Ranger, 1957). It must be emphasized that the division is artificial, for numerous septa span the fasciovenous plane. Nevertheless the division is used to advantage in the surgical removal of parotid tumors.

The deep relationships of the parotid gland are exposed in the dissection of the infratemporal region. The orbital aperture is studied in detail with the orbit. Proceed now to the scalp and removal of the calvaria.

Chapter 61

The Scalp and the Calvaria

The calvaria is the skull cap, the domelike superior portion of the skull. It is discussed along with the scalp because both of them must be taken into account in the applied anatomy of this region.

The basic plan of these two structures is presented in Figure 61-1. Figure 61-1B is useful because it is expanded to show the position of three important spaces, but Figure 61-1A is the one to be looked at closely because it shows that the spaces are not as wide open as the word "space" implies. Both the extradural and the subdural spaces are, indeed, potential spaces obvious only when they are occupied by fluid, usually

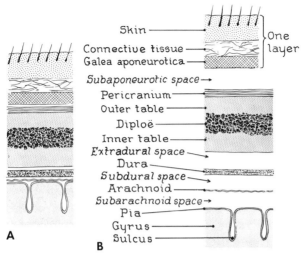

Figure 61-1. The layers and spaces between the skin of the scalp and the brain.

blood. The arachnoid is loosely apposed to the dura, which, in turn, is loosely adherent to the inner surface of the calvaria. It is worth repeating that the arachnoid is apposed to the dura. Why? Because it is common practice to talk of the pia-arachnoid; the arachnoid is connected to the pia by minute strands, trabeculae, similar to the strands of a spider's web (Fig. 61-2). Hence the name arachnoid; *arachne* in Greek means spider. Although Figure 61-2 shows the arachnoid and the pia mater adjacent on the summit of a gyrus, there are regions where the arachnoid and the pia are widely separated. The gaps so formed are termed cisterns because they contain cerebrospinal fluid but it should be

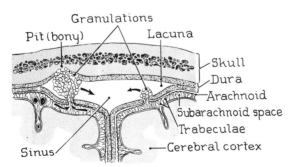

Figure 61-2. Coronal section of the superior sagittal sinus. Observe how an arachnoid granulation can protrude from a lacuna and occupy a pit in the calvaria. The pia and arachnoid are commonly identified as one tissue; the spaces between the trabeculae are then regarded as tissue spaces occupied by tissue fluid, the cerebrospinal fluid. The arrows indicate the direction of flow of cerebrospinal fluid from the subarachnoid space to the venous system.

realized that cerebrospinal fluid circulates through all the nooks and crannies, big or small, of the subarachnoid space and the fluid is not confined just to the cisterns. However, we are advancing too rapidly into fresh fields and we must return to a further consideration of the scalp.

ITEM 61-1. Scratch a line on the scalp from a point between the eyebrows to the external occipital protuberance. Incise the scalp through to bone along the entire length of the line you have just drawn. Elevate the edges of the incision and identify the layers illustrated in Figure 61-1. It is difficult, if not impossible, to separate the skin of the scalp from the subcutaneous tissue and the subcutaneous tissue from the galea. They form one layer separated from the pericranium by loose tissue that creates a plane of cleavage. Thus, when a person is scalped (as sometimes happens in industrial accidents) the entire layer separates from the skull. Now slide the tip of your curved scissors beneath the galea and open up the subaponeurotic space from the frontal to the occipital region. In doing so you will break emissary veins, which emerge from the skull, cross the subaponeurotic space, and drain into a venous plexus in the subcutaneous connective tissue.

ITEM 61-2. Next, at about the middle of the cranium make two lateral incisions at right angles to the anteroposterior incision you made first of all, and so establish four flaps that can be reflected to open up the subaponeurotic space more widely. Reflect the flaps and, in doing so, realize that in a very crude way you are doing what a neurosurgeon must do to expose the cranium. On each side, as you reflect the flaps you will expose the temporal fascia upon the temporalis muscle.

Read an account of the lymphatic drainage, the sensory innervation, and the veins and arteries of the scalp.

REMOVAL OF THE CALVARIA

It is recommended that the laboratory technicians be responsible for opening the skulls when the students are absent from the laboratory and that they use an autopsy saw. The dura must be left intact. In other words, only the skull, and not the dura, should be cut. This is not so difficult as it sounds because it is quite easy to "crack" the skull open. Proceed as follows:

Encircle the skull with a line placed about a finger's breadth superior to the superior margin of the orbits and similarly above the external occipital protuberance. On each side the line crosses the temporal fascia and the underlying temporalis muscle. Cut deep into the fascia and muscle to reach bone — the autopsy saw will not cut soft tissue. Using the saw, cut a groove in the outer table of the skull at the line. With experience one gets to know where to deepen the groove and where to leave it shallow. Then, with two T-chisels inserted into the groove, twist the chisels and so crack open the skull. Note that the bone beneath the temporalis muscle is thin, and therefore it is easily broken in a head injury.

THE CRANIAL EXTRADURAL SPACE

With the skullcap off, part of the cranial extradural space between the dura and the skull is exposed (Fig. 61-3). The space lines the entire internal aspect of the skull. Thus at present a considerable extent of the cranial extradural space remains unseen.

Normally the extradural space is a potential space because the dura is loosely adherent to the bone, but dura and bone can be separated to create an actual space. Separation may occur after a blow on the head; then the space is occupied by blood (extradural hemorrhage). It must be clearly understood that a blow on the head, even a slight blow, can easily produce an extradural hemorrhage. The hemorrhage is serious because it is an arterial hemorrhage, and grave because the hemorrhage is within the rigid confines of the cranium and soon causes a rise in intracranial pressure. Whatever the cause, a rise in intracranial pressure is dangerous and a prolonged rise in intracranial pressure can be mortal.

Treatment of an extradural hemorrhage is one of the most urgent emergencies in the practice of medicine. Briefly, the treatment is as

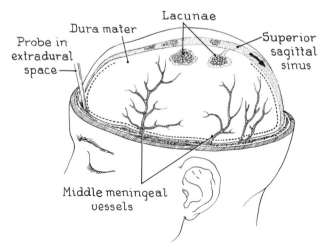

Figure 61-3. Part of the extradural space. The space extends over the entire internal aspect of the skull. The dotted line indicates where to make the incision to raise a flap of dura. The black arrow indicates the direction of blood flow in the sinus.

follows: The side on which the hemorrhage has occurred is determined. Then, approximately halfway between the external auditory meatus and the orbital aperture, a burr hole is made in the skull. Bone is nibbled away to enlarge the opening to obtain an adequate exposure of the bleeding artery. Once the skull is opened the situation is temporarily under control because excessive intracranial pressure has been alleviated. Blood spurts from the artery, but the bleeding stops once the artery has been cauterized.

ITEM 61-3. To demonstrate the proximity of the dura to the skull proceed thus. On each side, at a point halfway between the external auditory meatus and the orbital aperture, slip a probe between the dura and the skull (Fig. 61-3). In life, the brain is soft, so that the dura can be displaced fairly easily. In a cadaver, on the other hand, when the brain is properly embalmed, the brain is solid. Therefore, do not be misled by your present findings. In life, an extradural hemorrhage presses upon and may make a deep impression on the cortex of the brain; the consequences of such pressure must remain untold until you have studied further the anatomy of the central nervous system. However, the sources of an extradural hemorrhage can be sought now.

ITEM 61-4. An extradural hemorrhage may be arterial or venous—the former type is by far the commoner. Identify the arteries first. The right and left middle meningeal arteries are both conspicuous in the present dissection. Examine and compare the distribution of them both.

Each middle meningeal artery is a branch of the maxillary artery (Fig. 71-1). The meningeal artery enters the skull through the foramen spinosum, which should be identified now on a skull. Identify also the groove occupied by the artery in the floor of the middle cranial fossa and the point where the artery divides into anterior and posterior branches. Trace the grooves occupied by those branches. Next, on the cadaver, on both the right and left sides identify the branches of the middle meningeal arteries, sometimes lying quite deep in grooves in the skull. Sometimes, indeed, the middle meningeal artery is actually imbedded in the bone, between the inner and outer tables. Therefore, when the temporal bone is fractured, the middle meningeal artery is torn—resulting in an arterial extradural hematoma. The peripheral distribution of the branches across the external surface of the dura mater has already been examined.

Venous bleeding into the extradural space stems from a venous sinus torn in a fracture of the skull. The venous sinuses are incorporated in the dura; thus they are immediately related to the extradural space. The superior sagittal sinus should be observed next (Fig. 61-3), for it is a venous sinus that is commonly torn in a fracture of the skull. Observe how it arches from anterior to posterior, immediately related to the vault of the skull. Other sinuses elsewhere have a similar close relationship to the skull. All of the venous sinuses will be explored more carefully at a later stage of the dissection.

THE SUBDURAL SPACE

This space, another potential space, is immediately deep to the dura; hence it is called subdural. This space, too, lines the entire inside of the skull. To illuminate the significance of that fact it is worth interjecting that a subdural hemorrhage can occur at sites other than those to be exposed now. In other words, the student must visualize the subdural space in its entirety and not limit his vision to the part of it now to be examined.

ITEM 61-5. On both sides, carefully, leaving the subjacent arachnoid untouched, incise the dura as illustrated in Figure 61-3. Uncover the subdural space and the subjacent arachnoid by peeling each flap of dura toward the sagittal sinus. Proceed slowly as you approach the sinus and look for veins that penetrate the arachnoid; the veins lie for a short distance in the subdural space (Fig. 61-4). Then they join the superior sagittal sinus or a venous lake (lacuna); there are several of these venous lakes (lacunae) draining into the superior sagittal sinus. The student must recognize that a lacuna is simply a lateral extension of the superior sagittal sinus even though the channel between the sinus and the lacuna is quite narrow. Blood flows from the lacuna to the sinus.

In its brief course across the subdural space a cerebral vein may be

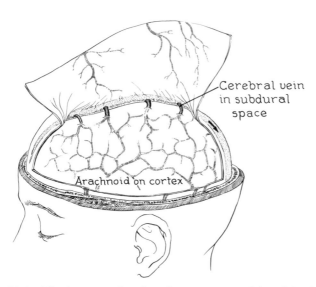

Figure 61-4.   The dura mater is reflected to expose part of the subdural space.

torn. The outcome, a subdural hematoma, is a curious phenomenon whose pathology and diagnosis cannot be discussed here, but the student can examine the anatomy of the space and observe how the cerebral veins pass through it. Subdural hematomas may develop as a result of a trivial blow and may remain undetected in elderly people. Perhaps there is a specimen in the dissecting laboratory. All the cadavers should be examined carefully for evidence of a subdural hematoma.

ITEM 61-6.   To see the termination of the cerebral veins proceed thus. Beginning at the frontal end and proceeding to the occipital end, slit open the superior sagittal sinus. The direction in which you are slitting the sinus is the direction in which blood flows. Flush out debris from the sinus. Trace at least one cerebral vein from the cerebral cortex to where it joins the superior sagittal sinus.

THE SUBARACHNOID SPACE

The membrane exposed when the dura is reflected is the arachnoid. The space deep to the arachnoid is the subarachnoid space, full, in life, of cerebrospinal fluid. The subarachnoid space surrounds the entire central nervous system (Fig. 64-1). Thus the central nervous system is totally immersed in cerebrospinal fluid. The circulation of cerebrospinal fluid is an important physiologic topic, one aspect of which can be dealt with here, namely the arachnoid granulations responsible for the transmission of cerebrospinal fluid into the superior sagittal venous sinus.

ITEM 61-7.   Examine a lacuna and observe an arachnoid granulation, a white granular structure, protruding into a lacuna (Fig. 61-2). The transmission of cerebrospinal fluid is a complex process but the gross anatomy is simple. The one question that usually confuses students is this: How can an arachnoid granulation protruding into a lacuna or into the superior sagittal sinus be related to a pit on the inside of the skull? The answer is given in Figure 61-2.

ITEM 61-8.   Peel off the arachnoid to open the subarachnoid space and to expose the cerebral arteries and veins lying in the space. In life, when the subarachnoid space is opened, cerebrospinal fluid leaks out because the cerebrospinal fluid is normally under pressure. After a surgical procedure it is not possible to close the subarachnoid space by suturing the arachnoid because the arachnoid is flimsy and transparent. Under those circumstances leakage of cerebrospinal fluid is prevented by carefully suturing the dura mater.

THE CEREBRAL HEMISPHERE

The characteristic feature of the cortex of the cerebral hemisphere is the presence of gyri and sulci. Many of the gyri and sulci have names; only a few of them are introduced in this text.

A single gyrus and its adjacent sulci or a group of gyri and sulci form an area of the cortex for which a specific function or group of functions has been determined. Those areas are not confined to the lateral surface of the hemisphere, the surface that is now exposed, but extend also onto the medial and the inferior surfaces. Thus, when the term cerebral cortex is used, it is an error to visualize only the lateral surface of the cerebral hemisphere.

ITEM 61-9. Carefully separate the cerebral hemispheres enough to expose the falx cerebri and to see at least some of the medial aspect of each hemisphere that lies adjacent to the falx. Next, carefully elevate the hemisphere anteriorly and posteriorly to demonstrate to some extent the inferior surface of the hemisphere. In the study of human neuroanatomy you will be able to examine these surfaces much more extensively. The purpose of the present incomplete demonstration is to awaken you to the extent of the cerebral cortex.

The close relationship of the medial surfaces of the cerebral hemispheres (they are separated only by the falx cerebri) is of more than a passing interest. It means that both hemispheres can be involved in the growth of a midline tumor, and, when the same functional areas of each hemisphere are so involved, identical signs will be produced on each side of the body. Further discussion of the clinical aspect of this example of applied anatomy must be withheld. Nevertheless, if it throws light on the proximity to each other of the medial surfaces of the cerebral hemispheres, it has served its purpose.

For descriptive purposes each cerebral hemisphere is divided into lobes: frontal, parietal, occipital, and temporal (Fig. 61-5). Fairly precise boundaries are described for each lobe, but it must be emphasized that these boundaries are purely anatomic. Knowledge of their existence must not create a concept of cerebral function restrained rigidly by boundaries. Obviously further discussion along these lines leads us into a discussion of the mystery of the human mind, which is beyond the scope of this text. Sufficient has been said, no doubt, to make the student

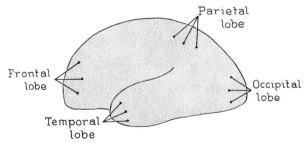

Figure 61-5. An indication of where the lobes of the cerebral hemisphere are located. The exact boundaries have been deliberately omitted to diminish their importance.

realize that he cannot split the function of the cerebral hemispheres into categories.

ITEM 61-10.   Identify the lobes of each hemisphere.

Orientation of the Hemisphere to the Skull

Obtain a skull with the skullcap off, more or less the same as in your cadaver. Look inside the skull and see that the floor of the skull is not flat but terraced. The anterior cranial fossa is at a higher level than the middle cranial fossa and the posterior cranial fossa is at a lower level.

Here one must interject the comment that the fossae are solitary structures. Thus each fossa extends from the right to the left side of the skull; it follows that each fossa has a solitary central zone and right and left extension from the central zone. That layout is particularly obvious in the anterior and the middle cranial fossae, but it is barely recognizable in the posterior cranial fossa. For ease in communication each lateral extension of the middle cranial fossa is usually referred to as *the* middle cranial fossa.

It is also important to establish now that the posterior cranial fossa is roofed by an incomplete sheet of dura, named the tentorium cerebelli because of its tentlike shape and its position superior to the cerebellum. The deficiency in the dura over the posterior cranial fossa is termed the tentorial notch. Thus each hemisphere is related to the anterior and middle cranial fossae and to the tentorium cerebelli.

Examine the skull more closely and establish that the floor of the anterior cranial fossa is also the roof of the centrally placed right and left nasal cavities and of both orbits.

Then establish that the central portion of the middle cranial fossa lies superior to the roof of the pharynx. The floor of each lateral part of this fossa is a slope. Posteriorly the slope is level with the superior margin of the external auditory meatus and is immediately superior to the petrous part of the temporal bone, wherein the middle ear and internal ear are placed. Anteriorly the floor of the middle cranial fossa is also the roof of the infratemporal fossa. Because of the stepdown from the anterior to the middle cranial fossa the contents of the lateral part of the middle cranial fossa lie directly posterior to the orbit.

The roof of the posterior cranial fossa, the tentorium cerebelli, has already been mentioned. The floor of the fossa contains the foramen magnum, through which the spinal cord passes and to which the inferior surface of the cerebellum is related.

THE PTERION

The sharp margin where the anterior cranial fossa changes abruptly to the middle cranial fossa is formed by the lesser wing of the sphenoid.

The lesser wing does not reach the side of the skull, but its companion, the greater wing of the sphenoid, forming part of the floor of the middle cranial fossa, does reach the side of the skull at the pterion. Many neurosurgical procedures are performed in the vicinity of these two wings, so the pterion is a significant landmark in selecting the correct site for a bone flap.

Examine the side of an intact skull and find the pterion. Four bones of the skull meet at the pterion, which is shaped like the letter H and is located at a point two fingerbreadths above the center of the zygomatic arch.

ITEM 61-11. Replace the skull cap on your cadaver and establish where the frontal, parietal, occipital, and temporal lobes of the brain lie in relation to the external surface of the skull cap. Remove the skull cap and confirm that each frontal lobe is superior to one of the nasal cavities and to an orbit; that each temporal lobe is superior to the infratemporal fossa, to the petrous part of the temporal bone, and to the tentorium cerebelli; and that each occipital lobe is related inferiorly to the tentorium cerebelli. On each side identify the pterion.

THE CORTICAL VESSELS OF THE CEREBRAL HEMISPHERE

In each sulcus of the cerebral hemisphere an artery and a vein lie immersed in cerebrospinal fluid. The arteries are branches of the principal arteries nourishing each cerebral hemisphere: the anterior and middle cerebral arteries, which are branches of the internal carotid arteries, usually, and the posterior cerebral artery, which is usually a branch of the basilar artery.

The approximate distributions of the cortical branches of each of the principal arteries are illustrated in Figure 61-6. There are also central branches of each of the principal arteries distributed to the internal regions of the hemisphere. Although the central branches are not illustrated here, they are as important as the cortical branches, if not more so in some respects. They will be studied in more detail in the course on neuroanatomy.

Figure 61-6. A lateral view of the left cerebral hemisphere to show the areas of cortex supplied by the anterior, middle, and posterior cerebral arteries. In the dissection, the middle cerebral artery is used to lead the dissector to the circulus arteriosus (the circle of Willis).

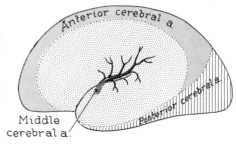

For descriptive purposes the veins of each cerebral hemisphere are divided into two groups, superficial and deep. In recent times the anatomy of both groups has been studied in depth in connection with the radiologic diagnosis of intracranial tumors. Because cerebral veins are connected to the cerebral arteries by fairly wide channels, a venous phase follows quite rapidly the arterial phase of cerebral angiography. Thus displacement of the veins, as well as displacement of arteries, has become an important feature to look for in the radiographic investigation of cerebral tumors (cerebral angiography). To name all the veins at this time would impose an unnecessary burden on the student. In time, however, he can expect to hear the cerebral veins dealt with in some detail.

The Ventricular System

Within each hemisphere there is a cavity named a lateral ventricle; it has a characteristic shape (Fig. 61-7). Each ventricle is connected to the solitary midline third ventricle by a foramen, the interventricular foramen (known also as the foramen of Monro). Within each ventricle there is a fringe of blood vessels, the tela chorioidea which is responsible for the production of cerebrospinal fluid. The cerebrospinal fluid leaves the ventricle through the foramen of Monro to enter the third ventricle. From there the cerebrospinal fluid enters the fourth ventricle, another solitary central cavity, which lies in the central nervous system in the posterior cranial fossa. The connection between the third ventricle and the fourth ventricle is a very narrow duct, the aqueduct of the midbrain. From the fourth ventricle cerebrospinal fluid reaches the subarachnoid space through certain apertures. How cerebrospinal fluid is transmitted to the venous circulation from the subarachnoid space has already been seen (p. 310). Although all this information is taking the student far in advance of the present stage of dissection, it is given here to point out that the cerebral hemisphere is not solid and to stress that each lateral ventricle is but a part of the entire ventricular system.

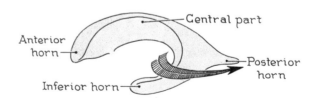

Figure 61-7. The cerebral hemisphere is not solid. The cavity within it, termed the lateral ventricle, is illustrated and its main features are named here. The foramen of Monro is not labeled. The arrow represents the sweep of the optic radiation.

The next chapter describes a method of hemispherectomy designed to give maximal exposure of the vessels and nerves at the base of the brain.

Chapter 62

Hemispherectomy

The purpose of hemispherectomy, the removal of one cerebral hemisphere, is to demonstrate the nerves and arteries at the base of the brain and not the successful removal of the cerebral hemisphere intact. Accordingly the cerebral hemisphere is removed piece by piece. On those occasions when the operator has attempted to remove the hemisphere intact some significant structure at the base of the brain has been slashed. During the removal of the hemisphere the student's attention will be drawn to major features of the hemisphere to be discussed in greater detail in neuroanatomy.

Occasionally in the dissecting room, evidence of the shift of one hemisphere across the midline is found. Examine your specimen very carefully by separating the cerebral hemispheres in the region of the falx cerebri to see if one or the other hemisphere is protruding underneath the archway of the falx, a protrusion spoken of clinically as a herniation. If herniation of a cerebral hemisphere beneath the falx cerebri has occurred, select the hemisphere that has not herniated for the next stage in the dissection.

DISSECTION

Separate the hemispheres sufficiently to reveal a broad solid bridge of tissue, the corpus callosum, connecting the two hemispheres. *On one side only*, through the hemisphere make a horizontal cut level with the superior surface of the corpus callosum. The plane of section lies immediately above the superior aspect of the lateral ventricle (Fig. 62-1). If the horizontal cut inadvertently opens the lateral ventricle and enters the corpus callosum, no harm is done as the next step will be a vertical cut through the corpus callosum. When this is done the portion of hemisphere sliced off will be released.

Dividing the corpus callosum presents no problem, but it must be done with care because you will be approaching a central region at the

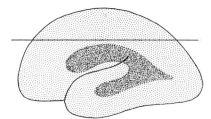

Figure 62-1. The line indicates the level of the first cut in hemispherectomy in a cadaver. The cut is immediately superior to the level of the corpus callosum and may enter the superior aspect of the lateral ventricle.

base of the brain where there are important structures. With a sharp knife, and always knowing exactly where the point of the knife has reached, cut the anterior end of the corpus callosum. Continue to cut this end, called the genu of the corpus callosum, until the optic chiasm is exposed. *Do not cut the chiasm.* Then cut the body of the corpus callosum and, finally, the posterior end of the corpus, which is known as the splenium. The pineal body is fully exposed once the splenium is cut.

Now separate the cut edges of the corpus callosum and peer down into the interval between them. If the corpus callosum cut was away from the midline—and it usually is—the septum lucidum (also known as the septum pellucidum) is seen. It is an anteroposterior, vertical, midline partition attached to the inferior surface of the corpus callosum and to the anterosuperior aspect of an elongated arched structure, the fornix. In addition to the septum lucidum you can see the superior surface of the thalamus, described in ordinary terms as a smooth round hump.

If the septum lucidum is seen in its entirety, you have opened the lateral ventricle. The septum lucidum is the medial wall of part of the lateral ventricle; the superior surface of the thalamus that is now exposed is the floor. The next slice off the hemisphere exposes more of the septum lucidum, opens up more of the lateral ventricle, and may cut off the superior surface of the thalamus.

Remove another slice of the hemisphere about 1 cm. thick and make a vertical cut into the thalamus to release the slice. More of the lateral ventricle is now open. Identify the anterior horn of the lateral ventricle, the central part of the ventricle, and the posterior horn. The inferior horn will be identified later.

Inside the ventricle a strip of granular material, the choroid plexus, is easily recognized. Trace the plexus anteriorly to where it leaves the ventricle at the interventricular foramen (the foramen of Monro). Also trace the plexus posteriorly and observe how it curves inferiorly to enter the inferior horn of the ventricle.

Break through the septum lucidum and realize that you have entered the lateral ventricle of the opposite side. At this level only the septum lucidum separates the two lateral ventricles.

Slip the tip of a probe through the foramen of Monro. The tip has entered a solitary midline cavity, the third ventricle, into which cerebro-

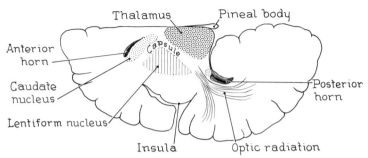

Figure 62-2. A horizontal section of the cerebral hemisphere to show certain features easily identified in the dissection. Study this figure and Figure 62-3 together. The tail of the caudate nucleus is not labeled.

spinal fluid drains from both lateral ventricles through both the right and left foramina of Monro.

With care, another slice may be taken from the hemisphere at the level of the pineal body. If the level of the slice has been well chosen several features are well seen (Fig. 62-2).

First, in this region of the hemisphere, there are several masses of gray matter of unusual shape (Fig. 62-3). Fortunately, a cross section of these masses is comprehensible and is visible in your present dissection (Fig. 62-2). The L-shaped zone of white matter, called the internal capsule (Fig. 62-2), includes fibers going to and from a substantial part of the cortex of the cerebral hemisphere. As a result there is such a concentration of nerve fibers in the internal capsule that minimal destruction there has widespread effects. One of the commonest disruptions in the internal capsule is due to the rupture of a very small artery; the result is paralysis of the opposite side of the body.

Second, at this stage of the dissection, the exact location of the inferior horn of the lateral ventricle can be demonstrated. Slide a probe or a matchstick into the inferior horn and confirm that the inferior horn lies in the temporal lobe posterior to the orbit. This relationship is taken advantage of in cerebral radiography. With the ventricular system full of air or with radiopaque fluid added to the cerebrospinal fluid, radio-

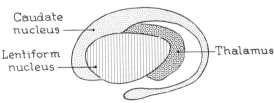

Figure 62-3. Lateral view of three masses of gray matter within the cerebral hemisphere. Study this figure and Figure 62-2 together.

graphs of the inferior horns of the lateral ventricles are taken through the orbits.

Third, the white matter immediately superior to the inferior horn of the lateral ventricle includes the optic radiation (Figs. 61-7 and 62-2). The radiation makes a wide sweep into the temporal lobe, and then narrows to a broad band of fibers lying apposed to the lateral aspect of first the inferior horn, and then the posterior horn.

Finally, observe how an area of the cerebral cortex lies deeper than the rest. The insula, as this area is called, lies deep to the lateral fissure. It is in the stem of the lateral fissure, in the region of the insula, that you will find the next important structure, the middle cerebral artery.

Identify the middle cerebral artery (Fig. 61-6). Be careful! In many cadavers the cerebral vessels are brittle as a result of calcification from arterial disease and embalming, so they break easily. By taking thin slices off the adjacent parts of the hemisphere, trace the artery toward its origin from the internal carotid artery. Observe how the middle cerebral artery, after it leaves the carotid artery, branches and branches again, giving the appearance of a spray of vessels. Examine closely the angles between the branches for evidence of berry aneurysm. An aneurysm looks like a little blister; it can rupture and give rise to a subarachnoid hemorrhage. Why is the hemorrhage described as subarachnoid?

Removal of the frontal lobe is next. In removing the frontal lobe it is necessary to preserve the anterior cerebral artery and the olfactory bulb and tract. Peel the anterior cerebral artery carefully off the medial aspect of what is left of the frontal lobe. Elevate the frontal lobe carefully so as not to disturb the olfactory bulb and tract. They lie in close relationship to the undersurface of the frontal lobe. Elevating the bulb off the cribriform plate on which it lies breaks the slender olfactory nerves passing through the plate to the nasal cavity. Every effort, therefore, must be made to leave the olfactory bulb and tract in situ while you remove piecemeal the frontal lobe.

Now examine the anterior cerebral arteries. Both of them can be found curving over the genu of the corpus callosum and continuing in a posterior direction on the superior surface of the corpus callosum. Trace each artery from its origin, the internal carotid artery, and observe how the anterior cerebral artery crosses superior to the optic nerve. Beyond the crossing point look carefully for a short artery, sometimes scarcely 1 mm. long, that joins the two anterior cerebral arteries. Although so short, this solitary artery, the anterior communicating artery, is frequently mentioned clinically because of the occurrence of aneurysms of its walls. The deep central location of the anterior communicating artery means that the surgical treatment of an aneurysm of that artery is difficult but not impossible.

If herniation of a hemisphere inferior to the free edge of the falx cerebri has occurred in your specimen, displacement of both anterior cerebral arteries to one side of the midline will have occurred. Such displacement is looked for on an anteroposterior view of a cerebral angiogram, as evidence of the presence of a space-occupying lesion that has displaced both hemispheres to one side of the cranium. However, the gap between the free edge of the falx and the corpus callosum decreases until there is no gap at all posteriorly. Thus, herniation of the medial surface of the hemisphere and displacement of the anterior cerebral arteries depend on the location of the space-occupying lesion.

In removing piecemeal the temporal lobe, observe how its pole extends anteriorly under the shelf created by the lesser wing of the sphenoid. As you remove the temporal lobe, look for evidence of herniation of its medial surface through the tentorial notch. It is not unusual to find that in some specimens it is necessary to lift the medial margin of each temporal lobe out of the posterior fossa over the taut edge of the tentorium cerebelli. Downward displacement of the medial aspect of each temporal lobe through the tentorial notch is a serious medical emergency. If tentorial herniation is present, it may have been the terminal cause of death because it causes midbrain compression.

Finally, on the medial aspect of the occipital lobe, elevate the arachnoid and then mobilize the posterior cerebral artery and trace it anteriorly while you remove the occipital lobe. Then carefully trim the cerebral peduncle until the vessels and nerves at the base of the brain are exposed.

Before you review the cranial nerves and arteries at the base of the brain, it is necessary to examine the dural folds, to cut the tentorium, to remove half of the cerebellum, and, finally, to identify the parts of the brain stem. These steps will be described in the next chapter.

Chapter 63

The Dural Folds and the Brain Stem

THE DURAL FOLDS

Both the falx cerebri and the tentorium cerebelli require more careful appraisal. In the intact skull they are tense, but in the present dissection much of that tension has been lost. Sufficient, however, remains for you to appreciate that in life both the falx and the tentorium are rigid partitions. The brain, then, is encased in a rigid container and is also fitted around rigid partitions. When space inside the container is taken up by something other than the brain (space-occupying lesion is the clinical term), the brain adjacent to a gap in the partition is pressed through the gap. Thus, herniation of the brain beneath the falx and into the tentorial notch occurs. It is not unusual to find examples of these changes in the dissecting laboratory.

Clinically, space-occupying lesions fall into two main categories, namely supra- and infratentorial. In brief, it is important to know that a tumor is either supra- or infratentorial, for on that basis the surgical approach is selected.

Another practical surgical aspect is the presence throughout the dural folds of venous sinuses. These venous sinuses are not named but they are well known to the neurosurgeon. They bleed freely when they are cut.

ITEM 63-1.   Examine the falx cerebri. Often it is not a complete sheet because of the presence of fenestrations. Its free edge is reinforced, contains the inferior longitudinal venous sinus, and lies some distance from the corpus callosum.

Examine the tentorium. Observe how it forms a roof for the posterior cranial fossa and acts as a support for the occipital lobes. Observe, too, how its superior surface is convex, declines laterally, and extends anteriorly to merge without interruption with the floor of the middle cranial fossa. Its central part is hoisted up by the falx cerebri so that the margin of the tentorial notch is not horizontal.

Select the midpoint of the exposed margin of the notch. Safeguard the trochlear nerve and the posterior cerebral artery. Cut the tentorium to create two flaps. Pull the anterior flap forward to open the cerebellopontine cistern, which is the gap posterior to the temporal bone, anterior to the cerebellum, and lateral to the pons. In life it is full of cerebrospinal fluid and is crossed by the seventh and eighth cranial nerves. This region is sometimes referred to as the cerebellopontine angle. Alert for the fourth cranial nerve, trim the anterior flap of tentorium close to the petrous temporal bone and the posterior flap close to the straight and transverse sinuses.

Safeguard the seventh and eighth nerves and carefully carve slices off the lateral lobe of the cerebellum. Almost the entire half of the cerebellum can be removed in this way to give a wide exposure of the other contents of the posterior cranial fossa.

THE BRAIN STEM (FIG. 63-1)

The brain stem comprises the midbrain, the pons, and the medulla. The midbrain is only 2 to 3 cm. long and about the same meas-

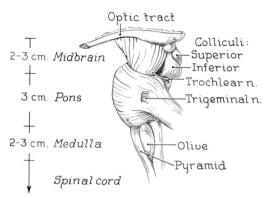

Figure 63-1.   Lateral view of the brain stem. For descriptive purposes, the cephalic end of the midbrain is level with the optic tract.

urement from side to side. Its posterior surface is easily identified by the presence of four small rounded eminences, the superior and inferior colliculi. The anterior aspect of the midbrain consists of two broad longitudinal masses, the two cerebral peduncles, separated from each other by the interpeduncular cistern. The midbrain occupies the tentorial notch but there is a significant short gap between the surface of the midbrain and the margins of the notch.

The pons is inferior to the midbrain and is slightly longer than the midbrain. Its anterior surface is easily identified; it consists of transversely arranged fibers with a characteristic forward bulge. The posterior surface of the pons is obscured by the cerebellum.

The medulla oblongata lies below the pons; it is 2 or 3 cm. long and tapers to meet the spinal cord at the foramen magnum. Its anterior surface is readily identified by paired elevations, the pyramids and the olives. The posterior surface of the medulla is obscured from view by the cerebellum.

ITEM 63-2.   Without breaking delicate structures, identify the main parts of the brain stem (Fig. 63-1).

The specimen is now ready for a review of the nerves and vessels at the base of the brain. The next chapter summarizes the bulk of information now to be met and is essential reading preliminary to the review.

Chapter 64

Basic Plan of Nerves, Arteries, and Veins at the Base of the Brain

NERVES

One of the basic features that requires emphasis is the occurrence of nerves in pairs. The complete description of the cranial nerves is always written in the singular, not the plural, and it is certainly much easier to describe a nerve in this way. The great disadvantage, known from experience, is that the junior clinical student, who has earnestly learned his anatomy as it is written, is sadly confused when he has to deal with the cranial nerves as pairs. This confusion is often demonstrated when he deals with the innervation of the extraocular muscles, but it is especially obvious when he deals with a central structure or region with a bilateral innervation.

For example, the muscles of the tongue are innervated by both the right and left hypoglossal nerves. If only one nerve is at fault only one half of the tongue is paralyzed. The muscles of facial expression are innervated by both the right and left facial nerves. Again, if one nerve is at fault only one half of the face is paralyzed. It is permissible to say that the muscles of the tongue or the muscles of facial expression are paralyzed, provided one realizes that the paralysis is unilateral. On the other hand, the muscular paralysis of a central structure may, indeed, be bilateral. Then both right and left innervations are involved. For example, the muscles of the entire soft palate may be paralyzed. Further discussion of this interesting aspect of the applied anatomy of the cranial nerves must be postponed. Sufficient has been said to make the student appreciate why a clinician establishes quickly whether a paralysis is unilateral or bilateral.

It is now appropriate to present a series of headings not only helpful in describing a nerve but also useful in clinical diagnosis. At each of the places indicated by one of the headings (Fig. 64-1C), the nerve pathway may be involved in some type of disorder. Whatever the process involving the nerve, the outcome is manifest in the distribution of the nerve, which is the sixth and last heading. A clinician retains the evidence he obtains on examination of the distribution of a nerve and goes back, in his mind's eye, along the nerve pathway to establish where the

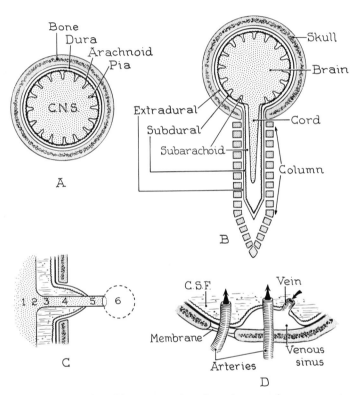

Figure 64-1. *A* and *B*. Diagrams to show how the central nervous system is surrounded by membranes, spaces and bone. *C*. Each nerve obtains a sleeve of dura-arachnoid-subarachnoid space. The length of the sleeve varies—the sheath of the optic nerve is the longest. The numbers are discussed in the text. *D*. How arteries reach the central nervous system. The vertebral artery penetrates a membrane. The internal carotid artery penetrates the skull; the winding course of this artery is ignored here.

breakdown in the transmission of impulses has occurred. This sounds like a laborious process, and it is, to a beginner. Yet once the method is familiar, the art of neurologic examination is born.

The headings are:
1. Central connections
2. Superficial origin
3. Intracranial course
4. "Intraosseous" course
5. Extracranial course
6. Distribution

Central Connections (Fig. 64-1C).   The nerve pathways within the central nervous system are dealt with in a separate study, neuroanatomy. That this is so is one of the most regrettable developments ever to occur in the teaching of anatomy. Ultimately, in clinical practice the student will find that nerve pathways are not in two parts, as they are in many a timetable. The central nervous system and the rest of the body are inseparable; a lesion in the former is recognized only by its manifestations in the latter. The student, faced with the separation of gross anatomy and neuroanatomy, often by a year in a curriculum, must integrate his knowledge of gross anatomy with his knowledge of neuroanatomy when that knowledge is eventually acquired.

Superficial Origin (Fig. 64-1C).   The superficial origin, i.e., the point where the nerve is obviously attached to the central nervous system, is the point where the nerve fibers first appear outside the central nervous system. It must be stressed that the fibers of which the nerve is composed have their origins elsewhere. This concept lessens the importance of the superficial origin, but not entirely. For example, rupture of the superficial origins of nerves can occur in association with high speed accidents. Certain nerves, because of the location, delicacy, and direction of the rootlets comprising their superficial origin, are more prone to rupture than others.

Intracranial Course (Fig. 64-1C).   The intracranial course extends from the superficial origin to the opening in bone through which the nerve passes. The course may be divided into two parts: All the cranial nerves pass through the subarachnoid space, the first part of the intracranial course, where they are bathed in cerebrospinal fluid. The length of nerve and its obliquity in the subarachnoid space vary from one pair of nerves to the next. The length of certain nerves and their obliquity, are significant in certain forms of intracranial disease because those nerves are vulnerable to shifts of the brain in relation to the skull and to the dural folds.

The second part of the intracranial course applies to a few cranial nerves only. Before the third, fourth, and sixth cranial nerves and the ophthalmic division of the fifth reach the superior orbital fissure where they enter the orbit, they leave the subarachnoid space and become intimately related to the cavernous sinus. In this second part of their intracranial course these nerves have a significant relationship to the internal carotid artery and other arteries.

The "Intraosseous" Course (Fig. 64-1C). The "intraosseous" course may be short or long and the opening in the bone may be narrow or wide. All cranial nerves are vulnerable in fractures when the boundaries of the intraosseous course are displaced. The classic example is the long winding course of the facial nerve through a narrow canal in the temporal bone. Certain fractures through the temporal bone injure the facial nerve. On the other hand, a shearing force across the very short and relatively wide superior orbital fissure may injure the nerves to the orbit.

Extracranial Course and Distribution. The extracranial course and distribution of each pair of cranial nerves are usually studied in more detail than is necessary. The student is reminded, therefore, that he must integrate his knowledge of neuroanatomy with his knowledge of gross anatomy so that without hesitation he can trace a nerve pathway from its beginning to its end (Fig. 64-1C).

ARTERIES

There are four sources of blood to the brain. On each side of the neck there is an internal carotid artery and a vertebral artery. Having entered the skull, each internal carotid artery branches into an anterior cerebral and a middle cerebral artery. In contrast to the branching of the carotid artery, the two vertebral arteries join to form the solitary basilar artery. After a short distance, however, the basilar artery divides into the right and left posterior cerebral arteries. How the internal carotid artery and the vertebral artery enter the skull is dealt with next.

As each artery destined for the central nervous system is separated from the central nervous system by bone (Fig. 64-1D), it must have an "intraosseous" course. Then each artery must puncture the dura and the arachnoid and cross the subarachnoid space to arrive on the surface of the central nervous system.

Each internal carotid artery has a winding course before it reaches the base of the brain. It passes first through the carotid canal, then through a dural venous sinus, the cavernous sinus, and finally through the arachnoid to enter the subarachnoid space (Fig. 64-1D). The easiest way to understand the winding path of the internal carotid artery is to see it on a specimen or to study angiograms of the cerebral arteries.

Each vertebral artery, on the other hand, does not pass through a long bony canal but passes through a gap between the skull and the vertebral column. Thus the vertebral artery has no true "intraosseous"

text continued on page 330.

Table 64-1. *Origin, Course, and Distribution of the Cranial Nerves*

CRANIAL NERVE	CENTRAL CONNECTIONS	SUPERFICIAL ORIGIN	INTRACRANIAL COURSE
I	For details concerning central connections a textbook of neuroanatomy should be consulted	On each side there are bundles of nerve fibers forming an olfactory nerve. The fibers are attached to an olfactory bulb connected to the brain by the olfactory tract.	The bundles pass briefly through the anterior cranial fossa.
II		For descriptive purposes each optic nerve begins at the optic chiasm. The optic pathway, however, extends from the retina of each eyeball to the occipital lobes.	At the junction of the anterior and middle cranial fossae, the optic nerve has a short but significant course in the cerebrospinal fluid, and is related to arteries.
III		On the medial aspect of the cerebral peduncle at the upper border of the pons.	It goes through the cerebrospinal fluid of the interpeduncular cistern to the wall of the cavernous sinus; passes near to several arteries.
IV		On the dorsal surface of the midbrain, immediately inferior to the inferior colliculus.	In the cerebrospinal fluid it runs inferior and parallel to the edge of the tentorial notch to circumvent the midbrain. Then the nerve enters wall of the cavernous sinus.
V		The middle of the lateral aspect of the pons, by a large sensory and a small motor root.	After crossing through the cerebrospinal fluid of the pontine cistern, the roots pass inferior to the superior petrosal sinus to a subdural location in the middle cranial fossa. The sensory root joins a ganglion; the motor root remains separate.
VI		On the lower border of the pons, immediately superior to the pyramid.	After ascending through the cerebrospinal fluid of the pontine cistern, the nerve enters the cavernous sinus where it lies lateral to the internal carotid artery.
VII		On the lateral aspect of the junction of the pons and the medulla, adjacent to the auditory nerve. The facial nerve has a motor component and an autonomic and sensory component, the nervus intermedius.	In the cerebrospinal fluid with the auditory nerve across the cerebellopontine cistern of the posterior cranial fossa.

INTRAOSSEOUS COURSE	EXTRACRANIAL COURSE	DISTRIBUTION	
Through perforations in the cribriform plate of the ethmoid. It is held that each bundle has its own sleeve of dura-arachnoid-cerebrospinal fluid.	Under the mucosa of the superior region of each nasal cavity.	To a small part of each nasal cavity.	I
Through the optic canal, in the wall of the sphenoidal air sinus.	Through the orbit in a sleeve of dura-arachnoid-cerebrospinal fluid which is in continuity with dura, etc., within the cranial cavity and the sclera of the eyeball.	To the retina of the eyeball.	II
Leaves wall of the cavernous sinus to pass through the superior orbital fissure.	Within the orbit.	To extraocular muscles — superior rectus (and levator palpebrae superioris), medial rectus, inferior rectus, inferior oblique: to intraocular muscles controlling pupil and lens.	III
Leaves wall of the cavernous sinus to pass through the superior orbital fissure.	Within the orbit.	To an extraocular muscle, the superior oblique.	IV
Ganglion gives off ophthalmic, maxillary, mandibular divisions. The ophthalmic lies in the wall of the cavernous sinus, then passes through the superior orbital fissure; maxillary — through the foramen rotundum; mandibular — through the foramen ovale.	Ophthalmic — through the orbit; maxillary — on the superior aspect of the maxilla; mandibular — in the infratemporal fossa.	Each fifth cranial nerve: Motor — muscles of mastication. Sensory — the skin of the face and scalp (Fig. 60-2), conjunctiva, mucous membrane of the oral and nasal cavities and of the nasal sinuses, teeth and gums, anterior two-thirds of the tongue, dura mater; temporomandibular joint. Autonomic — mucous glands in nasal and oral cavities.	V
Leaves the cavernous sinus to pass through the superior orbital fissure.	Within the orbit.	To an extraocular muscle, the lateral rectus.	VI
The intraosseous course begins at the internal acoustic meatus, then is long and changes direction through the temporal bone. The nerve is horizontal between the organ of balance and of hearing, is then related to the middle ear before descending vertically through the mastoid to the stylomastoid foramen.	Through the parotid gland to the face.	Each facial nerve: Sensory — taste. Autonomic — salivation. Motor — the frontalis, orbicularis oris, buccinator, and platysma, muscles of facial expression.	VII

Table 64-1. *Origin, Course, and Distribution of the Cranial Nerves* (Continued)

CRANIAL NERVE	CENTRAL CONNECTIONS	SUPERFICIAL ORIGIN	INTRACRANIAL COURSE
VIII		On the lateral aspect of the junction of the pons and the medulla adjacent to the facial nerve.	In the cerebrospinal fluid, with the facial nerve across the cerebellopontine cistern of the posterior cranial fossa.
IX		By rootlets attached in a groove posterior to the olive on the medulla.	Through the cerebrospinal fluid of the posterior cranial fossa.
X		On the medulla by rootlets between the olive and the inferior cerebellar peduncle. The rootlets are in line with those of the ninth and eleventh cranial nerves.	Through the cerebrospinal fluid of the posterior cranial fossa.
XI		The nerve has two components, spinal and cranial. The cranial part is dealt with in neuroanatomy. The spinal part is attached by several rootlets to the lateral aspect of the upper five cervical cord segments.	In the cerebrospinal fluid of the vertebral canal, the spinal accessory nerve ascends between the motor and sensory roots of the cord to enter the skull through the foramen magnum. Then the nerve travels through the posterior cranial fossa to the jugular foramen.
XII		By several rootlets to the medulla between the olive and the pyramid.	In the cerebrospinal fluid of the posterior cranial fossa anterolaterally, superior to the vertebral artery.

INTRAOSSEOUS COURSE	EXTRACRANIAL COURSE	DISTRIBUTION	
The nerve enters the internal acoustic meatus and proceeds in the temporal bone to the organs of balance and hearing.	None—the nerve ends in the temporal bone.	Organ of balance and organ of hearing.	VIII
Through the jugular foramen.	After leaving the jugular foramen the nerve passes onto the slender vertical stylopharyngeus to reach the level of the oropharynx, where it pierces the wall of the pharynx.	Sensory, from the back of the tongue, the region of the tonsil, the eustachian tube, the middle ear, the nasal and oral portions of the pharynx, the carotid sinus and body, the taste buds on the posterior third of the tongue; secretomotor fibers to the parotid gland; motor to the stylopharyngeus.	IX
Through the jugular foramen.	Neck, thorax, and abdomen.	Pharynx and gastrointestinal musculature down to the splenic flexure of the colon; larynx (sensory and motor); heart; bronchi; mucous glands of the gastrointestinal and respiratory systems. There is a significant sensory branch to the external acoustic meatus.	X
Through the jugular foramen.	From the foramen the nerve passes close to the internal jugular vein. through a cluster of lymph nodes, to enter the sternomastoid, which it supplies. Then the nerve crosses the posterior triangle of the neck embedded in fascia close to the skin to enter the trapezius, which it also supplies.	The sternomastoid and trapezius.	XI
Through the hypoglossal (anterior condylar) canal.	From the canal, the nerve proceeds laterally, then anteriorly, lying superficial to both the internal and external carotid arteries. The nerve occupies a characteristic location superficial to the "arch" of the lingual artery.	The muscles of the tongue are divided by a median sagittal septum into right and left halves. Each half is supplied by a hypoglossal nerve.	XII

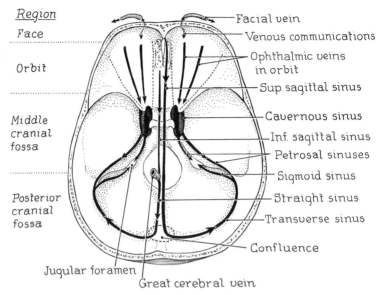

Figure 64-2. A plan of the principal venous sinuses and their relationship to the cranial fossae.

course in the skull. Furthermore, the vertebral artery does not meet a sinus in the dura. Thus it punctures dura and arachnoid immediately to enter the subarachnoid space (Fig. 64-1*D*).

VEINS

From the surface of the brain, veins leave to reach a venous sinus or venous system (Fig. 64-1*D*). Generally each vein goes to the nearest sinus or system. Each vein crosses the subarachnoid space and then penetrates the arachnoid and dura. That the vein crosses the subdural space was demonstrated when the dura was reflected. On each side all the venous sinuses eventually drain into the internal jugular vein, which begins at the jugular foramen at the base of the skull (Fig. 64-2).

Chapter 65

Review of the Intracranial Course of the Cranial Nerves, Cerebral Arteries, and the Dural Venous Sinuses

THE CRANIAL NERVES

The basic information is provided in the summary (Table 64-1). For each cranial nerve confirm the information under the headings Superficial Origin, Intracranial Course, and Intraosseous Course. Then, with a skull in hand, identify the foramina through which the nerves pass from both the inside and the outside of the skull.

The attachment of the spinal accessory nerve to the lateral aspect of the cervical cord cannot be seen well, but the nerve itself can be seen ascending through the foramen magnum. The glossopharyngeal nerve is easily spotted. It is separated from the vagus nerve by a tiny bridge of dura at the jugular foramen. The other cranial nerves are easily located.

THE INTRACRANIAL ARTERIES

There are numerous intracranial arteries, all of them significant because of the important parts of the central nervous system they supply. Occlusion of any one of these arteries produces a characteristic group of signs and symptoms (such a group is termed a syndrome, clinically). Experience in teaching indicates that knowledge of the arterial blood supply of the brain is more easily retained when it can be related to function. Accordingly, the more detailed study of the intracranial arteries should be postponed until the structure and function of the central nervous system have been studied. Meanwhile the cerebral and the cerebellar arteries can be observed.

ITEM 65-1. The Cerebral Arteries

Identify the internal carotid artery emerging from the cavernous sinus and piercing the arachnoid to enter the subarachnoid space, where it lies lateral to the optic chiasm. Identify the anterior and middle cerebral arteries, branches of the internal carotid artery. Observe how the anterior cerebral artery proceeds anteromedially as a superior relation of the optic nerve, and how the middle cerebral artery proceeds laterally. It continues laterally more or less parallel to the lesser wing of the sphenoid and buried in the depths of the lateral sulcus of the cerebral hemisphere.

Peer down into the posterior cranial fossa and see the vertebral artery puncturing the dura and the arachnoid to enter the subarachnoid space. Without mangling the cranial nerves in the fossa, follow the artery to where it joins its fellow from the opposite side to form the solitary basilar artery. Trace the basilar artery to where it branches. It is quite common in the dissecting laboratory to find arterial anomalies in this region; one of the posterior cerebral arteries may arise from the internal carotid artery.

The posterior cerebral artery and the internal carotid artery (or the middle cerebral artery) are connected to each other by the posterior communicating artery. Having identified these arteries, the student must now review the circulus arteriosus, the circle of Willis, consisting of the two posterior cerebral arteries, the two posterior communicating arteries, the two internal carotid arteries, and the two anterior cerebral arteries connected by the unpaired anterior communicating artery.

THE CIRCLE OF WILLIS

The common use of radiopaque injections to demonstrate intracranial blood vessels has confirmed the function and significance of the circulus arteriosus. For a long time, on the basis of its anatomic structure, the circle was regarded as a principal anastomosis, presumably of some importance. Today there is considerable proof that the anastomosis really is effective.

Having said that, we must stress that cerebral angiography and clinical experience reveal that there is considerable individual variation in the effectiveness of the anastomosis. For example, there are occasions when a radiopaque solution injected into the internal carotid system enters the anterior and middle cerebral arteries but does not flow through the posterior communicating artery to enter the posterior cerebral artery. On the other hand, sometimes the posterior communicating artery is incorporated in the posterior cerebral artery, which is then recognized as a branch of the internal carotid artery and not of the basilar artery. When this is so then a radiopaque injection into the appropriate internal carotid artery flows into the posterior cerebral artery also. Clearly the circulus arteriosus is yet another example of an anatomic region where basic descriptive anatomy is to be accepted merely as a guide and not as the absolute. Thus occlusion of any one of the internal carotid arteries or of the vertebral arteries may or may not deprive a part of the brain of sufficient blood to have serious consequences.

With the great developments in neurosurgical procedures, the circulus arteriosus is more significant today than ever before. The vessels forming the circle are prone to form aneurysms, the great majority of which are amenable to surgical treatment. That statement has no impact until you know that rupture of an aneurysm of a cerebral artery is suddenly dangerous to life because of the free flow of arterial blood into the limitations of the subarachnoid space within the confines of the cranial cavity.

Now that you see the location of the circulus arteriosus you can appreciate the dilemma of the neurosurgeon called upon to treat a subarachnoid hemorrhage. The cranium cannot be opened as widely as the abdomen, the thorax, the limbs, or the neck. Because the neurosurgical approach is limited it must be exact. The preoperative diagnosis must be precise. Yet any delay in controlling the hemorrhage may have a fatal result.

ITEM 56-2. Identify the vessels forming the circulus arteriosus in your specimen.

CEREBELLAR ARTERIES

When half the cerebellum was pared away to expose the brain stem the superior cerebellar artery was encountered, its branches spreading over the superior surface of the cerebellum.

There are two arteries on the inferior surface of the cerebellar hemisphere. The anterior inferior cerebellar artery, arising from the basilar artery, runs close to the seventh and eighth nerves and may be closely related to the internal acoustic meatus.

The posterior inferior cerebellar artery, a branch of the vertebral artery, is recognized immediately by its hairpin shape (sometimes a double hairpin). It is located close to the vagus and glossopharyngeal nerves on the lateral aspect of the medulla oblongata. It is the cerebellar artery most often mentioned clinically.

On each side, one tiny artery, the labyrinthine (also known as the internal auditory) artery, arising from the basilar artery, accompanies the seventh and eighth nerves into the petrous part of the temporal bone. Each tiny artery, scarcely visible in a cadaver, nourishes a labyrinth containing microscopic structures vital to the balance of the entire human frame.

The Dural Venous Sinuses

Several sinuses have been encountered in the course of the dissection so far, and there are many more. The number of venous sinuses can bewilder the student, but if he follows the arrows in Figure 64-2 he will soon appreciate that the blood flow in the sinuses is toward each internal jugular vein, which begins at the jugular foramen.

Some confusion occurs in the descriptions of the confluence of the sinuses (Fig. 64-2). It has long been recognized as a venous pool, fed by the superior sagittal sinus and the straight sinus and drained by the transverse sinuses. However, the confluence is not always present. The superior sagittal sinus may join one or the other transverse sinus and the same is true of the straight sinus. With the development and the progress in the use of cerebral angiography we have become much more aware that the confluence of sinuses, the so-called torcular Herophili (after Herophilus, circa 350 B.C.) is also subject to variation.

Guided by Figure 64-2, trace the dural venous sinuses in your specimen. It must be stressed again that in life blood flows freely through these sinuses. They are a surgical hazard at operation. Look, for example, at the superior petrosal sinus poised immediately superior to the sensory root of the fifth cranial nerve. Surgical procedures upon the fifth cranial nerve in this region must take this venous sinus into account, no matter how slender it seems in a cadaver. Furthermore, there are various pathologic conditions in which clotting of blood (thrombosis) occurs in the dural venous sinuses; the consequent venous congestion of the brain is usually fatal.

ITEM 65-3. Removal of the Other Hemisphere

There are several ways to proceed, all of them easy, successful, and instructive. The first way is to leave the hemisphere intact; then, selecting the appropriate procedures, continue the dissection of the head and neck. The end result is an excellent specimen typical of the specimens from which classic illustrations of a median sagittal section of head and neck have been drawn. The second way is to cut through the cerebral peduncle to release the hemisphere; in doing so the major arteries must be released from the hemisphere. The end result is a specimen similar to Figure 505 in *Grant's Atlas of Anatomy*. The third way is to repeat the method given in detail here. In our experience, most students choose the third way, mainly because they feel it reinforces knowledge already obtained.

Whatever your group elects to do, the next step, opening the fourth ventricle, must now be done.

Chapter 66

Opening the Fourth Ventricle

The fourth ventricle is the final part of the ventricular system. It lies anterior to the cerebellum and posterior to the pons and upper part of the medulla in the posterior cranial fossa. The ventricle is continuous with the aqueduct of the midbrain superiorly.

ITEM 66-1. To open the ventricle, identify the midline of the cerebellum. Keeping the knife blade strictly in an anteroposterior plane, cut into the midline of the cerebellum. While you advance carefully into the cerebellum, gradually separate the cut surfaces until you identify the cavity of the ventricle. Then extend the cut superiorly and inferiorly until the cavity is wide open.

In life, cerebrospinal fluid not only flows into the fourth ventricle through the aqueduct of the midbrain, but is also produced by the choroid plexuses, the granular structures protruding into the ventricle. Cerebrospinal fluid leaves the fourth ventricle through three apertures, one median and two lateral. The median aperture is located in the midline at the junction of the inferior aspect of the cerebellum and the medulla. It is usually obscured in the cadaver. Each lateral aperture is located at the extreme lateral corner of the lateral recess of the fourth ventricle. The boundaries of the opening are usually collapsed in a cadaver.

Review

The fourth ventricle is part of a hollow system located within the central nervous system. The other parts are the two lateral ventricles, the third ventricle, and the aqueduct of the midbrain. Cerebrospinal fluid, being produced continuously by the choroid plexuses, flows through the system. Most of the cerebrospinal fluid is produced by the choroid plexuses in each lateral ventricle and flows through each foramen of Monro into the third ventricle. Some more cerebrospinal fluid is produced in the third ventricle and the combined volume flows down the aqueduct of the midbrain into the fourth ventricle. A little more cerebrospinal fluid is produced in the fourth ventricle and the total volume leaves the ventricular system through the median and the two lateral apertures to enter the subarachnoid space around the cerebellum and the medulla. Those three apertures are the only openings through which cerebrospinal fluid flows from the ventricular system to the subarachnoid space.

That those three small apertures are nearly always fashioned to perfection is one of the mysteries of human development. Occasionally the orifices fail to develop, and then C.S.F. accumulates within the ventricular system. The result is one variety of hydrocephalus, a condition offering nothing but despair until recent times, when modern medical science has developed ways of draining the ventricular system. In the course of these recent developments, many questions have been raised regarding the pathogenesis of hydrocephalus. Accordingly, neither the mode of origin of hydrocephalus nor its surgical treatment is discussed further here, but you should look closely at the anatomy of the fourth ventricle with reference to the entrance and exit of cerebrospinal fluid.

Chapter 67

The Cavernous Sinuses and the Hypophysis Cerebri

On each side of the midline of the skull, the third, fourth, and sixth cranial nerves, the ophthalmic division of the fifth cranial nerve, and the internal carotid artery have an intimate relationship with the cavernous sinus. The hypophysis cerebri lies in the midline between the two cavernous sinuses. It has already been pointed out that the sinus is less than the size of the tip of a little finger; it is indeed small and difficult to dissect.

ITEM 67-1. Begin with the third and fourth nerves. By careful dissection with a blunt-ended probe, trace them through the roof of the cavernous sinus as far as the superior orbital fissure.

The sixth nerve lies inside the sinus. To expose the sixth cranial nerve, carefully open the superior aspect of the wall of the cavernous sinus, displace the ophthalmic division of the trigeminal nerve laterally, and flush out the debris in the sinus. The sixth nerve lies on the lateral aspect of the internal carotid artery. Observe how the sixth nerve ascends through the subarachnoid space of the posterior cranial fossa before bending to pierce the dura to enter the cavernous sinus. Trace the nerve to the superior orbital fissure.

Observe the winding shape of the internal carotid artery, a shape now commonly referred to as the carotid siphon.

THE HYPOPHYSIS CEREBRI

Between the cavernous sinuses lies the hypophysis cerebri, measuring 8 by 10 by 15 mm. It is difficult to believe that the influence of such a small structure penetrates so deeply into the function of the entire human frame. Two main parts of the gland are recognized, an anterior lobe, hailed as the mastermind of the endocrine system, and a posterior lobe which has several functions, the most widely known of which is the prevention of secretion of an excessive amount of dilute urine. To touch briefly upon all of the functions of the hypophysis cerebri without knowledge of its histology and cytology as well as of the functions of the other endocrine glands and of the kidneys will only lead to confusion. Furthermore, as modern research has revealed, the functions of the actual lobes of the hypophysis cannot be divorced from the functions of its stalk and of the adjacent part of the brain. The amount of minute research, in recent times, into this small region can only be described as colossal. Therefore, it is a relief to say that the gross anatomy of the hypophysis cerebri is simple. The relevant facts are dealt with here, as follows:

(1) Like all endocrine glands, the hypophysis has a profuse blood supply. On each side of it are the cavernous sinuses; anteriorly and posteriorly these sinuses are connected by intercavernous sinuses. Venous blood drains from the hypophysis into all of these sinuses by numerous thin-walled veins. In life, therefore, the hypophysis cerebri virtually sits in a pool of blood.

Numerous minute arteries reach the hypophysis and its stalk from the circulus arteriosus lying on the superior aspect of the diaphragma sellae.

(2) The superior surface of the anterior lobe is related, first, to the diaphragma sellae and then to the posteroinferior surface of the optic chiasm. To emphasize the significance of that relationship it is stated without explanation or qualification that the chiasm incorporates fibers responsible for vision in both the right and left temporal fields. Pituitary tumors compressing the chiasm ultimately reduce vision in both temporal fields.

(3) The hypophysis lies in the hypophyseal fossa, the sella turcica. The precise measurements of the sella are known and radiologists consider these measurements very carefully when they are called on to assist in the diagnosis of an early tumor, for erosion of the sella is commonly seen in pituitary tumors.

(4) The sphenoidal air sinus separates the hypophyseal fossa from the nasal cavities, which lie anteroinferiorly.

(5) Posterior to the posterior wall of the sphenoidal air sinus the hypophyseal fossa is separated from the roof of the pharynx by a 1 cm. thickness of bone.

The last two points will be readily apparent when the head is divided (p. 407). It is worth stating now, however, that the anterior lobe of the hypophysis is developed from the region of the embryo that ultimately becomes the roof of the pharynx.

ITEM 67-2. Identify the stalk (also known as the infundibulum) connecting the hypophysis to a region of the base of the brain termed the hypothalamus. Tilting the optic chiasm toward the midline reveals the stalk, but it may also easily break the stalk. If the stalk does not break, cut it to reveal more clearly how it goes through the diaphragma sellae to join the hypophysis. Observe the numerous little arteries reaching the stalk and the close proximity of the cavernous sinuses. Snip away the diaphragma sellae to expose the hypophysis, which may have changed beyond all recognition because of postmortem autolysis. Establish the relationship of the hypophysis to the optic chiasm.

Chapter 68

The Orbital Opening

There are several openings in the bony walls of the orbits, most of them transmitting significant structures, but the orbital openings are the largest of them all. Leading into the sockets for the eyes, they dominate the front view of the skull. Sometimes the orbital opening is referred to as the orbital aperture and, rarely, as the aditus orbitae. The soft tissues within the margin of the opening are often referred to as "the eye."

Exercise

In life, the most obvious features of "the eye" are the eyelids and the anterior pole of the eyeball.

The relationship of the pole to the orbital margin is of great practical importance. Obtain a skull and examine the orbital margin. It is nearly square in shape, but the sides of the square are not on the same plane. Confirm that fact by viewing the skull from the side. The superior part of the orbital margin overhangs the opening, while the lateral part of the margin is swept back. From the same view point, observe how the frontal process of the maxilla and the nasal bone are built forward to form the root of the nose.

Now, on both sides of your own face, place the tip of the index finger on the extreme lateral margin of the orbital opening. With a light touch press medially to demonstrate how much each eyeball protrudes beyond the margin. At least one third, perhaps a little more, of each eyeball is palpable.

To vivify these facts, proceed thus. With both eyes open, and without moving the head, look as far to the left as possible. Then bring the tip of the right index finger from a posterior position forward toward the lateral margin of the right orbital opening. The tip of the finger reaches the opening without being seen. Imagine that the tip of the finger is the prong of a pitchfork wielded vigorously by a companion while your gaze is concentrated elsewhere. Clearly the eyeball, poised in the orbital opening, is vulnerable on the flank.

As a further demonstration, look straight ahead and close one eye — for example, the left eye. Continue to look ahead and observe how the root of the nose obscures vision to the left while vision to the right is quite extensive. Under normal circumstances vision beyond the temple is sufficient to protect the individual from danger. The range over which the eye can see in all directions when the eye gazes forward is referred to as the visual field. The perimeter of the visual field can be mapped out by special techniques, and its precise determination is an important part of ophthalmology. If the student refers to a textbook of physiology he will find illustrations of each visual field and he will see that the nasal side is indented whereas the temporal side is round. Why?

THE ANTERIOR POLE OF THE EYEBALL

Looking more closely at the eyeball, one can easily identify the iris diaphragm, in the center of which is the pupil, a circular space of variable diameter. Anterior to the iris and the pupil is, first of all, a space, the anterior chamber, occupied by a fluid, the aqueous humor, and second, the cornea. Thus, when you view the iris and pupil of a healthy eye you view them through the cornea and aqueous humor.

The Greek word for cornea was keras; hence the term *keratitis*, meaning inflammation of the cornea; the prefix kerato is frequently used in pathologic terms referring to the cornea.

Part of the anterior surface of the lens of the eyeball is exposed within the pupil but the lens, too, is transparent. Between the posterior surface of the iris and the remainder of the lens is a slit-like interval, the posterior chamber, which also contains aqueous humor.

REFRACTION

Light rays entering the eyeball pass through three media, first air, then the cornea and aqueous humor (considered together), and finally the lens; the cornea, the anterior chamber, and the lens are millimeters in depth. Refraction is the bending of rays of light as they pass through the interface between one medium and another; the purpose of the interface here is to redirect light rays to a focal point on the retina. The refractive index of the cornea and aqueous humor is static, whereas that of the lens is variable, in keeping with its function, to focus. Even so, the lens is only responsible for a quarter of the total refraction. Thus, to save the cornea is an urgent need when its surface and its structure are in peril.

The white of the eye is the sclera. What is not generally appreciated at a first glance is that the white sclera is seen through a very thin, delicate membrane, the conjunctiva, which is transparent. Furthermore, the junction of the sclera and the cornea, known clinically as the limbus, is not visible under normal circumstances.

Figure 68-1 shows how the conjunctiva is reflected from the posterior surface of each eyelid on to the adjacent part of the sclera to form a recess called a fornix. Having spread over the entire anterior surface of the sclera, the conjunctiva continues in a modified form over the anterior aspect of the cornea. The change occurs at the limbus. The conjuctiva is discussed further with the lacrimal apparatus.

ITEM 68-1. If the eyeballs of the cadaver are collapsed they are easily restored by injecting water.

On a cadaver, on one side only, open the eyelids and expose the anterior pole of the eyeball. Identify the conjuctiva covering the sclera. The conjunctiva will be examined more thoroughly in a moment. Identify the limbus. The cornea, opaque in a cadaver, is easily identified.

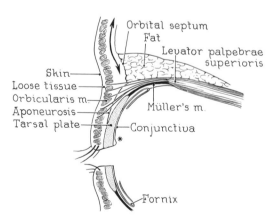

Figure 68-1. Section of the eyelids to show the principal features. The tarsal glands and the ciliary glands have been omitted. The arrows indicate a plane of cleavage in continuity with the subgaleal space of the scalp. The asterisk indicates a gutter (not as deep as this on every specimen); the gutter is a common place for foreign bodies, such as grit, to lodge.

Carefully, with the point of a sharp scalpel, incise the cornea at the limbus. An outflow of aqueous humor indicates that the anterior chamber has been entered. Continue the incision along the limbus until the cornea is completely detached.

Examine the iris, the pupil, and the exposed part of the lens. The cadaveric lens is opaque.

Slip the tip of a probe posterior to the iris and anterior to the lens to enter the slit-like interval, the posterior chamber.

At this time a jelly-like substance usually flows out from behind the lens. This substance is the vitreous humor, which occupies almost the entire eyeball and must be distinguished from the aqueous humor located in the extremely small anterior and posterior chambers.

THE EYELIDS

To shield the eyeball from injury, to keep dust and obnoxious fumes off the cornea and the conjunctiva, and to guard the retina from blinding light are the functions of the eyelids. Reinforced by plates of dense fibrous tissue, loosely suspended across the orbital opening, and controlled by the swiftly moving orbicularis oculi muscle, as quick as a wink the eyelids afford considerable protection to the structures at the orbital opening and within the orbit. Close your eyes tight and observe how the tissues at the orbital openings become so quilted that it is not possible to identify the eyeballs. Furthermore, it is known that when the eyes are closed the eyeballs rotate so that the pupils are directed superiorly. Thus it is the inferior part of the eyeball, usually the sclera, not the cornea, that bears the brunt of an injury.

The gap between the eyelids is the palpebral fissure (palpebra means eyelid). Canthus, from the Greek word *kanthos*, meaning corner of the eye, is the clinical term for the medial and lateral extremities of the palpebral fissure. Epicanthic, a descriptive term meaning upon the canthus, is applied to a fold of skin across the medial canthus, a fold that is said to be typical of the Mongoloid race.

A more characteristic feature of the Mongoloid facies, however, is the absence of the upper lid fold, known to some as the orbitopalpebral sulcus; in other words, in the Mongoloid the skin of the eyelid does not slip beneath the shelter of the superior orbital margin but continues flat to the forehead. A surgical procedure involving the muscle, the levator palpebrae superioris (Figure 68-1), can create the fold. A similar fold is present on the lower lid.

A feature that gives character to the face and yet is not usually noticed is the hollow between the root of the nose and the eyelids. The tip of the index finger can skulk deep in the hollow and not be seen by the other eye. Once these bilateral hollows are flattened by a blow, the victim looks like a frog, but, perhaps, more pugnacious. Demonstrate the hollow, known as the concavity of the medial canthus, upon yourself.

When the eyes of a normal person are open, the upper margin of each iris is overlapped by the upper lid while the lower margin of the iris is touched by the lower lid. Not too much of the sclera, the white of the eye, is seen. Widening or narrowing of one or both palpebral fissures is of importance in clinical medicine. In widening of the fissure, all the iris is exposed and the white of the eye is conspicuous; a momentary appearance of this sort is associated with fear; a persistent appearance suggests that the eyeball is protruding from its socket, hence the term exophthalmos; the term opposite to exophthalmos is enophthalmos.

There is a tendency to overlook the significance of the loose thin skin of the eyelids, until a severe burn destroys the skin to such a degree that the eye cannot close. Fortunately, modern treatment can do much to remedy the anguish of this dreadful condition. Observe that even in an embalmed cadaver the skin of the eyelid is lax.

The significance of the orbicularis oculi in keeping the eyelids close to the eyeball has already been emphasized when the muscles of the face were examined (p. 299).

The levator palpebrae superioris is the muscle that raises the upper lid. The movement is particularly obvious when the eyes look up and the head does not move. Indeed, the muscles elevating the eyeballs and the levatores palpebrae superioris act together. Figure 68-1 shows how the levator muscle comes anteriorly to the eyelid from the posterior region of the orbit to end in an aponeurosis that inserts into the anterior aspect of the tarsus as well as into the skin, and also how a deep portion of the muscle inserts into the superior edge of the tarsal plate. This deep sheet of muscle, known as Müller's muscle, is controlled by the sympathetic nervous system. Similar muscle fibers are found in the lower lid.

The eyelid was known to the Greeks as the blepharon, hence the term blepharitis, meaning inflammation of the eyelids.

ITEM 68-2. In a cadaver it is easier to examine an eyelid after it has been cut, so make a vertical incision to cut each eyelid in half. Carefully controlling the knife or the scissors, continue to cut until you reach the orbital margin. Examine a cut edge of the upper lid and identify the following layers: loose thin skin, loose connective tissue, the orbicularis oculi muscle, the aponeurosis of the levator palpebrae superioris (to be explained shortly), the tarsal plate and orbital septum (also to be explained shortly), and the conjunctiva. All these layers are illustrated in Figure 68-1.

Note that the posterior edge of the lid margin is sharp, quite different from the anterior edge, which is round. Alignment of the sharp edge is a challenge that must be met in emergency surgery. Furthermore, the posterior surface of the eyelid adjacent to the edge is slightly concave; the concavity is a common site for foreign bodies (Fig. 68-1).

The aponeurosis of the levator palpebrae superioris can easily be distinguished from the orbital septum. Identify the superior aspect of the anterior surface of the tarsal plate; the aponeurosis immediately adjacent to that surface belongs to the levator palpebrae superioris.

Identify the orbital septum which is very thin but identifiable. How the septum ascends to its attachment at the orbital margin is seen in Figure 68-1.

The Glands of the Eyelids

On the lid margin there are two or three rows of eyelashes, usually curving outward, but not always. The sebaceous glands opening into the follicles of the eyelashes are rudimentary. And the sweat glands of the eyelid are also rudimentary. Their openings are located between the lashes. A stye, recognized by its location on the lid margin, is an acute inflammation of one of these small glands.

On the deep surface of the tarsal plate lie 20 or more tarsal glands. Described by Hendrik Meibom, a German anatomist, the tarsal glands are often referred to as Meibomian glands. Swelling of one of these glands is termed a Meibomian cyst, and is recognized by its location on the orbital surface of the lid, where it is obscured from view by the tarsal plate.

ITEM 68-3. Examine the lid margin. Where are the lashes located? What is their shape? Evert the eyelid and look on its deep surface for the tarsal glands, parallel yellowish streaks, at right angles to the lid margin. Then examine the lid margin closely immediately anterior to its sharp edge and see if you can detect the orifices of the tarsal glands.

The Tarsal Plate and the Orbital Septum

Between each tarsal plate and the adjacent orbital margin extends a thin sheet of fascia, the orbital septum (also called the palpebral fascia), which is so flimsy in an embalmed elderly cadaver that the young dissector usually breaks through it before he realizes he has done so. This contingency must not cause the dissector to ignore the orbital septum; it is an important factor in keeping the eyelids and the eyeball in apposition. Proceed, therefore, as follows and it should be possible to demonstrate part of the septum easily.

ITEM 68-4. Examine the lid margin carefully and see if you can see a gray line, which is used clinically to indicate the plane of cleavage you are about to enter between the orbicularis oculi and the tarsal plate. It is possible to separate the orbicularis oculi easily from the tarsal plate. Indeed, clinically, fluid may accumulate between them, for example, fluid that has gravitated from the galeal space of the skull (Fig. 68-1).

To elevate orbicularis oculi, your partner must pull the lateral half of the upper lid firmly inferiorly to stretch and tighten the tissues as much as possible. While he does this, you reflect the muscle off the plate with a sharp knife until you reach the orbital margin. The change from the dense tarsal plate to the flimsy orbital septum is usually obvious.

The orbital septum is an anatomic landmark, a barrier separating the structures of the actual orbit from those of the orbital opening. Accordingly orbital fat is retained within the orbit by the septum but often in elderly people a small fragment of orbital fat protrudes through the septum and forms a visible "tag" on the lid. This is especially common on the medial half of the upper lid where the orbital septum is less well defined.

ITEM 68-5.   Continue to reflect the orbicularis oculi off the tarsal plate and the orbital septum. Pull the plate strongly medially and scratch off all muscle in the region of the lateral canthus to expose the lateral palpebral ligament, which is a reinforcement of the orbital septum attached to the lateral palpebral tubercle. A similar ligament exists at the medial canthus. Unfortunately, the medial palpebral ligament is not always easily demonstrated in an elderly cadaver. The ligament consists of anterior and posterior layers that are attached to the anterior and posterior lacrimal crests to complete the enclosure for the lacrimal sac (Fig. 68-2).

Exercise

On your own face use the left index finger and press the flat of the nail on the lateral aspect of the left eyeball while the tip presses on the internal aspect of the middle of the lateral orbital margin. The lateral palpebral tubercle (Whitnall's tubercle) is readily felt; although it is small, it is prominent. Also identify the tubercle on a skull.

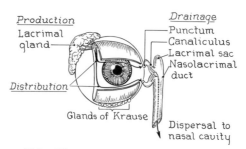

Figure 68-2.   The components of the lacrimal apparatus.

Then, in a similar manner, press inferomedially through the lower lid at the medial limit of the inferior orbital margin and identify a tiny knob, no bigger than the tip of a blunt pencil, located where the anterior and posterior lacrimal crests begin their ascent. Also identify this little knob without a name and the anterior and posterior lacrimal crests upon a skull.

THE ORBITAL FASCIA

Because names have been given to many parts of the orbital fascia the student conceives the fascia as a series of individual structures. On the contrary, the fascia is all oné tissue. Thus the orbital septum and the medial and lateral palpebral ligaments are one. Other parts yet to be met in this continuous fascial system are Tenon's capsule, the ligament of Lockwood, the muscle sheaths and check ligaments, and the more specialized lateral and medial horns of the aponeurosis of the levator palpebrae superioris. The fascial system obtains a firm attachment to the entire orbital margin, especially to the lateral palpebral tubercle and the lacrimal crests.

LACRIMAL APPARATUS (FIG. 68-2)

In addition to the mechanical protection of the eyelids, the eyeball is protected by a thin film of fluid. Everyone has experienced at some time or other watering of the eye from exposure to dust, obnoxious fumes, or fluid, but in addition to its flushing and neutralizing actions, lacrimal fluid possesses certain chemical properties, one of which is particularly important in quelling bacteria and controlling viruses. Thus the function of the lacrimal fluid commands your attention and it is true to say to the future physician that the lacrimal apparatus through which the fluid flows is a significant anatomic system throughout all the ages of man, from the womb to the grave.

The components of the lacrimal apparatus are:
(1) The lacrimal gland, its ducts, and the glands of Krause
(2) The conjunctival sac
(3) The lacrimal punctum (one on each lid)
(4) The lacrimal canaliculus (one in each lid)
(5) The lacrimal sac
(6) The nasolacrimal duct

The components may be grouped according to function with reference to the lacrimal fluid (Fig. 68-2): production, distribution, and drainage.

Production of Lacrimal Fluid

The lacrimal gland, which secretes lacrimal fluid or tears, is located within the orbit. Therefore, first obtain a skull. Examine the upper and outer region of the orbital opening. Then slide a fingertip from within the orbit to cross the tip of the orbital margin at the region you have just examined. In most skulls one senses a shallow fossa; in life it is lined by periosteum adjacent to which is the lacrimal gland. In addition to lying in the shelter of the orbital margin, the lacrimal gland lies deep to the orbital septum, as you will now see.

ITEM 68-6.   Examine the lateral half of the upper lid of the cadaver and pull the tarsal plate inferiorly to put tension on the orbital septum. Incise the septum parallel to the orbital margin. Separate the cut edges and expose the lacrimal gland. It is clear that the gland lies posterior to the orbital septum and is, therefore, excluded from the orbital opening. Nevertheless it is an essential part of the lacrimal apparatus. The gland is completely exposed when the orbit is opened.

Distribution of Lacrimal Fluid

The conjunctival sac is responsible for the distribution of lacrimal fluid. Such a prosaic statement conveys nothing of the imaginative research of Wolff (1946), who plotted the currents and plumbed the depths of the lacrimal fluid like an oceanographer surveying the seas. Wolff found that the lacrimal fluid is not a thin film swept from the superior fornix to the medial canthus with every blink of the eye, but that the fluid accumulates at the posterior margins of the lids; thence the fluid reaches the puncta. He also reported how the oily secretions of the glands of the lid form protective films over the cornea. The full account makes fascinating reading.

The neck of the conjunctival sac is the palpebral fissure, and at the part at which the conjunctiva is reflected from the lid to the sclera a recess, called a fornix, is formed (Fig. 68-1). Thus a superior and an inferior fornix are recognized.

ITEM 68-7.   Using a blunt probe, manipulate the eyelids and explore the fornices with the tip of the probe. Slide the tip through the entire length of each fornix.

No doubt you appreciate that in life the conjunctival sac does not gape as it is shown in most illustrations. The eyelids are in fact closely applied to the eyeball, and the fornices are potential spaces.

Some ten or more tiny ducts from the lacrimal gland open into the lateral part of the superior fornix. To look for them is time-consuming.

In addition to the definitive lacrimal gland, small accessory lacrimal glands, the glands of Krause, are found elsewhere related to the fornices. Although these glands are described as accessory, they secrete as much fluid as the lacrimal gland itself.

Drainage of Lacrimal Fluid

Examine the medial canthus. Observe how the eyelids alter shape and form sides to the lacus lacrimalis. This portion of the eyelid is named the lacrimal portion to distinguish it from the ciliary portion supporting the eyelashes (cilium is another name for eyelash). The "bottom" of the lake is uneven and features the plica semilunaris and the lacrimal caruncle.

ITEM 68-8.   Examine the junction of the lacrimal and ciliary portions of the lid by everting both the upper and lower lids. This maneuver brings both lacrimal papillae out of the groove between the plica and the caruncle and exposes the lacrimal punctum, a tiny opening on the tip of the papilla. So important is the relationship of the punctum to the conjunctival sac that it is worth repeating the maneuver not only on the cadaver but also on yourself with the aid of a mirror. The inferior punctum faces both superiorly and posteriorly; the superior punctum faces both inferiorly and posteriorly. Only the slightest pressure is necessary to bring each punctum into view. The very slight pressure required to do so is an indication of the critical relationship normally in existence between the punctum and the sac. If the relationship is altered one way or the other it must be restored by a surgical procedure that must be just so accurate.

From the punctum a tiny duct leads to the lacrimal sac. The duct, called a canaliculus, is measured in millimeters and is not straight. The first part of the canaliculus of the upper lid ascends vertically for a short distance, and the canaliculus of the lower lid descends likewise. The second part of each canaliculus is horizontal. Both parts terminate in the lacrimal sac (Fig. 68-2). With a sharp pointed knife it is possible to open a canaliculus.

The lacrimal sac is the blind upper end of the nasolacrimal duct. It can be exposed by skillful dissection with a sharp pointed knife. The surgeon, exposing the lacrimal sac, encounters the orbicularis oculi muscle and the medial palpebral ligament. However, at this stage the quickest way to establish the location of the lacrimal sac and the nasolacrimal duct is to examine a skull.

On a skull identify the lacrimal bone and the groove in which the sac lies. Then slip a slender matchstick into the nasolacrimal canal and observe in the nasal cavity where the match emerges. What is the direction of the canal?

How lacrimal fluid enters the drainage system is the subject of debate, and there is little to be gained by reviewing the debate. One fact is agreed upon: blinking does disperse excess lacrimal fluid.

One point concerning the drainage system must be stressed. The duct system must be patent for drainage to be successful. Sometimes in newborn children the duct system is blocked and the blockage does not clear with time. Then it is necessary to probe the ducts to establish drainage. At that time a knowledge of the precise anatomy of the drainage system becomes supremely important, for otherwise the duct can be damaged beyond repair.

Review

Review the anatomy of the lacrimal apparatus under the three headings referring to the lacrimal fluid, production, distribution, and drainage.

Chapter 69

The Contents of the Orbit

Introduction

The only way the undergraduate can see the contents of the orbit easily is to dissect away its walls. Beforehand, therefore, he must obtain a skull and review the walls of the orbit.

The orbit is pyramidal in shape; the orbital opening is the base; the optic canal and the superior orbital fissure are at the apex. That the long axis of the orbit is directed laterally as well as anteriorly from apex to base is of great significance because the action of two of the extraocular muscles running parallel to that axis is affected accordingly (p. 358). Examine the orbit and observe each wall with some care.

The medial wall possesses two distinctive features. The first, the lacrimal fossa for the lacrimal sac, is easily identified. The second is the orbital plate of the ethmoid bone, which is not so easily identified except by the sutures connecting it to adjacent bones. The smooth surface of this aspect of the ethmoid is very different from the medial aspect, where air cells abound. Most of the ethmoid bone consists of air cells that communicate with the nasal cavities (Fig. 69-1). The most anterior ethmoidal air cells are medial to the lacrimal fossa, a relationship well known to the ophthalmic surgeon.

The floor of the orbit is the roof of the maxillary air sinus, and the roof of the orbit is the floor of the anterior cranial fossa. Included in the roof is part of the frontal air sinus. The bone separating any of these air sinuses from the orbit may be so thin that pus from the sinus can erode through the bone to enter the subperiosteal space of the orbit; the periosteum separates the pus from the orbital contents.

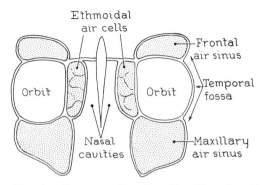

Figure 69-1. The air cells surrounding the orbits. The sphenoidal air sinuses are posterior to the ethmoidal air cells.

At the apex of the orbit observe the optic canal. Slip a match through the canal and establish its cranial orifice medial to the anterior clinoid process at the junction of the anterior and middle cranial fossae. Medial to the optic canal is the sphenoidal air sinus, a close relationship not generally appreciated. Lateral to the optic canal is an oblique cleft called the superior orbital fissure, which connects the middle cranial fossa with the orbit.

The lesser wing of the sphenoid forms the superior boundary of the superior orbital fissure. That fact has no impact upon the student's mind until he reads that the wing is a common site for a certain type of tumor. As the tumor grows it invades the orbit.

When the roof and the lateral wall of the orbit are removed, and removing them is the next step, further details will become apparent.

The structures to be identified in the orbit are (1) the superior, inferior, medial, and lateral rectus muscles, forming a muscle cone; (2) the superior and inferior oblique muscles; (3) the levator palpebrae superioris; (4) the nerves that supply those muscles; (5) the ophthalmic artery; (6) the ophthalmic veins; (7) the ciliary nerves and vessels; (8) the optic nerve in its sheath and the eyeball; (9) the lacrimal gland; and (10) the branches of the ophthalmic division of the fifth cranial nerve proceeding to their peripheral distribution. These structures are arranged in a very simple manner around the optic nerve. Unfortunately, the simplicity of this arrangement is not evident to a student dissecting the orbit for the first time. It is necessary for him to proceed at random from one small structure to another because of the limited space within the orbit. Therefore, once he has examined the structures of the orbit individually, he should view them collectively system by system and note their relationship to the optic nerve as an axis.

ITEM 69-1.   To open the orbit proceed as follows: Identify the level of its floor and cut through all soft tissue on the lateral aspect of the zygomatic bone at that level; continue the cut posteriorly into the temp-

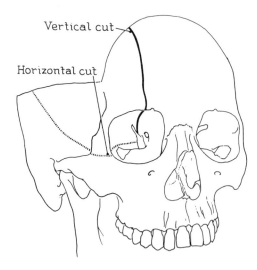

Vertical cut

Horizontal cut

Figure 69-2. The two saw cuts to open the orbit.

oralis (Fig. 69-2). Then with an autopsy saw make a horizontal cut through the frontal process of the zygomatic bone and continue the cut posteriorly to end level with the lesser wing of the sphenoid.

Next palpate the supraorbital notch on the superior margin of the orbital opening. With an autopsy saw make a vertical cut into the frontal bone immediately *lateral* to the supraorbital notch (Fig. 69-2).

Finally, from inside the skull — and do not cut deeply because the bone is very thin — continue the vertical cut posteriorly through the roof of the orbit to the *lateral* side of the optic canal.

To release the fragment you have just outlined with the saw, tap the anterior part of the fragment firmly with a mallet. Once the fragment is loose, turn it forward to open the orbit. The fragment peels off easily because the periosteum, called the periorbita when it covers the bones of the orbit, is only lightly attached to bone. In anticipation of the next step, it must be emphasized that periorbita is very thin.

ITEM 69-2. All the structures connected with the eyeball lie within the confines of the periorbita. Therefore make a longitudinal incision into the superolateral aspect of the periorbita. Reflect and remove periorbita.

ITEM 69-3. The orbital fat, packed closely around the structures of the orbit, has to be dispersed in the course of the dissection. To see the structures in the orbit adequately it is necessary to remove as much fat as possible.

ORBITAL FAT

The orbital fat is selected for comment because it is regarded as a nuisance in the dissection of the cadaveric orbit, when the main purpose is to demonstrate the many small structures hidden by the solidified fat. During surgery the orbital fat is found to be semifluid, troublesome to manipulate, and prone to leak if its globules are ruptured. The fat must not be allowed to leak extensively, for otherwise the orbital contents lose their natural support and the very precise mechanism for moving the eyeball is impaired.

ITEM 69-4. Identify the lacrimal gland and mobilize it sufficiently to establish its connection with the conjunctival sac. It is curious how the lacrimal gland straddles the lateral edge of the levator palpebrae superioris.

ITEM 69-5. Lying imposed upon the orbital fat are the frontal and lacrimal nerves and the two branches of the ophthalmic nerve. The third branch, the nasociliary nerve, is hidden meantime.

The frontal nerve is easily identified as a narrow white strap proceeding anteriorly to the region of the supraorbital notch.

To identify the lacrimal nerve, pull the lacrimal gland gently anteriorly and superiorly. This maneuver elevates the lacrimal nerve, which has a cutaneous distribution on the eyelid and, in addition, supplies the autonomic fibers to the lacrimal gland. The latter reach the lacrimal nerve by a devious route we need not explore, but they are significant fibers nonetheless because they bring the lacrimal gland under the control of the autonomic nervous system. Thus the lacrimal gland is not an isolated organ, master of its own function.

ITEM 69-6. In this approach to the orbit the lateral rectus muscle is the gate, and it is necessary to open the gate to enter the orbit. Identify the lateral rectus muscle and slide a probe or the tip of blunt-ended scissors down the medial side of the muscle. Slide the scissors anteriorly and posteriorly to mobilize the muscle. Cut the muscle vertically in the middle to create two flaps. Turn the anterior flap toward the eyeball and mobilize the flap until its attachment to the eyeball is clearly seen.

At this time it is easy to demonstrate how a sleeve of fascia extends along the lateral rectus muscle. The sleeve is continuous with a layer of fascia (Tenon's capsule) lying upon the sclera of the eyeball. Similar sleeves of fascia are present on the other extraocular muscles; the sleeves, also known as sheaths, are essential for the smooth action of the muscles and therefore must be preserved in surgery of the extraocular muscles. At the same time, note where the tendon of the lateral rectus is attached to the eyeball. The tendon is attached posterior to the limbus, at a distance measured in millimeters. This is so for the tendons of all the extraocular muscles. The exact distance is extremely important to the ophthalmic surgeon when he moves the attachment of a tendon to correct strabismus (in other words, a squint, cross-eyes, or wall-eyes).

Next peel the posterior flap of the lateral rectus posteriorly. To get the flap back to the posterior attachment of the muscle, it may be necessary to use bone forceps to nibble tiny fragments of bone away from the vicinity of the superior orbital fissure. Then the lateral rectus can be turned back to expose the sixth cranial nerve. Observe how the nerve enters the medial surface of the muscle between its posterior and middle thirds.

Making a clean dissection and obtaining an adequate reflection of the lateral rectus muscle is the key to the entire dissection of the orbit.

ITEM 69-7.   The next procedure is to reflect the frontal nerve and the levator palpebrae superioris in order to improve access to the remaining contents. Tie the frontal nerve in two places with a thread. Cut between the ties. Reflect the cut ends clear of the superior surface of the levator palpebrae superioris.

ITEM 69-8.   Carefully mobilize the levator close to the eyeball. Then cut across the muscle about its midpoint. Elevate and mobilize the anterior part of the muscle and demonstrate its connection with the upper eyelid. The muscle fibers of the levator run parallel to the long axis of the orbit, but this has little effect upon its action because the aponeurosis of the levator widens anteriorly to be attached medially and laterally to the orbital margin. Demonstrate these attachments by pulling the aponeurosis.

ITEM 69-9.   Once the levator palpebrae superioris is reflected the superior surface of the superior rectus muscle is exposed. Make sure that you see the muscle clearly and observe the direction of its fibers. They run laterally as well as anteriorly from their posterior to their anterior attachment, and the significance of this fact will be brought out when the action of the extraocular muscles is discussed.

A Functional Unit

Although all of the muscles have not yet been seen, it is appropriate at this stage to stress that the levator palpebrae superioris and the superior rectus are a functional unit with a common nerve supply. The eyelids are retracted when the eyes look up. What is the nerve supply of these two muscles?

ITEM 69-10.   Now move to the floor of the orbit to identify the inferior rectus and inferior oblique muscles. At the level of the floor of the orbit, pick away orbital fat. If you work with a light touch it is permissible to "pick blindly"—orbital fat comes away easily, whereas definite structures offer resistance. (This technique, mark you, is a technique confined to the dissection of an embalmed cadaver.)

Establish definitely the inferior rectus muscle and find, on its lateral margin, the inferior division of the oculomotor nerve. Gently mobilize the nerve and carefully trace it anteriorly to where it enters the inferior oblique muscle. In doing so you begin the destruction of the ligament of Lockwood.

THE LIGAMENT OF LOCKWOOD

This ligament may be described as a hammock of fascia slung between the lateral orbital tubercle and the vicinity of the lacrimal crest. The support it provides the eyeball is demonstrated clinically when the bony floor of the orbit is eliminated in the removal of the maxilla. If the ligament of Lockwood is left intact the eyeball does not sag.

The ligament is a significant part of the fascia of the orbit, a fascia artificially subdivided into Tenon's capsule, muscle sheaths, and check ligaments. The ligament is scarcely recognized by the undergraduate when he exposes the inferior oblique muscle in this present dissection. Yet the ligament is a well-known surgical landmark, thick and easily identified; it is vascular and is a likely source of a troublesome hemorrhage.

ITEM 69-11.   Elevate and rotate the eyeball carefully to obtain a good view of the inferior oblique. Trace the muscle to its insertion on the sclera; the insertion is close to the site of the macula lutea of the retina.

ITEM 69-12.   Trace the inferior division of the oculomotor nerve posteriorly. If the lateral rectus muscle has been turned back sufficiently, the division can be traced to the point where it communicates with the ciliary ganglion. The ganglion is a relay station in the autonomic nervous system, and from it emerge the short ciliary nerves going to the eyeball. In this present dissection, the ganglion, although it is measured in millimeters, is easily found and is often recognizable by its pinkish red color, which has never been satisfactorily explained.

ITEM 69-13.   The ciliary ganglion also communicates with the nasociliary nerve. Find the nasociliary nerve and trace it medially, superior to the sheath of the optic nerve. The long ciliary nerves arise from it.

ITEM 69-14.   Immediately superior to the nasociliary nerve, the superior division of the oculomotor nerve can be found ascending to enter the superior rectus muscle, which it supplies, and then the levator palpebrae superioris, which it also supplies. The nerve is the link in this functional unit (p. 352). All these structures are easily and quickly identified if the lateral rectus muscle is reflected far enough posteriorly.

ITEM 69-15.   Medial to the ciliary ganglion lie the ophthalmic veins. The ophthalmic veins are usually empty in a cadaver and, because of their thin walls, they are usually destroyed inadvertently. They drain all the tissues of the orbit and terminate in the cavernous sinus. Their communication with the veins of the face has already been referred to (p. 297). Some veins also leave the orbit through the inferior orbital fissure.

THE CENTRAL VEIN OF THE RETINA

The central vein of the retina also drains into one of the ophthalmic veins. The central vein has a significant crossing through the subarachnoid space, where its thin wall is subject to the pressure of the cerebrospinal fluid (Fig. 69-3). When the vein is compressed the effect upon its field of drainage is the same as the effect of compressing the veins of the forearm. The changes seen in the optic disc and the retina with the aid of an ophthalmoscope are termed papilledema.

ITEM 69-16. The ophthalmic artery may be poorly filled, but it can be easily identified at its source, the internal carotid artery. Examine the carotid artery medial to the anterior clinoid process and find the ophthalmic artery. At this point you are in the subarachnoid space. Trace the ophthalmic artery distally to where it leaves the space. If necessary nibble open the optic canal with bone forceps.

The ophthalmic artery supplies all the tissues of the orbit. Of its many branches, one solitary artery and one group of arteries are really significant, namely the central artery of the retina and the anterior and posterior ciliary arteries. The central artery is illustrated in Figure 69-3. The posterior ciliary arteries can be seen in this present dissection as minute vessels accompanying the ciliary nerves. The anterior ciliary arteries branch off the small arteries in the extraocular muscles to enter the sclera.

All the ciliary arteries, both anterior and posterior, ultimately anastomose in the vicinity of the corneoscleral junction. In the living, they may be seen there when they are congested with blood. The appearance of congestion of the ciliary arteries, known as ciliary flush, is very characteristic and can be readily distinguished from congestion of the conjunctival vessels.

ITEM 69-17. Cut the superior rectus muscle, reflect the two flaps, and remove orbital fat to expose the sheath of the optic nerve. Slit the sheath and expose the nerve. Demonstrate that the sheath is continuous with the dura within the cranium and with the sclera.

ITEM 69-18. Continue to remove orbital fat until you see clearly how the superior oblique muscle becomes tendinous and how its tendon and accompanying synovial sheath pass through a pulley, the trochlea,

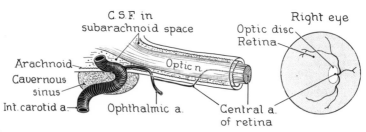

Figure 69-3. The central artery of the retina and its accompanying veins inevitably cross the subarachnoid space. A rise in cerebrospinal fluid pressure compresses the thin-walled veins and gives rise to changes in the optic disc termed papilledema. How would you examine an optic disc?

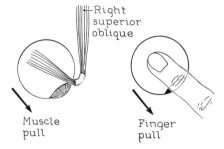

Figure 69-4. With the aid of a ball the principle of the action of the superior oblique is easily demonstrated.

bend acutely, and are inserted into the posterolateral aspect of the sclera (Fig. 69-4), beyond the equator of the eyeball.

Next find the fourth cranial nerve entering the muscle. Finally identify the medial rectus muscle and, if possible, the branch of the oculomotor nerve supplying the muscle.

Review

The eyeball and the optic nerve are central to the other structures of the orbit. The four rectus muscles grouped around the eyeball and nerve form a muscle cone with its apex at the apex of the orbit; the muscles are named according to their anatomic positions, i.e., superior, inferior, medial, and lateral. To augment the action of the four rectus muscles there are two oblique muscles, superior and inferior. The sixth cranial nerve supplies the lateral rectus muscle, and the fourth cranial nerve supplies the superior oblique muscle. The third cranial nerve supplies the medial, inferior, and superior rectus muscles and the inferior oblique muscle as well as the levator palpebrae superioris muscle, which is not a muscle of the eyeball but of the upper eyelid.

Orbital fat occupies the spaces between the centrally placed optic nerve and eyeball and the muscles grouped around them.

The ophthalmic vessels are widely distributed throughout the orbital fat; the ophthalmic artery enters the orbit in the optic canal; the ophthalmic veins leave the orbit through the superior and inferior orbital fissures. Ciliary nerves also are embedded in the orbit fat. The ciliary nerves, accompanied by the posterior ciliary blood vessels, lie parallel to the optic nerve and pass through the posterior aspect of the sclera. The anterior ciliary vessels pass through the sclera where the tendons of the extraocular muscles join the sclera. The sixth and the fourth cranial nerves enter their respective muscles almost immediately. The branches of the third cranial nerve, however, travel through the fat to their destination. The frontal nerve proceeds through the orbit and is sensory to the eyelid. The nasociliary nerve is sensory to the skin of the nose as well as to the cornea. It is held that no lymphatic vessels or nodes are present in the orbit.

Although the central artery and veins of the retina are extremely small, they are extremely important. They can be seen with the aid of an ophthalmoscope.

Chapter 70

The Action of the Extraocular Muscles

Vision is such a complex process combining central factors, i.e., factors within the central nervous system, and peripheral factors, i.e., those in the orbits, that it takes years of study and experience to master all that is involved in perfect sight. That this is so is worth stressing because this chapter is but an introduction to the action of the extraocular muscles, the muscles that move the eyeball or oculus; all the other factors involved in perfect vision are ignored. The intention of this commentary is to prevent any false impressions one might obtain from reading simplified statements of the action of the extraocular muscles.

The anatomic attachments of the extraocular muscles and the direction of their fibers give no indication of the real function of the muscles, because all the muscles are involved simultaneously in movements of the eyeballs. Moreover, simultaneous active relaxation of the muscles defined as antagonists is as important as active contraction of the muscles defined as prime movers.

The eyeball is almost a perfect sphere, free to rotate on a cushion of fat that serves as a lubricant. Rotation is controlled by the extraocular muscles, acting with a precision that never ceases to amaze even the most experienced eye surgeon. The muscles are the four recti, which form a muscle cone already observed in the dissection of the orbit; the actions of the four recti are augmented by the two oblique muscles whose function is a fascinating study but which can only be touched upon briefly in this text.

The movements of the eyeball are named according to the direction in which the anterior pole of the eyeball turns. Turning the eyeball so that the pupil is directed toward the nose is adduction; a turning away from the nose is abduction. Directing the pupil toward the ceiling without tilting the head back is elevation; the opposite of elevation is depression. The medial and lateral rectus muscles, primarily responsible for adduction and abduction and hence called adductors and abductors, are also referred to clinically as the horizontal recti; this is a puzzling term because, anatomically, the broad surfaces of the muscles face medially and laterally—the term horizontal refers to their function. A similar explanation applies to the superior and inferior recti, the elevators and depressors, described clinically as the vertical recti because of their function.

Each eye muscle, including the oblique muscles, has subsidiary actions concerned with the rolling of the eyeball around its anteroposterior axis. This rolling, known clinically as torsion, is of real significance in eye surgery, but its complexity places it beyond the scope of this text, except to say that movement of the 12 o'clock position on the perimeter of the iris is used to distinguish intorsion from extorsion. When the position moves toward the nose, intorsion occurs. The opposite movement is extorsion.

MONOCULAR MOVEMENT

In proceeding further, let us consider only one eyeball and let us deal with horizontal movements first because they are relatively simple. When the left eyeball is abducted, i.e., the pupil moves away from the nose, the left lateral rectus contracts and the left medial rectus actively relaxes. When the left eyeball is adducted, then the left medial rectus contracts and the left lateral rectus actively relaxes.

Vertical movements of the eyeball are not so simple as horizontal movements. Simplified statements on the action of the vertical recti mislead the student and bring him into conflict with his clinical tutor. Accordingly the vertical movements are described here in some detail. Vertical movements are controlled primarily by two elevator muscles that work together and two depressor muscles that also work together. For the left eye the elevators are the left superior rectus and the left inferior oblique; the depressors are the left inferior rectus and the left superior oblique. The alert student will have observed the combination of a superior with an inferior muscle. This is fact, even if it seems strange. The action of the oblique muscles can be readily demonstrated in principle on a ball marked with a circle to indicate the anterior pole (Fig. 69-4).

In elevation both elevators contract while their antagonists, both depressors, actively relax. In depression the opposite is true. However, in either elevation or depression, the degree of abduction or adduction of the eyeball determines the responsibility or the efficiency of each elevator or depressor muscle. How the change of responsibility comes about is dealt with next.

Figure 70-1 shows that the orbital axis of the left orbit does not

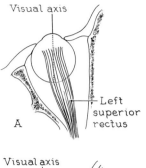

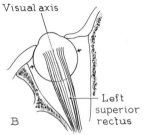

Figure 70-1. The superior (and inferior) rectus muscle lies parallel to the orbital axis. The muscle is in its optimal functional position when the eyeball is abducted. The arrows indicate the axis around which the eyeball rotates when the visual axis coincides with the orbital axis.

coincide with the visual axis of the left eyeball when the eyeball is in its primary position. But the figure shows also that the two axes do coincide when the eyeball is abducted. In this position the fibers of the superior rectus are at right angles to the horizontal axis, around which the eyeball will rotate. The superior rectus, now in its optimal functional position, acts as the principal elevator, and is assisted slightly by the inferior oblique.

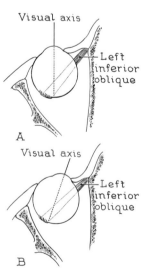

Figure 70-2. When the eyeball is adducted, the visual axis and the fibers of the inferior oblique are nearly parallel. This is the optimal position for the muscle to act as an elevator.

As the left eyeball moves from the position of full abduction toward a position of adduction, the efficiency of the left superior rectus diminishes until it reaches the position of full adduction, when the muscle is least efficient. However, as Figure 70-2 shows, this is the position in which the visual axis and the direction of the inferior oblique now almost coincide; the fibers of the muscle are almost at right angles to the axis around which the eyeball rotates to elevate the pupil. Thus it is in adduction that the inferior oblique is the more efficient elevator. Clearly, in the intermediate positions of the left eyeball between full abduction and full adduction, elevation is shared by both the left superior rectus and the left inferior oblique.

The function of the left inferior rectus and the left superior oblique can be interpreted in a similar way.

BINOCULAR MOVEMENT

So far only monocular movements have been considered. Now we must consider binocular movements (Latin *bini* — two); they are the perfectly coordinated movements of both eyes together, movements that are necessary for normal stereoscopic vision.

Binocular movements are complex, but they can be reduced to an abstract (Fig. 70-3). The arrows represent the direction of the main actions of the right and left extraocular muscles as they occur in fully coordinated movements. To prevent confusion, it must be pointed out that the actions indicated differ from the actions given in many anatomic texts, in which the action of each muscle, isolated and not in conjunction with other muscles, is considered. The diagram is one to which an ex-

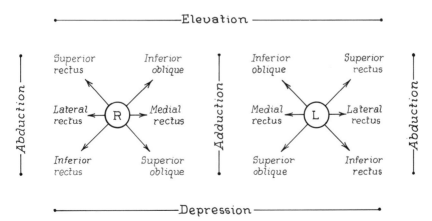

Figure 70-3. R and L refer to the patient's eyes. The reader is the clinician examining the patient's ocular movements.

perienced ophthalmic surgeon constantly refers when he is analyzing the more complex problems involving the extraocular muscles.

Examining Figure 70-3, consider the muscles employed when the subject looks to his right, which is a simple horizontal movement of both eyes. The right lateral rectus and the left medial rectus contract, while the right medial rectus and the left lateral rectus actively relax.

What muscles are involved when the subject looks up and to the right without tilting his head? The answer is in the footnote below.

Some Clinical Applications

The functional anatomy discussed in this chapter is the basis of several clinical applications, of which three are chosen for comment: double vision, head posture, and the selection of muscles to be treated surgically in event of muscular weakness or paralysis of one or more of the extraocular muscles.

Double Vision

Failure of muscular coordination because of weakness or paralysis of one or more of the extraocular muscles results in a breakdown of binocular vision and the patient sees two images, a distressing if not a fearful experience. The patient is aware that the two images are not always the same distance apart. He sees the images farthest apart when he looks in the direction in which the weak muscle would normally pull the eyeball. The separation of the images is minimal when he looks in the opposite direction. It is only natural that the patient will do what he can to be rid of the double images. One common method of doing so is described next.

Head Posture

Keeping the eyeballs in the direction opposite to the direction in which the weak muscle normally acts reduces or eliminates double vision. Subconsciously many patients adopt a head posture that assists the maintenance of this unusual position of the eyeballs. For example, a patient with a weak left lateral rectus avoids looking to the left and prefers to keep looking to the right. To achieve his preference, when he has to look straight ahead he turns his head to the left. In other words, his face is turned toward the side of the paralyzed muscle (Fig. 70-4).

Answer to the question above: The right superior rectus and the left inferior oblique contract, while the right inferior rectus and the left superior oblique actively relax. The answer, however, is not complete because there is a lesser contribution by the other elevators and depressors (Fig. 70-3).

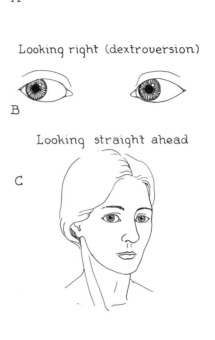

Attempting to look left   (levoversion)

A

Looking right (dextroversion)

B

Figure 70-4. Head posture is an important clue to weakness or paralysis of one or more of the extraocular muscles. In this instance, which lateral rectus muscle is paralyzed?

Looking straight ahead

C

Thus head posture may be a clue to an extraocular muscle paralysis, and by carefully analyzing the posture of a patient's head an ophthalmologist can determine which muscle is paralyzed. This curious yet physiologic link between the eyes and the head must be remembered because an abnormal head posture in a child can all too easily be attributed to the neck instead of to the eyes.

Surgical Treatment

The student will have realized by now that a study of the extraocular muscles must take into consideration all 12 muscles, six in each orbit; the action of any one muscle cannot be isolated from the action of the others. However, rather than group the muscles according to the orbit in which they lie, the student reviewing the extraocular muscles should group them according to their major function, i.e., group together those turning the eyes in directions to the right (dextro group) and those doing likewise to the left (laevo group) (Table 70-1). The junior student need only learn the principle embodied in the grouping; the ophthalmic surgeon must know the grouping in detail.

Finally, this text has dealt in simplified terms with the main actions

Table 70-1. *Eye Movements*

This table shows the names of the coordinated eye movements and the pairs of muscles that impart these movements. The table refers to the patient's eyes. The reader is the examiner viewing the patient. The table should be studied in conjunction with Figure 70-3.

Dextro elevation	Right superior rectus Left inferior oblique	Left superior rectus Right inferior oblique	Laevo elevation
Dextroversion	Right lateral rectus Left medial rectus	Left lateral rectus Right medial rectus	Laevoversion
Dextro depression	Right inferior rectus Left superior oblique	Left inferior rectus Right superior oblique	Laevo depression

of the extraocular muscles. There are, however, secondary and tertiary actions in addition to these actions. For example, the main action of the superior rectus is elevation; its secondary action is adduction; its tertiary action is intorsion. These subsidiary actions may be of great importance in planning the surgical treatment of a squint.

Chapter 71

Dissection of the Infratemporal Fossa

There is on each side of the skull an interesting little region called the infratemporal fossa. The fossa is on the medial side of the ramus of the mandible and directly inferior to the middle cranial fossa. It is of interest not only to the dentist but also to the doctor. For example, the posterior superior alveolar nerves are sufficiently accessible in the fossa that they can be anesthetized; the same may be said of the inferior alveolar nerve. In medicine, electroencephalograms of the activity of the temporal lobe of the brain can be obtained by thrusting sphenoidal electrodes into the depths of the infratemporal fossa. The mandibular nerve and, through the foramen ovale, the trigeminal ganglion are accessible for certain methods of treatment. The major vessels and nerves in the fossa must be borne in mind in reconstructive surgery of the mandible. Clearly the infratemporal fossa deserves to be called interesting even though it is little, as you will now see.

Obtain a skull with the mandible in place and locate the infratemporal fossa on the medial side of the mandible and inferior to the middle cranial fossa. Examine the mandible and note on the superior margin of the ramus of the mandible, from anterior to posterior, the coronoid process, the mandibular notch, and the neck and head of the mandible. Move the mandible far enough to be able to appreciate the shape of the head, then the corresponding shape of the mandibular fossa on the skull. Observe that the anterior boundary of the mandibular fossa is a protuberance projecting inferiorly. This protuberance, known for long as the articular eminence, is now called the articular tubercle.

Return to the mandible and identify the anterior border of the ramus. Slide the tip of an index finger up and down the border. In a normal, well-formed mandible this vertical border is sharp, concave inferiorly, and convex superiorly. Observe superiorly the position of the coronoid process in relation to the zygomatic arch.

Take off the skull cap. From inside the skull insert a matchstick into the foramen ovale; then peer through the mandibular notch and see the location of the foramen in relation to the notch. What is the distance of the foramen from the outer aspect of the zygomatic arch?

If the mandible is attached to the skull by springs allowing the mouth to open, open the mouth and insert the tip of an index finger to explore the medial aspect of the ramus. Slide the fingertip posteriorly from the anterior border over a ridge that Grant and Basmajian (1965) term the strengthening buttress and dentists term the temporal crest. Stop halfway between the anterior and posterior borders. Palpate in that region at the level of the cusps of the molar teeth and identify the lingula projecting posteriorly over the mandibular foramen. Now remove the mandible from the skull and examine the location and level of the foramen and lingula more closely. One can also see the mylohyoid groove running anteroinferiorly from the mandibular foramen.

A few more features of significance remain to be identified on the skull. Examine the posterior surface of the maxilla. On it you will find two or more minute foramina, the posterior superior alveolar foramina — more about these later. Slide the tip of a finger superiorly on this surface so that the tip comes to rest in the inferior orbital fissure. Slide the tip posteromedially along the inferior orbital fissure to reach a vertical cleft, the pterygomaxillary fissure. From this fissure slide the finger posteriorly onto the lateral pterygoid plate. Then move to the medial side of this plate and identify the medial pterygoid plate, unmistakable in a first class skull because of the hamulus, a hooklike projection at the lower end of the plate. The space between the plates is termed the pterygoid fossa. The medial pterygoid plate, however, is incorporated in the pharyngeal wall and is excluded from the infratemporal fossa by a small muscle, the tensor palati (p. 413).

The roof of the infratemporal fossa is also the floor of the middle cranial fossa. In the roof the foramen ovale and the adjacent foramen spinosum are easy to identify. Having done so, slide the tip of an index finger laterally on the roof until you feel a fairly distinct edge, the infratemporal crest, where the direction of the skull changes abruptly from the infratemporal to the temporal fossa.

The bony contours of the infratemporal fossa have now been examined. They will, however, be referred to again in the course of the dissection, so it is advisable to keep a skull at the dissecting table.

THE LATERAL PTERYGOID MUSCLE

In each infratemporal fossa the dominant feature is the lateral pterygoid muscle, horizontally disposed, 1.5 cm. thick, and filling almost the entire fossa. Thus nerves and vessels passing through the fossa must pass over, through, or under this muscle. Once this simple fact is realized, much of the anatomy of the fossa becomes clear. The attachments of the muscle will be seen in the course of the dissection. Briefly they are anterior to the lateral pterygoid plate and an adjacent part of the base of the skull, and posterior to the neck of the mandible.

ITEM 71-1.   Dissect One Side Only

Remove the remains of the parotid gland and the masseteric fascia to expose the masseter. The muscle slants obliquely inferoposteriorly from the zygomatic arch to the mandible. By blunt dissection with closed, blunt-ended scissors, demonstrate the anterior and posterior borders of the muscle. What is the relationship of the posterior border to the neck of the mandible?

With an autopsy saw make two vertical cuts into the zygomatic arch, one cut at its posterior border and the other cut at the anterior border of the zygomatic attachment of masseter. In the next step the neurovascular bundle to the masseter will be encountered for a short time before the bundle is ruptured. Mobilize the bony fragment, with masseter attached, and gently peel it inferoposteriorly in the direction of its fibers. The neurovascular bundle to the masseter emerges superior to the lateral pterygoid, passes through the mandibular notch, and enters the deep surface of masseter close to the neck of the mandible. This nerve must be safeguarded in surgical procedures involving the neck of the mandible. Break the bundle and peel the masseter right to its attachment on the angle of the jaw.

THE TEMPOROMANDIBULAR JOINTS

These joints, hinging the mandible to each side of the skull, are of great significance to both the doctor and the dentist. For example, the joints are synovial (p. 270) and therefore are subject to the types of diseases to which synovial joints are prone. Another example is the care that must be taken to avoid dislocation when the mouth is opened wide in general anesthesia or during the passing of a "scope" into the esophagus or the trachea. In dentistry the temporomandibular joints are supremely important, especially in orthodontics.

Orthodontics itself now has many branches but, in general, it may be said that orthodontics is concerned with occlusion. Occlusion is defined as "the relation of the maxillary and mandibular teeth when in functional contact during activity of the mandible."* Activity, or movement, of the mandible occurs at the temporomandibular joints. Because of the great importance of orthodontics, the anatomy of the temporomandibular joint requires detailed and careful study. However, a summary, even a lengthy one, of all the factors involved in the activity of the mandible is not within the scope of this text. The presence or absence of teeth, the part played by sensory receptors, the muscles moving the mandible, the tongue and other factors must all be considered not just separately but together. Accordingly, here, only the basic anatomy of the joint is demonstrated to serve as a foundation for a more detailed study with the aid of a larger, more comprehensive text. †

ITEM 71-2. Dissection of the Temporomandibular Joint

The capsule of the temporomandibular joint is not substantial except laterally, where the fibers of the lateral ligament reinforce the capsule. It is time-consuming to try to clean the lateral ligament on a cadaver. The significant facts are: first, that the fibers of the lateral ligament are directed posteroinferiorly from the zygomatic arch to the neck of the mandible and, second, that they are strong.

Open the joint with the aid of an autopsy saw. Keeping the blade of the saw parallel to the ramus of the mandible, slice off the lateral aspect of the joint (Fig. 71-1). All the principal features of the joint are exposed in this way. By pushing the mandible away from the skull, two synovial cavities can be demonstrated, one superior to and the other inferior to the articular disc. Examine the disc.

ITEM 71-3. With the zygomatic arch removed, a good view of the tendinous attachment of the temporalis is obtained. The temporalis was cut in half when the skull cap was removed. The student should observe the full extent of the muscle, and then observe how the tendinous fibers of the temporalis are attached to the entire length of the coronoid process. The thickness of the temporalis muscle also requires your attention. The muscle is about 1.5 cm. thick; its superficial zygomatic fibers blend with the deep fibers of masseter, and its deep temporal fibers blend with the fibers of the lateral pterygoid.

The buccal nerve is of significance to dentists and can be found closely applied to, if not embedded in, the tendinous fibers of the temporalis on the medial side of the coranoid process.

---

*Dorland's Illustrated Medical Dictionary, Philadelphia, W. B. Saunders Company, 1965.

†See Sicher, H.: Oral Anatomy. St. Louis, C. V. Mosby. 4th ed., 1965.

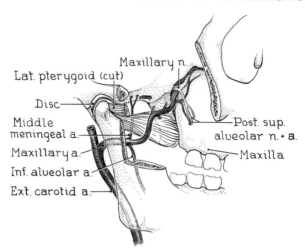

Figure 71-1.   An extensive dissection of the infratemporal fossa after removal of the zygomatic arch. The maxillary artery in its course through the fossa supplies the teeth and gives off the middle meningeal artery. In a cadaver, the artery is usually obscured from view by the pterygoid plexus of veins.

ITEM 71-4.   The next step is to remove the ramus of the mandible. First, with an autopsy saw cut horizontally the neck of the mandible. Second, estimate the level at which the mandibular foramen is located. It is about midway between the lowest point of the mandibular notch and the lower border of the mandible. Immediately above that level and with care, make a horizontal cut through the mandible. Deep to the mandible at this point lie important nerves and vessels.

A segment of bone is now loose. Peel it superiorly, slowly, until the buccal nerve is released from the temporalis. Then pin the temporalis clear of the region. This procedure removes the lateral wall of the infratemporal fossa and exposes the lateral pterygoid muscle.

ITEM 71-5.   Because the lateral pterygoid muscle is a major landmark, it must be identified now, although it is often obscured from view by veins yet to be removed. To demonstrate the lateral pterygoid muscle, which is attached to the neck of the mandible as well as to the articular disc, grasp the neck and the disc with strong toothed forceps. Pull posteriorly and observe the fibers of the lateral pterygoid.

ITEM 71-6.   Sometimes in the cadaver the infratemporal region is obscured by a plexus of veins, solid, distended and adherent to the muscles and to the maxillary artery. Under those circumstances, dissection of the region is not easy and requires sharp dissection to isolate the maxillary artery from the venous plexus. Remove as much of the venous plexus as you can, and then trace the maxillary artery toward the lateral pterygoid muscle. The destination of the artery will be seen shortly.

ITEM 71-7.   To make the lower border of the lateral pterygoid more obvious, identify the inferior alveolar and the lingual nerves. Elevate them gently and trace them toward the skull until they disappear deep to the lower border of the lateral pterygoid. Slide the tip of curved, blunt-ended scissors about 1 cm. deep to the border. Open and withdraw the scissors. Proceed in that fashion until the muscle is mobilized and the lower border is obvious. The muscle should now be sufficiently mobile for you to demonstrate its action as follows: Pull the head of the mandible and the articular disc posteriorly. The lateral pterygoid muscle fibers are stretched. Push the head of the mandible and the disc anteriorly. The muscle fibers buckle. One may deduce that in life the lateral pterygoid muscles, acting together, pull the mandible anteriorly. A pterygoid muscle acting alone pulls its side of the jaw forward so that the chin moves to the opposite side.

ITEM 71-8.   To demonstrate the superior border of the lateral pterygoid muscle slide the tip of curved, blunt-ended scissors immediately inferior to the infratemporal crest, which is the ridge between the infratemporal and the temporal fossa. By twisting the scissors slightly, opening them, and then withdrawing them, you should reveal the cleavage between the muscle and the skull. The muscle fibers of the lateral pterygoid are horizontal and should not be confused with the vertical fibers of the temporalis, some of which may still be in the dissector's field. The deep temporal nerves can usually be located at this time.

ITEM 71-9.   The maxillary artery supplies certain important areas, namely the lower jaw, the upper jaw, the nasal cavity, the meninges, and the eardrum. Branches to the eardrum are never seen in a routine dissection, and dissection of the arteries of the nasal cavity is rarely successful. The nasal cavities are recognized by everyone as very vascular regions; the clinician who has seen an inflamed eardrum is aware that it, too, is vascular.

The inferior alveolar artery, the posterior superior alveolar arteries, and the middle meningeal artery can be identified now.

Carefully cut the capsule of the temporomandibular joint to release the disc and the head of the mandible. Then peel the lateral pterygoid muscle completely out of the fossa. The more complete the removal of the muscle the easier it is to see the remaining structures.

The inferior alveolar artery accompanies the nerve of the same name. The middle meningeal artery ascends to the foramen spinosum. The posterior superior alveolar arteries accompany nerves of the same name, but those nerves, mark you, are branches of the maxillary division of the trigeminal nerve (Fig. 71-1). The posterior superior alveolar arteries and nerves enter foramina already identified on the posterior surface of the maxilla. Identify all these structures.

ITEM 71-10.   The mandibular nerve is now accessible. Push the tip of a probe through the foramen ovale and confirm the relationship of the nerve to the middle cranial fossa. If the trigeminal ganglion is still intact, confirm the connection of the nerve with the ganglion and trace the nerve from the ganglion through the foramen ovale to the infratemporal fossa. Reconsider the position of the foramen with reference to the lateral pterygoid muscle. The foramen is medial, so the branches of the mandibular nerve pass over under or through the muscle (Fig. 71-2).

ITEM 71-11.   The auriculotemporal nerve has not been mentioned so far. It usually arises by two roots from the mandibular nerve. The roots embrace the middle meningeal artery, a characteristic formation that identifies them both almost immediately. Identify the nerve and trace it for a few centimeters to show that it lies medial to the neck of the mandible before ascending to cross the lateral aspect of the zygomatic arch.

ITEM 71-12.   The chorda tympani (Fig. 71-3) is a nerve with a time-honored place in the history of medicine. In 1864 Claude Bernard cut the chorda tympani of a cat and observed the effect upon the submaxillary gland. The chorda tympani is still of great interest today for quite different reasons. It may or may not be injured in fractures of the mastoid region. Furthermore it may have to be sacrificed in surgical procedures in the vicinity of the tympanic membrane.

The chorda tympani is found by tracing the lingual nerve toward the foramen ovale. Sometimes the chorda is quite long and, therefore, easily found. Sometimes, however, it joins the lingual nerve close to the foramen ovale.

ITEM 71-13.   In the present dissection the medial pterygoid muscle is the last of the big muscles to be identified. Observe how the medial pterygoid fibers are directed obliquely inferoposteriorly from the medial side of the lateral pterygoid plate to the medial side of the angle of the jaw; these fibers are parallel to those of the masseter muscle; hence the two muscles have essentially the same action.

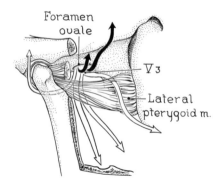

Foramen ovale
V3
Lateral pterygoid m.

Figure 71-2. Part of the lateral pterygoid muscle cut away to show the location of the foramen ovale medial to the muscle. The white arrows represent the four sensory branches of the mandibular nerve. Identify them. The black arrows represent the nerves to the masseter and temporalis. The nerves to the medial and lateral pterygoid muscles are not shown.

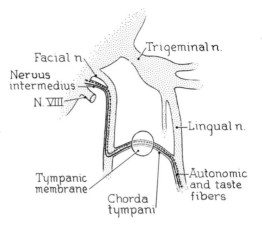

Figure 71-3. Diagram to explain the chorda tympani and its link with the nervus intermedius. The tympanic membrane is the "drumskin" of the tympanum, which is the middle ear. Tympani means *of the tympanum*.

THE MUSCLES OF MASTICATION

By definition the muscles of mastication are the paired medial and lateral pterygoids, the temporalis and the masseter muscles. They are responsible for moving the mandible in chewing. In addition, however, the suprahyoid muscles make a significant contribution by stabilizing the hyoid bone and the floor of the mouth. Therefore, to restrict the term muscles of mastication to the four pairs of muscles named here is unrealistic, but useful nevertheless because it encompasses only those muscles supplied by the motor root of the trigeminal nerve. Read an account of the four paired muscles of mastication. Clinically they are quickly tested by asking the patient to clench his teeth. The masseters and the temporalis muscles are subcutaneous and can be easily seen and felt.

Exercise

Place the fingers over each masseter (or temporalis) and clench the teeth. Both masseters are felt to tighten.

To test the lateral pterygoids, ask your partner to jut his jaw forward so that the lower teeth are anterior to the upper teeth. Ask him to keep his jaw in that position while you attempt to push it posteriorly. The push is resisted by the lateral pterygoids.

The relationship of the infratemporal fossa to the oral cavity is of prime significance to dentists. The relationship should be reviewed when the oral cavity is examined.

Chapter 72

Introduction to Trigeminal Neuralgia

Trigeminal neuralgia is a dreadful affliction characterized by episodes of excruciating pain in the face, usually precipitated by a seemingly trivial stimulus on one part of the face, which is described as the trigger point. The cause of trigeminal neuralgia is unknown. The pain of trigeminal neuralgia is experienced in one or more of the cutaneous areas supplied by the sensory divisions of the trigeminal nerve.

A physician dealing with pain in the face realizes that there are many possible causes, so the diagnosis of true trigeminal neuralgia is not as simple as this commentary may suggest. Let us assume, nevertheless, that the diagnosis has been confirmed and that the patient experiences such anguish that surgical treatment must be undertaken even though it has inevitable and undesirable consequences. Basically, surgical treatment of trigeminal neuralgia is interruption of the appropriate sensory pathway, namely one or more of the divisions of the trigeminal nerve, but that means that other modalities of sensation, not pain alone, are destroyed. Most of us have experienced numbness of the teeth tongue and face for a brief time following a dental anesthetic and can imagine the hardship of more extensive, permanent anesthesia of a region of the face and mouth. Accordingly much research has been done to establish more accurately where pain fibers are located in the trigeminal nerve. Even so surgical treatment of trigeminal neuralgia is still a drastic measure, not to be undertaken lightly. With these grave facts in mind, proceed to examine the trigeminal nerve more closely.

ITEM 72-1. Inspect the attachment of the trigeminal nerve to the lateral aspect of the pons (Fig. 72-1). The attachment is fully exposed in the present dissection, but remember that normally the attachment lies inferior to the tentorium. Therefore, normally it is not immediately accessible from the supratentorial aspect; nor is it easy to reach by the infratentorial approach because of the cerebellum. Thus the surgical approach to the pontine attachment of the trigeminal nerve is difficult.

ITEM 72-2. Identify the very small motor and the very large sensory root. In a surgical procedure, when the sensory root is cut the motor root, which goes to the ipsilateral muscles of mastication (p. 369), is spared.

370

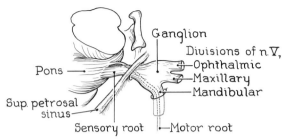

Figure 72-1. Scheme of the parts of the trigeminal nerve, which is discussed in Chapter 72, Introduction to Trigeminal Neuralgia.

It is believed that the pain fibers of all three divisions of the nerve congregate in the lateral part of the sensory root close to the pontine attachment. Although the pain fibers cannot be seen, examine the attachment.

Nearer to the ganglion, the fibers for all modalities of sensation are regrouped according to the divisions of the nerve. Thus the fibers of the ophthalmic division come to be medial, and with them, it must be stressed, are fibers concerned with the sensation and, therefore, the preservation of the cornea. On this basis the medial margin of the sensory root may be spared when the sensory root is cut close to the ganglion. Examine the medial margin, even though there is no evidence of regrouping into divisions, or of the corneal fibers.

Next observe the relationship of the superior petrosal sinus to the sensory root (Fig. 72-1). The sinus is a surgical hazard in obtaining adequate exposure of the root. The subarachnoid space extends anteriorly below the sinus to form a recess named the cavum trigeminale or Meckel's cave (after a German anatomist, Meckel). Slip the tip of a pair of curved, blunt-ended scissors immediately inferior to the sinus in order to identify the cave.

In the examination of the ganglion and the three divisions of the trigeminal nerve, remember that the temporal lobe of the brain has been removed and that you have before you an anatomic, not a surgical, exposure. The surgeon reaches the ganglion by opening the skull in the temporal region. He does not incise dura but strips it off the middle cranial fossa, thus elevating the temporal lobe. The middle meningeal artery crosses his field of view from the skull to the dura, so he coagulates and divides the vessel. Continuing to strip off dura, he soon exposes the mandibular division of the trigeminal nerve at the foramen ovale. Using the division as a guide, and taking further surgical steps, he reaches the ganglion and then the sensory root.

ITEM 72-3. Do likewise. Strip off all dura from the middle cranial fossa until the trigeminal ganglion and the ophthalmic, maxillary, and mandibular divisions of the trigeminal nerve are seen. Finally cut out a portion of the superior petrosal sinus. All being well, you should have before you an excellent demonstration of the trigeminal nerve from its pontine attachment to the superior orbital fissure, the foramen rotundum, and the foramen ovale. Somewhere between those points may lie the mysterious factor responsible for trigeminal neuralgia.

The proximity of the semilunar ganglion to the foramen ovale is of some practical significance. It is possible to push the tip of a needle, inserted through the skin surface, into the foramen ovale. In this way it is possible to reach the mandibular division of the trigeminal nerve either with an anesthetic or a destructive agent. The technique requires a very detailed description that is out of place here.

Chapter 73

The Basic Plan of the Neck

To set out for the first time on an anatomic dissection of the neck without reviewing the lay of the land is to enter a jungle blindfolded. On the other hand, with a plan of the neck in mind, the student can advance through some very intricate anatomy without being trapped in an undergrowth of fine detail. The plan is presented in this chapter. Study it thoroughly before you dissect. You should know, perhaps, that some experienced anatomists have criticized the content of this chapter as too elementary. That may be so, but in my experience the plan has smoothed the way for too many students for this chapter to be omitted.

In the neck, the proximity of so many vital structures means that every step in a surgical dissection is important. Thus, surgical procedures demand proficiency to a degree the novice cannot appreciate, for in the operating room structures are not exposed to the same extent as in the anatomy laboratory. The surgeon, therefore, views the anatomy of the neck differently from the anatomist and many clinicians. The surgeon is concerned with the anatomy of surgical approaches—exactly where to make the correct incision to reach a specific region. Once the procedure has begun he looks for surgical landmarks. They serve not only as indicators of depth but also as pointers to the whereabouts of other significant structures. To stray beyond one of those pointers is to enter an entirely different surgical region from a direction that may be unusual, difficult, and dangerous.

It would seem to be a natural consequence to teach the anatomy of the neck on a regional basis. Indeed, for generations the anatomy of the neck was taught in this way. Today the need is different. It is the continuity of major structures, such as the internal jugular vein, seen in so many different regions of the neck, that is important to the student about to face the challenge of clinical diagnosis. Therefore, the following basic plan of the neck was devised. Having grasped the principle laid down in the plan, the student may choose to concentrate on the anatomy of two regions of the neck, namely the carotid triangle (Fig. 74-1) and the root of the neck (p. 395). Excluding thyroid surgery, 90 per cent of surgery in the neck deals with these two regions.

ORIENTATION OF THE VERTEBRAL COLUMN AND SKULL

The correct orientation of the skull to the cervical vertebral column is the first requirement. To appreciate the orientation quickly, one can draw two vertical lines and one horizontal line on a lateral view of the head and neck (Fig. 73-1). Admittedly, the lines are unrealistic because the head and neck are rarely held in such a rigidly upright posture. Nevertheless, the lines bring forth dimensions that would otherwise remain unseen.

Horizontal Line (1, Fig. 73-1)

The external acoustic meatus, the external occipital protuberance, and the floor of the orbit lie approximately on the same horizontal line. The external acoustic meatus is approximately halfway between the external occipital protuberance and the anterior margin of the orbit. In anthropology this horizontal line is drawn with precision through exact points and is then known as the base line of the skull. One must not, however, confuse the base line with the base of the skull. The base of the skull is not horizontal; both the occiput and the maxillae project inferior to the baseline. The occiput and the left maxilla are illustrated but not labeled in Figure 73-1.

Intermediate Vertical Line (2, Fig. 73-1)

Observe that the external acoustic meatus and the tips of the upper three cervical transverse processes are in a vertical line. The tip of the first cervical transverse process is not only directly inferior to the external acoustic meatus but is also palpable anterior to the mastoid process (Fig. 73-1). The transverse processes of the first three cervical vertebrae and of the remaining four cervical vertebrae lie on a curve, in keeping with the curvature of the cervical spine.

Posterior Vertical Line (3, Fig. 73-1)

The spinous process of the first thoracic vertebra (T1) is directly inferior to the external occipital protuberance. This relationship de-

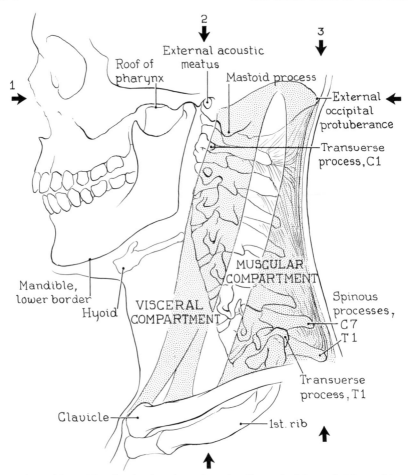

Figure 73-1. Line drawing based on a lateral radiograph of the neck. The position of the bony landmarks in relationship to each other are discussed in the text. 1 (arrows) — horizontal line. 2 (arrows) — intermediate vertical line. 3 (arrows) — posterior vertical line.

pends absolutely on the posture of the individual. The spinous processes of the vertebrae above T1 lie on a curve anterior to this line. In the midline, the interval between the skin of the back of the neck, the spinous processes above T1, and the occiput are occupied by the ligamentum nuchae. Once the ligamentum nuchae is taken into account in drawing a cross section of the neck (Fig. 73-2), it is interesting how much the perspective of the drawing improves.

TWO BASIC COMPARTMENTS OF THE NECK

The intermediate vertical lines (right and left) divide the neck into two compartments, a muscular compartment posteriorly and a visceral

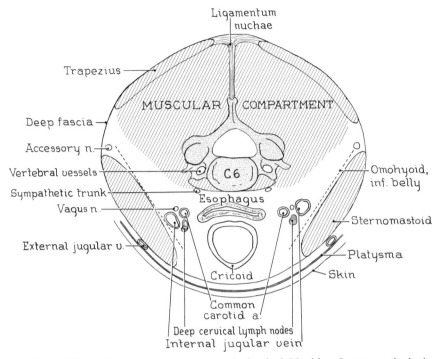

Figure 73-2. Schematic cross section at the level of C6 with reference to the basic plan of the neck. Observe that the cricoid cartilage, an easily identifiable subcutaneous landmark, is level with C6. The dotted lines indicate the plane of the omohyoid muscles. The thyroid gland and phrenic nerves have been omitted.

compartment anteriorly (Figs. 73-1 and 73-2). The bodies of the cervical vertebrae, projecting anterior to the transverse processes, occupy a central part of the visceral compartment. Deep in the central part of the muscular compartment lie the vertebral canal and the spinal cord.

The advantage of dividing the neck this way for descriptive purposes and of defining a muscular compartment is that details of all the muscles in the compartment need not be learned. Such details serve no useful purpose in clinical practice. The student, then, can devote his time to a study of the anatomy of the visceral compartment.

The Superior Boundary of the Neck

The superior boundary of the neck may be divided into two parts. The superior boundary of the posterior compartment is the occiput. The superior boundary of the anterior compartment is not the mandible, as you might expect; the mandible forms the boundary of the floor of the oral cavity. The anterior compartment extends superoposterior not only to the floor of the oral cavity but also to the oral cavity itself and to the nasal cavities. The roof of the pharynx (Fig. 73-1) indicates the location of the superior boundary of the visceral compartment of the neck. The roof is inferior to the body of the sphenoid bone. It is this region that is frequently referred to clinically as "the base of the skull."

The Inferior Boundary of the Neck

The obvious boundaries are created by the clavicles and the scapulae. However, the first ribs must be taken into account. Along with the vertebral column and the manubrium, the first ribs form the boundary of the thoracic inlet. Each rib separates the thoracic inlet from the intermediate part of each cervicoaxillary canal (Fig. 81-1). Thus the inferior boundary of the neck is the thoracic inlet and the right and left cervicoaxillary canals.

THE SIX PLANES OF THE ANTERIOR COMPARTMENT OF THE NECK

The structures of the anterior compartment are arranged in six planes that are easily identified even though some of the planes are far from being a complete sheet (Fig. 73-2). The planes are as follows:

(1) Skin
(2) Platysma and underlying superficial venous plane
(3) Sternomastoid and deep fascia
(4) Strap muscles
(5) Deep venous and lymphatic plane
(6) Arterial plane

The skin of the neck cannot be dismissed without comment. The beauty of the skin of the neck complements the beauty of the skin of the face, as every woman knows. Every surgical procedure of the neck is planned to preserve the appearances of the skin, to avoid an obvious, ugly scar. What is not generally realized is the significance of the next plane or layer, the platysma, in maintaining the natural appearance of the skin of the neck. The significance is apparent when the platysma is paralyzed, for then the skin of the neck droops in wrinkles and the elegance of the neck is marred.

In all surgical approaches to the visceral compartment of the neck, one or both the platysma muscles are incised. The skin is not usually dissected off the platysma; skin and platysma are treated as one layer. In closing the incision, however, the platysma is recognized as a particular layer, and its edges are sutured carefully together to prevent gaping of the skin incision. The external jugular veins (p. 382) representative of the superficial venous plane lie deep to the platysma.

The third layer in the approach to the anterior compartment of the neck is composed of the sternomastoid and the deep fascia. Conspicuous in action, the stermomastoid spans the side of the neck. Its superior attachment is posterior, overlying the posterior belly of the digastric muscle and the muscular compartment (Fig. 73-1). Its inferior attachment is anterior, overlying the inferior belly of the omohyoid muscle and the visceral compartment (Fig. 73-1). The slant of the sternomastoid, its curve toward the angle of the jaw, and how its elevation provides shape while swathing the side of the neck are severe tests of artistic skill; the length and breadth of the muscle provide an extensive obstacle in anatomic dissections, and yet the muscle is an excellent surgical landmark in most surgical procedures on the neck.

The stermomastoid and the trapezius are incorporated in a sheet of deep fascia investing the neck (Fig. 73-2). The fascia extends across the front of the neck from one sternomastoid to the other. It is this sheet of fascia that braces forward the sternomastoid muscles; once the fascia is incised parallel to the anterior border of the sternomastoid, the muscle can be retracted a significant distance posteriorly.

The investing layer of fascia extends from the sternomastoid to the trapezius (the interval between these two muscles is referred to as the posterior triangle of the neck) and provides a "crosswalk" for the accessory nerve (p. 329). In this location this important nerve, now the nerve to trapezius, is dangerously close to the surface of the body (Fig. 73-2). If it is necessary for a surgeon to operate in the upper half of the interval between sternomastoid and trapezius, he is very conscious of the presence of the accessory nerve.

The fourth plane is that of the strap muscles. The term strap muscles is usually applied to the muscles in close relationship to the thyroid gland. Here, the term has been extended to include both the posterior belly of the digastric and the inferior belly of the omohyoid. Superiorly, deep to the sternomastoid, the posterior belly of the digastric straps the carotid arteries, the internal jugular vein and related lymph nodes, and the vagus nerve to the sidewall of the pharynx (Fig. 73-3). Except for superficial veins and nerves, all neurovascular structures related to the posterior belly of the digastric run deep to that belly, and this statement includes the external carotid artery and the facial artery at its origin from the external carotid artery. At the root of the neck, in the same plane as the posterior belly of the digastric, the inferior belly of the omohyoid lies like a strap across the brachial plexus, the internal jugular vein, the common carotid artery, and the vagus nerve (Fig. 73-2). Normally the central tendon of the omohyoid lies anterior to the internal jugular vein at the level of C6.

In addition to the two muscle bellies, the posterior belly of the digastric and the inferior belly of the omohyoid, in this fourth plane there is a sheet of fascia of limited extent between the omohyoid and the clavi-

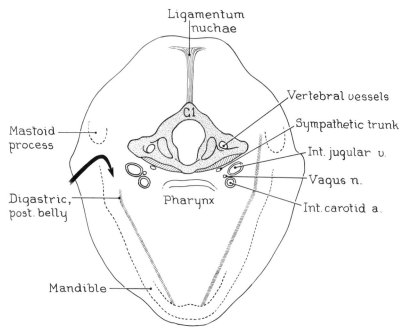

Figure 73-3. Scheme to show the immediate anterior relationships of C1 with reference to the basic plan of the neck. The positions of the mandible and of the posterior belly of the digastric are indicated. In an actual cross section at this level very little of the mandible and digastric is seen. Examine Figure 73-1. The black arrow indicates a space between the medial aspect of the ramus of the mandible and the sidewall of the pharynx. The space is occupied by muscles and other structures.

cle. This fascia provides the sling through which the central tendon of the omohyoid operates.

The fifth plane is termed the venous and lymphatic plane, and consists of the internal jugular vein, its tributaries, and the chain of deep cervical lymph nodes related to the entire length of the jugular vein. The internal jugular vein, at the base of the skull, is an immediate posterior relation of the internal carotid artery and an immediate anterior relation of the transverse process of C1 (Fig. 73-4). At the end of its course the vein is an anterior relation of the arterial system (Fig. 73-4). Throughout its course the vein gradually passes lateral to the arterial system, and so it comes about that the common carotid artery is an immediate anterior relation of the transverse process of C6 (Fig. 73-4). Most of the significant venous tributaries to the internal jugular vein pass lateral to the arterial system. In other words, the veins of the neck are superficial to the arteries.

The sixth plane is the arterial plane, adjacent to the pharynx, esophagus, and trachea. In addition to some small but significant arteries at the root of the neck, the principal arteries are the carotids. The

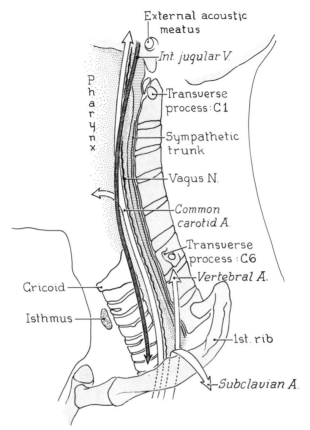

Figure 73-4. Lateral view of the neck with white arrows representing major arteries and the black arrow representing the internal jugular vein. The positions of the vagus nerve and the sympathetic trunk are indicated. Observe the posterior, lateral, and anterior relationships of the internal jugular vein to the carotid system.

common carotid artery branches into the internal and external carotid arteries. The first two arteries are more or less in line, and it is most unusual for them to have any branches. Thus they form a stem from which the external carotid artery arises. The external carotid artery is largely responsible for the distribution of blood to the regions deep and adjacent to the arterial plane.

THE CORE

Finally, it must be recognized that the pharynx and esophagus (Figs. 73-1 and 73-2) are the core of the visceral compartment of the neck.

The pharynx and esophagus may be likened to an air vent on the deck of a ship or on the roof of a barn (Fig. 73-5), except that the margin

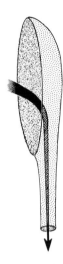

Figure 73-5.   A highly diagrammatic representation of the pharynx and esophagus.

of the opening of the pharynx is irregular in its attachment to the skull
and the surface of the pharynx is uneven.

The opening of the pharynx is posterior to the nasal cavities, the
oral cavity, and the larynx. Hence for descriptive purposes the pharynx
is divided into nasal, oral, and laryngeal parts (Fig. 73-6). At the level of
C6, the pharynx joins the esophagus.

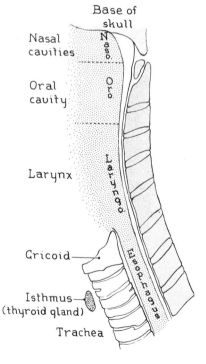

Figure 73-6.   Diagrammatic lateral view
of the pharynx.

Review the basic plan of the neck, beginning with the pharynx and the esophagus and proceeding plane by plane, anteriorly, laterally, and posteriorly to the skin.

Chapter 74

Dissection of the Neck

ITEM 74-1. The platysma muscles are useful landmarks for skinning the neck. The muscles spread inferiorly across the clavicle and were encountered when the skin was reflected from the anterior chest wall. Begin at the cut edge of skin that runs parallel to the clavicle, and, on both sides of the neck, peel the skin off. Go slowly until you are sure you have identified the platysma. Remain superficial to the platysma; its brownish, slender bundles are very characteristic and they are beautifully illustrated in *Grant's Atlas of Anatomy*, Figure 526. Having identified the plane between the skin and the underlying platysma muscle, proceed to reflect the skin superiorly as far as the mandible. When and where necessary, make cuts in the skin to create flaps. Continue to reflect the skin from the entire neck, proceeding carefully after you leave the posterior border of the platysma muscle. Keep the point of the knife directed toward the skin and remove skin entirely from the posterior aspect of the neck as well. In some cadavers the neck is very short. The shoulders are elevated and there is a heavy deposit of subcutaneous fat interwoven with tough fibrous tissue. In such a cadaver skinning the neck is toil. It requires the assistance of all the dissectors at the table to position the neck in such a way that it is as easy as possible for the dissector to reflect skin.

ITEM 74-2. Removal of the Platysma Muscle

Dissect the lower end of the platysma muscle from the clavicle and carefully reflect the platysma superiorly as far as the mandible. It is worthwhile to establish a correct plane of cleavage before proceeding rapidly with the reflection. The external jugular vein, lying immediately deep to the platysma (see Fig. 73-2) is an excellent guide. Leave the vein undisturbed on the sternomastoid muscle. As you approach the jaw, look out for the branch of the facial nerve to the platysma. If the parotid gland has already been dissected, the nerve to the platysma will have been found close to the angle of the jaw.

THE EXTERNAL JUGULAR VEINS

Always included in the physical examination of the cardiovascular system is an inspection of the external jugular veins, which are easily seen on the side of the neck, where they are deep only to the skin and platysma. The veins join the deep venous system so close to the right side of the heart that under certain circumstances their fullness with blood reflects the fullness of the terminal part of the deep venous system. In other words, the external jugular veins serve as indicators of venous pressure. Your clinical tutors will teach you certain fundamental steps to be taken in the assessment of venous pressure by examining the external jugular veins. Here only the anatomy counts, and the following points are pertinent. It is unusual, but it occasionally does happen that both external jugular veins are absent; sometimes one is absent. Consequently, before any conclusions regarding venous pressure are made, the presence of external jugular veins must be verified. Each vein lies across the sternomastoid muscle on a line from the angle of the jaw to the middle of the clavicle. Piercing the deep fascia, the external jugular vein joins the subclavian vein in the vicinity of the junction of the subclavian and internal jugular veins.

The external jugular vein is classified as a superficial vein. As such it must pierce deep fascia (p. 7) to join the deep venous system, a fact that can be demonstrated now.

ITEM 74-3.   Dissection of the External Jugular Vein

Divide the external jugular vein on the surface of the sternomastoid. Grasp the cut end of the vein, the end that is nearest to the clavicle, and peel the vein toward the clavicle. Observe how the vein penetrates the investing layer of the fascia of the neck that lies between the sternomastoid and trapezius.

Scattered along the length of the external jugular vein are some of the superficial cervical lymph nodes. The superficial cervical lymph nodes require special consideration, and it is convenient to consider them now.

THE SUPERFICIAL LYMPHATIC DRAINAGE OF THE HEAD AND NECK

For a long time it has been recognized that lymph from the skin of the scalp, the auricles, and the face drains into a ring of lymph nodes named according to their anatomic location. Thus, occipital, retroauricular, superficial parotid, submandibular, and submental (*mentum*, in Latin, means chin) groups are recognized. They lie at the junction of the back of the neck and the skull, behind and in front of the auricle, and under the margin of the mandible and the chin.

Although the submandibular and submental lymph nodes have been mentioned here, it must be understood that those two groups are not superficial, but are deep because they are found beneath the deep fascia. Therefore the lymph vessels from the face, beginning as superficial vessels, penetrate the deep fascia (p. 8) at the margin of the jaw to reach their destination.

In addition to the ring of lymph nodes just described, on each side there is a vertical group of superficial lymph nodes scattered along the length of the external jugular vein.

Lymph nodes in any of the groups mentioned above are rarely found in the cadaver, but this does not mean they are unimportant. Like lymph nodes elsewhere in the body, these nodes react to disorders, such as infection, in their field of drainage. Accordingly, when one or more of these lymph nodes is found to be enlarged it is imperative to survey their entire field of drainage, and the survey must include the skin of the scalp.

The lymphatic drainage of the head and neck is discussed further on p. 384 when the deep cervical nodes are considered.

REFLECTION OF STERNOMASTOID

ITEM 74-4. Slide the tip of a pair of blunt-ended, curved scissors posterior to the inferior end of the sternomastoid and, by blunt dissection, mobilize the end of the muscle from the underlying tissues. Cut the entire muscle close to the sternum and to the clavicle. Holding the superior cut edge of the muscle firmly with a toothed forceps or a hemostat, begin to peel the muscle toward the mastoid process. When the anterior jugular vein is present (it passes posterior to the sternomastoid muscle), it is a useful indicator of depth. The anterior jugular vein and its relationship to the sternomastoid is demonstrated in *Grant's Atlas of Anatomy*, Figure 542. Begin to peel the sternomastoid muscle off the side of the neck. In elevating the muscle, small but significant arteries entering its deep surface will be ruptured. Be on the lookout for the spinal accessory nerve (p. 329). The nerve leaves the posterior border of the sternomastoid muscle at its midpoint and then crosses in the deep fascia of the neck (Fig. 73-2) to reach the trapezius.

Several cutaneous nerves to the skin of the neck will be encountered at the middle of the posterior border of the sternomastoid. They are usually well illustrated in atlases and textbooks, and their anatomy needs no emphasis at the present time. These nerves are cutaneous branches of the cervical plexus and are of some interest to the anesthetist who may wish to anesthetize the skin of the anterior aspect of the neck over the thyroid gland. Their chief significance, however, is in referring pain to the shoulder from the upper abdomen. For example, pain may be experienced in the left shoulder following rupture of the spleen or when the pleura on the diaphragm is inflamed (diaphragmatic pleurisy).

ITEM 74-5. Once the accessory nerve is identified as it leaves sternomastoid, proceed to find it entering sternomastoid as follows: Turn the muscle back and continue to mobilize it toward the mastoid process. In doing so, separate the muscle from the remains of the parotid gland, a procedure that may require some very vigorous dissection because in a cadaver the muscle and the gland are usually found stuck together by tough fibrous tissue. Emerging anterior or posterior to the internal jugular vein and entering the sternomastoid, the accessory nerve cannot be mistaken for anything else. It may well be obscured from view by a cluster of lymph nodes.

With the sternomastoid muscle reflected off the side of the neck, the next plane, the plane of the strap muscles, is now in view. Because the posterior belly of the digastric muscle and the inferior belly of the omohyoid are so slender, they scarcely obscure the venous and lymphatic plane. For a reason that will become clear in the next commentary, the lymph nodes are considered now.

THE DEEP CERVICAL LYMPH NODES

On each side of the neck, lymph nodes are clustered along the entire length of the internal jugular vein, even to the base of the skull. The nodes are classified as deep (p. 7) because they are deep to the deep fascia, in contradistinction to the superficial nodes, which lie superficial to the deep fascia of the neck (Fig. 73-2), in which the trapezius and the sternomastoid muscles are incorporated. The deep cervical nodes, like deep nodes elsewhere in the body, receive lymph from their corresponding superficial nodes. Thus lymph from the superficial nodes, which you have just examined (p. 382), drains ultimately into these deep cervical nodes. In addition to receiving the superficial lymphatic drainage, the deep cervical nodes have additional sources of lymph. In fact, it may be said that the right and left deep cervical nodes receive lymph from the entire head and neck. Consequently, when one or more of the deep cervical nodes becomes enlarged and some underlying pathologic process suspected, the tissues of the entire head and neck must be carefully examined. The examination will include the scalp, the orbital apertures, the nasal cavities, the pharynx, the tonsils, the oral cavity, both external auditory meatuses, the auricles, the esophagus, the larynx, the trachea, the thyroid gland, the teeth, the gums, the salivary glands — in fact it means an examination of every tissue in the head and neck.

On each side of the neck, two of the lymph nodes of the deep cervical chain are distinguished from the rest. They are named the jugulodi-gastric lymph node and the juguloomohyoid lymph node. The jugulodi-gastric lymph node lies at the point where the digastric muscle crosses the internal jugular vein. This lymph node is so frequently enlarged, for example, in infections such as tonsillitis, that it has become a landmark in physical examination of the neck. The other node, the juguloomohyoid node, lies at the point where the omohyoid muscle crosses the internal jugular vein.

From the lower end of the deep cervical lymph nodes, a jugular lymph trunk emerges and joins the deep venous system somewhere in the vicinity of the junction of the internal jugular and subclavian veins. On the left side, however, the jugular lymph trunk may join the thoracic duct. The jugular trunks are rarely seen in a cadaver.

It has already been stated (p. 329), but it is worth stating again that the accessory nerve, before it enters the sternomastoid and, after it leaves the muscle to proceed to the trapezius, is surrounded by lymph nodes. When these lymph nodes become involved in disease the accessory nerve is in peril.

ITEM 74-6. Identify the deep cervical lymph nodes. In particular, identify the jugulodigastric node and observe its location with reference to the jaw. Also identify the juguloomohyoid node and its location with reference to the root of the neck.

The Ansa Cervicalis

This structure is dealt with, not because it is especially important, but because it is a confusing little item in the dissecting laboratory. The following brief description should be sufficient to prevent the student from spending time unnecessarily searching for details of the ansa cervicalis. On the anterior aspect of the internal jugular vein, there is usually present a U-shaped formation from which nerves to three muscles of the strap muscle group emerge. Do not be surprised if the U lies posterior to the internal jugular vein. It often does. One limb of the U descends from the cervical nerve plexus, and is therefore called the descendens cervicalis. The other limb of the U descends from the hypoglossal nerve, and is therefore called the descendens hypoglossae. At a point that varies from cadaver to cadaver, the two limbs meet. Calling this meeting a loop leads many students to think that the nerve fibers descend in one limb and ascend in the other. No so. After their descent in one limb or the other, the nerve fibers proceed through the part where the two limbs meet and then go on to their destination, a muscle. From the ansa cervicalis, nerves proceed to the omohyoid, sternothyroid, and sternohyoid muscles.

ITEM 74-7.   Identify the ansa cervicalis and trace one limb back to the hypoglossal nerve and the other to the cervical plexus. Clinically, it is not an important structure except that it is encountered in an operative procedure termed a radical neck dissection, in which a large segment of the jugular vein is removed.

THE COMMON FACIAL VEIN

This vein, a surgical landmark, is ligated and cut in the surgical approach to the carotid triangle in which the bifurcation of the common carotid artery lies (Fig. 74-1). The vein will now be identified.

ITEM 74-8.   The external jugular vein has been cut already and its terminal part traced to its junction with the subclavian vein. Now trace the cranial part of the external jugular vein to its junction with the retro-mandibular vein (Fig. 60-3). Trace the anterior branch of the retro-mandibular vein to its junction with the facial vein. This junction is the beginning of the common facial vein. Trace this vein to where it joins the internal jugular vein. Ligate the common facial vein at its beginning and end. Cut the vein between the ties. Other branches of the internal jugular vein will be identified and cut at a later stage in the dissection.

Sectioning the Omohyoid and Digastric

ITEM 74-9.   Tie two ligatures around the tendon of omohyoid and cut the tendon. Next slit the omohyoid fascia close to the inferior muscle belly and reflect the muscle posteriorly. Use the ligature to keep the

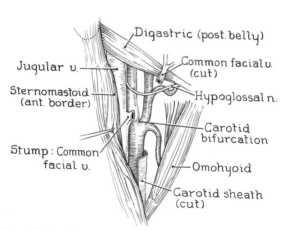

Figure 74-1.   The surgical landmarks of the carotid triangle.

muscle clear of the field of view. Then reflect the superior belly to its attachment to the hyoid bone.

ITEM 74-10.   Now observe how the tendon of the digastric is held by a sling of fascia to the hyoid bone and how a slender muscle, the stylohyoid, runs parallel to and overlaps the superior edge of the posterior belly of the digastric. Slip a ligature around the stylohyoid and the posterior belly of the digastric as close to the hyoid bone as possible. Cut the tendon of the digastric and the attachment of the stylohyoid to the hyoid bone. Peel back those two muscles as far as possible toward the skull. It is important to do this well in order to get a full exposure of the structures lying deep to the muscles. In the neck of a cadaver there is tissue that would ordinarily be scarcely seen during a surgical procedure and, if seen, would likely be swept aside, but with embalming this soft tissue gains substance. You must learn to ignore such tissue in the cadaver while you seek the structures named. Use the ligature around the posterior belly of the digastric to keep the muscle clear of the dissector's field. Having reflected the posterior belly of the digastric and the omohyoid, you have arrived at the venous and lymphatic plane represented by the internal jugular vein and the deep cervical lymph nodes that have been considered.

THE INTERNAL JUGULAR VEINS

These two veins, one on each side, drain blood from almost the entire head and neck. They are classified as deep veins because they lie deep to the deep fascia investing the neck (Fig. 73-2). Thus they are similar to deep veins elsewhere in the body (p. 7); accordingly a superficial vein such as the facial vein penetrates the deep fascia to reach the jugular vein.

There is, however, this difference. The internal jugular veins are so close to the thorax that they are more sensitive to the pressure changes within the thoracic cavity than deep veins elsewhere in the body. Thus when the jugular vein is cut open, there is a great danger that air will be sucked into the vein and form an air embolus.

The result of air embolus depends on the amount of air and where the embolus eventually lodges, whether it remains on the venous side or reaches the arterial side. In the former, air is carried to the lungs where large amounts of air are tolerated and eventually absorbed. Therefore pulmonary air embolism is not necessarily fatal. On the arterial side, however, 1 cc. of air may bring instant death if the air lodges in a coronary or a cerebral artery. Today, air is most likely to enter the left side of the circulation during cardiac surgery. Cardiac surgeons are extremely cautious in order to prevent this disastrous complication. Air may also reach the left atrium and, therefore, the left side of the circulation, from a pulmonary air embolism when large amounts of air are absorbed into the pulmonary circulation. There is some doubt that air may be transmitted from the right to the left side through a patent foramen ovale because of the pressure differences between the left and right atria.

The student can judge from the size of the internal jugular vein the volume of blood normally flowing through the vein. The hemorrhage upon laceration of the internal jugular vein can be massive.

Finally, each internal jugular vein is in such close relationship to the deep cervical lymph nodes that diseased lymph nodes can easily become adherent to the vein. When the lymph nodes are removed surgically in a procedure called a radical neck dissection, a segment of the jugular vein is also removed in much the same way as in the following description.

ITEM 74-11. In the cadaver the internal jugular vein usually obscures "everything." Remove the vein as follows: Tie two ligatures around the internal jugular vein close to its termination. Be careful not to include the vagus nerve in the ligatures. Cut the vein between the ligatures and, peeling the vein toward the skull, identify and cut two of its tributaries, the middle thyroid vein and the superior thyroid vein.

The next tributary will probably be the common facial vein, a surgical landmark of the carotid triangle. This vein has already been identified and cut. Why it is necessary to distinguish this particular vein in surgical procedures in this region becomes more apparent as the dissection reaches a deeper level. The common facial vein may have several significant branches, e.g., the lingual vein and the superior thyroid vein.

Continue to mobilize the jugular vein. However, it is not possible to mobilize the jugular vein right to the base of the skull because the vein lies deep to the styloid process, but observe, if it is possible to do so, how the internal jugular vein, traced toward the base of the skull, gradually goes posterior to the internal carotid artery and become an anterior relation of the transverse process of C1.

The arterial plane of the neck is now in view and may be considered under two headings, the vessels proceeding directly to enter the cranium and the vessel proceeding to the face and the rest of the head and neck. The former are represented by the common carotid and the internal carotid arteries and the latter is the external carotid artery.

A student who is fortunate enough to obtain a copy of *Clinical Symposia*, Volume 14, No. 4, by the Ciba Company, will find in it a well-illustrated account of radical neck dissection. All the structures that the student has encountered so far in this dissection of the neck of a cadaver are shown clearly in a clinical setting in that symposium.

Chapter 75

The Hypoglossal and Vagus Nerves and the Sympathetic Trunk in the Neck

THE HYPOGLOSSAL NERVE

This nerve, more or less horizontally disposed, lies between the venous and arterial planes and is a surgical landmark in the carotid triangle.

In the summary of the cranial nerves, p. 329, it was stated that the hypoglossal nerve, having left the anterior condylar foramen, proceeded inferiorly and laterally to adopt a characteristic position on the lateral aspect of the internal carotid, external carotid, and lingual arteries. You now have the opportunity to identify the hypoglossal nerve in the characteristic situation just described.

ITEM 75-1. Identify the nerve and its relationships and trace it proximally to where it disappears toward the anterior condylar foramen. Then trace it distally for a short distance in the direction of the tongue. Each hypoglossal nerve supplies one half the musculature of the tongue.

THE VAGUS NERVES

Almost all the fibers belonging to the cranial outflow of the parasympathetic system enter the vagus nerves to wander far and wide through the neck, thorax, and abdomen. *Vagare*, in Latin, means to wander. Although the vagus nerves are spread so extensively, their anatomy is quite simple. On the other hand, their function is complicated and requires careful study, for the functions controlled by the vagus nerves are very significant in so many aspects of medical practice. The following are some of the more significant anatomic points.

(1) At the base of the skull, each vagus nerve receives a sensory branch with fibers coming from parts of the auricle, the external auditory meatus, and the tympanic membrane. Few anatomists have seen this nerve, but all practicing physicians bear it in mind. Even slight stimulation of the area supplied by the auricular branch of the vagus nerve may induce, through the rest of the vagus nerve, reflex coughing, vomiting, and even fainting.

389

(2) A pharyngeal branch to the pharyngeal plexus is usually easily found.

(3) Laryngeal branches to the voice box, as it is known to the layman, require particularly careful consideration because the larynx is a central structure, and therefore its nerve supply must be visualized in its bilateral form. Figure 78-7 should be studied carefully. The internal laryngeal nerves supply the mucous membrane of the larynx down to the level of the vocal cords. Below that level, the mucous membrane is supplied by the recurrent laryngeal nerves. Each external laryngeal nerve supplies a cricothyroid muscle, shown but not labeled on Figure 78-7. The recurrent laryngeal nerves are the most important nerves to the larynx because they supply all the small muscles responsible for vocalization within the framework of the thyroid cartilage (p. 423).

(4) Cardiac branches are rarely seen well in the undergraduate human dissection laboratory. Their significance is doubtful, but they must be kept in mind in the experimental laboratory when the heart of a dog, for example, is being completely denervated for experimental purposes.

ITEM 75-2.   Each vagus nerve descends within the carotid sheath adjacent first to the internal carotid artery and then to the common carotid artery before the nerve crosses the subclavian artery to enter the thorax. The carotid sheath is a surgical landmark, but it is not easy to distinguish the true carotid sheath in an embalmed cadaver because embalming solidifies tissue that would ordinarily not be seen or would be swept aside by a sponge during an operative procedure. Slit the tissue around the carotid artery and free the vagus nerve. To identify the branches of the vagus nerve, begin inferiorly and , on each side, identify the vagus nerve and its recurrent laryngeal branch. Near its termination that branch has a close relationship to the inferior thyroid artery, a relationship that will be explored more carefully when the thyroid gland is examined.

ITEM 75-3.   Then trace each vagus nerve superiorly. Hold the carotid artery well anteriorly; gently but firmly hold the vagus nerve posteriorly, superiorly, and laterally. This maneuver elevates the superior laryngeal branch of the vagus before the branch runs deep to the carotid arteries. The division of the superior laryngeal nerve into its branches occurs at a variable distance from the vagus nerve. Grasp the superior laryngeal nerve and pull it firmly toward you while you examine the thyrohyoid membrane to see the internal laryngeal nerve disappear through the membrane. Identifying the superior laryngeal nerve and its branch, the internal laryngeal nerve, is no real problem. But to identify the external laryngeal nerve is a problem at the present time because the nerve is very slender, is easily broken, and is closely applied to the side of the pharynx. However, the nerve is in close relationship to the superior thyroid artery and the upper pole of the lateral lobe of the thyroid gland, so it can be easily identified when the thyroid gland has been dissected.

ITEM 75-4.   Next identify the pharyngeal branch of the vagus nerve. This branch passes between the internal and external carotid artery to reach the pharyngeal plexus.

Last, do not look for, but do not forget the auricular branch of the vagus nerve.

THE SYMPATHETIC TRUNK IN THE NECK

On each side of the neck, immediately posterior to the carotid sheath, the sympathetic trunk is found. It is recognizable as one or more, usually more, strands of nerve fibers interrupted by one or more ganglia. Forthwith it is essential to establish that the impulses in the sympathetic trunk in the neck travel in the direction of the skull. That, then, is the direction of the sympathetic trunk in the neck. The nerve fibers in the trunk are the cervical part of the thoracolumbar outflow of the autonomic nervous system.

Three ganglia are usually recognized on the sympathetic trunk in the neck, the inferior, middle, and superior cervical ganglia. The inferior ganglion is often blended with the first thoracic ganglion (p. 460). The middle ganglion lies about level with the transverse process of C6, where the vertebral artery enters the foramen transversarium. In contrast to the insignificant size of the middle cervical ganglion is the demonstrable size of the superior ganglion. It is elongated and pointed at both ends, and is indeed a useful anatomic landmark in the identification of the sympathetic trunk in the neck. Before discussing briefly the branches of the cervical sympathetic trunk, it is worth pointing out that the inferior thyroid artery wends its way through the sympathetic trunk at the level of the sixth cervical vertebra. When there is a tendency to divorce the structures of this region widely from each other, this simple fact concerning the inferior thyroid artery emphasizes the proximity of the structures not only to each other but also to the vertebral column.

Fibers of the sympathetic trunk, in the neck and elsewhere in the body, reach their destination in three ways (Fig. 75-1).

(1) Via the surface of an artery

(2) Via other nerves

(3) Directly

ITEM 75-5.   Identify the inferior cervical ganglion. When the upper limb is dissected you will be asked to look for branches from the ganglion to the brachial plexus to demonstrate the second way that sympathetic nerve fibers reach their destination. Ignore the middle cervical ganglion and proceed to identify the superior one. At a later stage in the

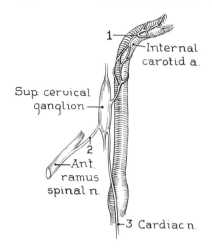

1—Internal carotid a.

Sup. cervical ganglion—

2

—Ant. ramus spinal n.

—3 Cardiac n.

Figure 75-1. Sympathetic fibers reach their destination in three ways, (1) on the surface of arteries, (2) by joining anterior rami, and (3) directly. Thus the thoracolumbar outflow is diffused throughout the body.

dissection, you will find the carotid nerves that pass from the superior cervical ganglion on to the external aspect of the internal carotid artery. In this way sympathetic nerve fibers enter the skull. Sympathetic nerve fibers also enter the skull on the surface of the vertebral arteries. Finally, do not delay to look for cardiac nerves; they are not easily found in a cadaver. Nevertheless, they must be kept in mind.

Horner's Syndrome

In 1869, Dr. Johann Friedrich Horner, a Swiss ophthalmologist, wrote a clinical description of the face of a patient, Frau Anna Brandli. This description, known to be the first of its kind, is brilliant in its execution, fascinating to read (see Fulton, 1929) and, what is more, remains unchallenged. Today, Horner's syndrome is summarized in terse medical terms, ptosis, enophthalmos, myosis, and anhidrosis, so that reading the original account (found in Fulton, 1929) is a refreshing experience.

Horner's syndrome is the outcome of the paralysis of the cervical sympathetic trunk, a fact that has been proven by Claude Bernard's experiments on a dog eight years before Horner wrote his clinical report. The syndrome is explained more fully as follows: Although some of the impulses traveling from the thoracolumbar outflow into the cervical sympathetic trunk are destined for the upper limb, most of them proceed to the head and neck. Thus, if the cervical sympathetic trunk is interrupted, no impulses can reach the upper limb or the head and neck. On p. 3 it was pointed out that the sympathetic system maintains the small arteries of the body in a state of moderate vasoconstriction and that when the sympathetic system is inactive the arteries dilate. Furthermore, it was pointed out that the sympathetic system promotes sweating; thus, after sympathectomy, the skin in the area affected becomes red, warm, and dry, and, if it is the cervical sympathetic trunk that is involved, it is the skin of one half of the face and neck that becomes red, warm, and dry. To quote Horner (see Fulton, 1929), "the boundary of the redness and warmth was exactly in the midline."

In addition, however, the cervical sympathetic system is responsible for dilation of the pupil as well as assisting in elevating the upper eyelid. To the student this must seem like a remote possibility, but it is true; without sympathetic innervation the pupil contracts and the upper eyelid droops. It is contraction of the pupil, drooping of the upper eyelid, and congestion of the conjunctival and nasal vessels, as well as redness, warmth, and dryness of one half of the face and neck, that constitute a complete Horner's syndrome. The causes of the syndrome are many, but they all have one thing in common, one way or another impulses through the cervical sympathetic trunk are blocked.

Chapter 76

The Common and Internal Carotid Arteries, the Vertebral Arteries, and the External Carotid Arteries

THE COMMON AND INTERNAL CAROTID ARTERIES

The right common carotid artery, a branch of the brachiocephalic artery, leaves that artery at the level of the right sternoclavicular articulation. The left common carotid artery arises directly from the arch of the aorta. At the level of the upper margin of the thyroid cartilage, both the right and left common carotid arteries branch at the carotid bifurcation into the internal and external carotid arteries. The carotid bifurcation is a surgical landmark. The internal carotid artery is in line with the common carotid artery, so one may describe the external carotid artery as branching off a straight arterial stem consisting of the other two carotid arteries, extending from the root of the neck to the base of the skull. Furthermore, usually neither the common carotid artery nor the internal carotid artery has any major branches in the neck, whereas the external artery is a series of branches.

The concept of the straight arterial stem must not exclude certain features of the carotid bifurcation that are of vital significance to the cerebral circulation. First, the lower end of the internal carotid artery is slightly distended; the distension, known as the carotid sinus, may extend inferiorly to incorporate the superior end of the common carotid artery. Second, in the fork between the internal and external carotid arteries is a minute body, measured in millimeters, called the carotid body or the glomus caroticum; occasionally a tumor of the carotid body occurs. The carotid sinus is sensitive to changes in arterial blood pressure, while the carotid body is sensitive to changes in the level of arterial oxygen. It is these two small nondescript structures, located on each side of the neck, that maintain the pressure and oxygen content of the all-important cerebral circulation. The carotid sinus becomes sensitive to pressure in some older people so that pressure on the carotid sinus from a hard collar, for example, causes them to faint.

ITEM 76-1. Cut the common carotid arteries at the root of the neck. Slit open both arteries lengthwise and examine their intima. It is a curious fact, revealed by modern methods of clinical investigation, that a small patch of arterial disease in the intima of one or both common carotid arteries close to their bifurcation may be sufficient to reduce cerebral blood flow to an inadequate level. The narrowing is termed stenosis by vascular surgeons.

The student will get the opportunity to see the internal carotid artery in the carotid canal when the petrous part of the temporal bone is dissected. The terminations of the internal carotid arteries have already been seen.

Proceed now to review the two vertebral arteries that are of no less importance than the carotid arteries in sustaining the cerebral circulation.

THE VERTEBRAL ARTERIES

Each vertebral artery is considered in four parts, for descriptive purposes, according to the following locations:

(1) The vertebral triangle
(2) The transverse processes of the upper sixth cervical vertebrae.
(3) The suboccipital triangle.
(4) Inside the skull.

The Vertebral Triangle. The so-called triangle in which the vertebral artery lies is bordered medially by the longus cervicis and laterally by the scalenus anterior. The apex of the triangle is the transverse

process of C6. The base of the triangle is debatable; probably the subclavian artery, from which the artery arises, is the most appropriate.
   ITEM 76-2.   Investigate the boundaries of the triangle *(Grant's Atlas of Anatomy,* Figs. 536, 536A, and 536B) and observe how the inferior thyroid artery loops across the apex of the triangle. Along the medial border of the triangle the sympathetic trunk emerges from the thorax and ascends on the longus cervicis muscle. The inferior cervical ganglion is a posteroinferomedial relation of the vertebral artery while the tiny, inconspicuous middle cervical ganglion is an anterior relation at the apex of the triangle. The vertebral vein occupies a variable position in the triangle, and, on the left side, the thoracic duct crosses the vertebral triangle in a variable location. In a surgical procedure, to expose the vertebral artery adequately, it is necessary to detach scalenus anterior from the first rib. Immediately posterior to scalenus anterior is the brachial plexus, a surgical landmark. In a cadaver it is easier to cut the common carotid artery to expose the vertebral artery to better advantage. This has already been done.
   The Transverse Processes.   This part ascends through the foramina transversaria of the upper six cervical vertebrae until it emerges from the transverse process of C1. It will be recalled that the transverse process of C1 projects laterally *anterior* to the mastoid process. Examine a skeleton and confirm these facts, but take a closer look at the lengths of the transverse processes of C1 and C2. The transverse processes of C1 project further laterally than those of C2. The vertebral arteries conform to this increase in length and proceed laterally as well as superiorly before they turn medially to enter their respective suboccipital triangles. The lateral displacement of each vertebral artery is of more than passing interest, and will be commented upon once the remaining parts of the vertebral artery have been dealt with.
   The Suboccipital Triangle.   The third part of the vertebral artery lies in the suboccipital triangle. To understand the anatomy of the triangle and the course of the vertebral artery through it, it is necessary to digress to a basic description of the junction of the column to the skull.
   The Junction of the Column to the Skull.   Examine an atlas and you will recognize that it is a ring (Fig. 76.1A). Examine the external aspect of the occiput (Fig. 76-1B). It, too, may be described as a ring. The two rings are held together by a muscular cuff and a membranous cuff; a diagram to illustrate this point is included (Fig. 76-1C).
   Now examine the superior surface of the atlas and the inferior surface of the occiput. You will observe corresponding articular facets at the margins of the bony rings. The facets form the atlantooccipital joints, and the capsules of those joints are incorporated in the membranous cuff (Fig. 76-1 *A* and *B*). You see in Figure 76-1*A* that the membranous cuff is subdivided into solitary anterior and posterior atlantooccipital membranes and the capsules of the two atlantooccipital joints.

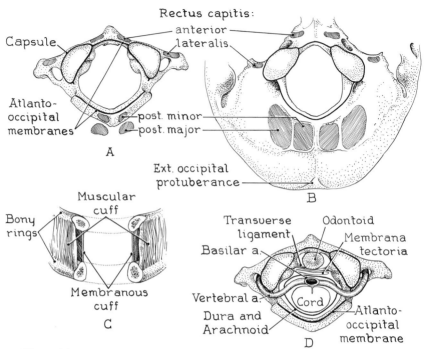

Figure 76-1. These diagrams are referred to in the section on Junction of the Column to the Skull, p. 395.

The muscular cuff, which is external to the membranous cuff, is by no means complete, represented as it is by several pairs of small muscles. Most of these muscles are vertical (hence the word rectus) and, being attached to the head, the caput, they are referred to as "capitis." The attachments of these muscles are shown in Figure 76-1 *A* and *B*. Rectus capitis posterior major, unfortunately, spoils a nice concept by being attached to C2, not C1.

On each side of the suboccipital region there are, in addition to the vertical muscles, two oblique muscles, both of which are attached to the transverse process of the atlas. One oblique muscle is attached to the skull, the other to the spine of C2, so that along with rectus capitis posterior major they form a triangle, the suboccipital triangle (Fig. 76-2). Each triangle lies more or less in a horizontal plane not in a vertical plane. It is, unfortunately, usually illustrated in a vertical plane (Fig. 76-2), but this is so only when the skull is tilted anteriorly into a position possible only in the dissected cadaver. To confirm the normal position of the triangle, palpate on yourself the external occipital protuberance, the spine of C2, and the transverse process of C1.

With these facts in mind we can now return to the vertebral artery.

The Suboccipital Triangle. Having passed through the foramen

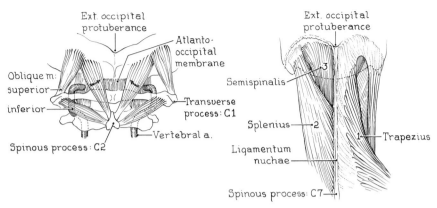

Figure 76-2. In a cadaver the suboccipital triangle is exposed by reflecting (1) the trapezius, (2) the splenius capitis, and (3) the semispinalis capitis. Further instructions are given on p. 398.

transversarium of the atlas, each vertebral artery turns medially, skirts the atlantooccipital articulation, enters the suboccipital triangle, penetrates the posterior atlantooccipital membrane, pierces the dura and arachnoid, and enters the subarachnoid space (Fig. 76-1*D*). In the space the fourth part of the artery has already been seen.

The Applied Anatomy of the Vertebral Artery at the Base of the Skull. The curves in the vertebral arteries as they thread their way from the vertebral column into the skull are of little significance in the normal person. The curves become extremely significant when the blood flow through the arteries is reduced by narrowing of the artery, not necessarily in the vicinity of the skull. Under those conditions, the turning of the head may be sufficient to reduce the blood flow even more, even to a degree that cerebral function is affected. To the layman the medical history sounds like lunacy: "Every time I take the car out of the garage I get spots before my eyes." To the physician the history suggests that blood flow through one of the vertebral arteries is being further impaired by a rotation of the head and neck to a degree that warrants further investigation. Angiography of the vertebral artery is difficult because of the location of the first, second, and third parts of the vertebral artery. Accordingly, vertebral angiograms are usually obtained by introducing a radiopaque fluid into the blood stream of the arch of the aorta. Thence the branches of the arch and their branches can be visualized.

ITEM 76-3. Dissection of the vertebral arteries in the suboccipital triangles may be omitted if the neck of the cadaver is thick with fat, the muscles heavy, and the fibrous tissue tough. Dissection under those circumstances is unrewarding and time consuming. Usually, in a large laboratory, several good specimens are available and, if the following instructions are obeyed, dissection of the suboccipital triangles is soon done.

The suboccipital triangles do not involve much dissection if the object is simply to expose the vertebral arteries. Three pairs of superficial muscles must be reflected first (Fig. 76-2). Begin with the trapezius. Detach each trapezius from the skull, then from the ligamentum nuchae. Next detach each splenus capitis (Fig. 76-2) from the ligamentum nuchae and the thoracic spines. Reflect it as far laterally as possible. Finally, to detach the semispinalis capitis, first identify the spinous process of C2. Then, by blunt dissection with the fingers or blunt-ended, curved scissors between the semispinalis capitis muscles, expose the small muscles attached to the spine of C2. Having partly exposed those small muscles, cut both semispinalis capitis muscles from the skull and pull them inferiorly (i.e., toward the thorax) to expose the small muscles entirely. The semispinalis muscle is much broader and thicker than the student expects; it is a common error not to cut it entirely.

ITEM 76-4. Quickly identify the muscles of each suboccipital triangle (Fig. 76-2). Within each triangle is a meshwork of veins supported in fairly dense fascia. Scratch away the veins and fascia, using horizontal sweeps of the scissors. The horizontal posterior arch of the atlas is easily identified. Superior to it lies the vertebral artery. Boldly clear away tissue to expose as much of the artery as possible. Do so on both sides. Then turn the head of the cadaver from side to side and observe what happens to the vertebral arteries.

Because of the difficulties met with in an embalmed cadaver, dissection of the suboccipital region may give the feeling of venturing into an unexplored wilderness. To correct that impression the student should know that surgical procedures are performed in this region. For example, the posterior arch of the atlas may be bound to the laminae and spine of C2 to stabilize this part of the vertebral column. Again, when an arteriovenous fistula (i.e., a false connection) develops between the vertebral artery and the suboccipital venous plexus it is necessary to ligate the fistula. Thus the anatomy of this small region is not insignificant. Most of the surgical procedures in this region, however, are done through a midline approach, where the ligamentum nuchae provides a relatively bloodless plane of cleavage between the mass of muscle on each side.

ITEM 76-5. Return to the origin of the vertebral artery. Slit open the subclavian artery near the origin of the vertebral artery, and then slit the vertebral artery. Flush out all debris and examine the intima at the orifice of the vertebral artery and nearby. It is known that arterial disease in the vicinity of the orifice of the vertebral artery may be sufficient to reduce blood flow along the rest of the vertebral artery. If the arterial disease is not too extensive it is often removed by one of several operative procedures designed to restore the blood flow through the vertebral artery to an adequate level.

THE EXTERNAL CAROTID ARTERY

The names of the branches of the external carotid artery are self-explanatory. They are the superior thyroid artery, the lingual and facial arteries, the occipital and posterior auricular arteries, and a small ascending pharyngeal artery, and two terminal branches, namely the superficial temporal and the maxillary arteries. These names alone indicate the extensive distribution of the external carotid artery to a large part of the head and neck. The student, however, may not realize that the maxillary artery, whose branches ramify around the maxilla, eventually supplies blood to the teeth of the upper jaw, the hard and soft palates, and the floor of the orbit, as well as to the lateral wall of the nasal cavity and the nasal septum. The blood supply of the nasal cavities is copious.

ITEM 76-6. Grasp the origin of the external carotid artery and pull the artery strongly away from the neck. Keeping the artery under tension, free 1 or 2 cm. of each branch by blunt dissection. There are usually no problems with the superior thyroid, lingual, and facial arteries. The occipital and posterior auricular arteries should be easily found if the posterior belly of the digastric (and the associate stylohyoid) is reflected clear of the dissector's field. The ascending pharyngeal branch is so small that it scarcely deserves attention; if you look for it, it is found medial to the main carotid vessels—between them and the pharynx. Of the two terminal branches, the superficial temporal artery is easily found crossing the zygomatic arch, but the maxillary artery is difficult to locate at the present stage of the dissection. The maxillary artery disappears deep to the ramus of the mandible to reach the maxilla. Deep to the ramus, in a cadaver, the maxillary artery is so often tightly embedded in a dense venous plexus. Time is saved if the demonstration of this artery is left until the ramus of the mandible is removed (p. 366).

The terminations of the branches of the external carotid artery will be encountered when the remaining regions of the head and neck are dissected.

Review

Draw a diagram to show the arterial blood supply of the cerebrum from the arch of the aorta to the circle of Willis (circulus arteriosus). Indicate significant bony landmarks.

Chapter 77

The Thyroid and Parathyroid Glands

Although the thyroid gland and the parathyroids have different functions, they are considered together because of their close anatomic relationship, which must be borne in mind in all surgical procedures on the thyroid gland. Indeed, the glands are so intimately related that, in the last half of the nineteenth century, the findings on experimental removal of the thyroid gland were confusing to the scientists because they were unaware of the significance of the parathyroid glands. Moreover there was a species difference to add to the confusion; what happened in the dog upon total thyroidectomy did not happen in the rabbit. Eventually the anatomic distinction between the thyroid and the parathyroid glands was made, their respective functions established, and ultimately extracts of their secretions were purified. Thyroid hormone is responsible for development and growth in the infant and the regulation of basal metabolism throughout the span of life. Parathyroid hormone plays a significant role in the balance of the calcium and phosphorus content of the entire human frame. The pertinent facts concerning the anatomy of the thyroid gland are dealt with first.

THE THYROID GLAND

In life, although the normal thyroid gland is sometimes visible, especially in a woman's neck, it can scarcely be felt because it is soft. A thyroid gland found to be as firm in a patient as it is in a cadaver would be considered abnormal. Whether or not such a gland should be removed is a decision only an expert can discuss.

The physician stands behind his patient to palpate the thyroid gland (Fig. 77-1) so that he can make use of the most sensitive parts of his fingers, the pulps. When the gland is palpable, "more palpable than usual," the decision he must make, is the gland normal or abnormal, is by no means an easy one, even in the hands of a physician with great experience with the thyroid gland.

The thyroid gland moves with the trachea and larynx on swallowing. Swallowing, therefore, is used clinically to distinguish tumors of the thyroid gland from other swellings in the neck. The findings of this test, like those of other clinical tests, must be interpreted with care, as you will learn from your clinical instructors.

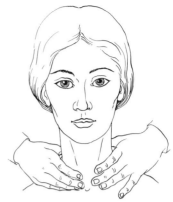

Figure 77-1. Clinical examination of the thyroid gland.

Exercise

Place the tip of a finger on your thyroid cartilage and keep it there while you swallow. What did you observe?

The thyroid gland has two lobes connected by an isthmus. Each lobe tapers from a somewhat rounded, fairly broad inferior pole (another word for "end") to a slender upper pole; its external surface bulges at its broadest part; thus when the thyroid gland is visible in the neck each lobe looks like a small pear, but the deep surface of the gland is not round. It is concave because it is molded to the anterolateral aspect of the trachea.

The isthmus lies anterior to the second, third, and often the fourth ring of the trachea. It is only the upper poles that are related to the thyroid cartilage. Most of the gland lies inferior to the cartilage and is therefore related to the cricoid cartilage and trachea, while the lower poles are close to the thoracic inlet.

Each lobe is related to the larynx and trachea, the pharynx and esophagus, and the carotid sheath enclosing the common carotid artery. On the deep surface of each lobe lie the parathyroid glands. Two pairs of nerves, the recurrent laryngeal and the external laryngeal nerves, are also related to the thyroid gland. These and other anatomic relationships will be seen in the dissection of the gland.

ITEM 77-1. Dissection of the Thyroid Gland

The skin and platysma have already been reflected from the front of the neck, and the investing layer of deep fascia between the anterior borders of the sternomastoid muscles was disrupted when the sternomastoid muscles were reflected. These three layers are taken into consideration in the surgical approach to the thyroid gland. The two sternohyoid muscles, adjacent to the midline, are now fully exposed, and deep to them are the margins of the sternothyroid muscles. Observe on the anterior surfaces of the sternohyoid muscles the anterior jugular veins.

Trace the veins inferiorly to the level of the suprasternal notch where each vein turns laterally deep to the sternomastoid muscle, and, at the same level, is connected medially to its fellow by the jugular arch. In operations on the thyroid gland, the strap muscles are usually retracted to each side, but, sometimes, in order to increase the exposure of the gland in a difficult procedure, the sternohyoid and sternothyroid muscles are cut transversely. Do the same here. Cut the sternohyoid and sternothyroid near their superior attachments and reflect the larger portion of the muscles inferiorly. Do likewise with the omohyoid muscles. The thyroid gland is now exposed.

Examine the isthmus. Where is it located in relation to the rings of the trachea? Is there a pyramidal lobe present? If so, is the pyramidal lobe attached to the hyoid bone?

It is appropriate to consider the anatomy of the isthmus in more detail with reference to an emergency procedure termed tracheostomy, but before that is done it is helpful to distinguish between tracheostomy and tracheotomy. This means distinguishing between two Greek words—*stoma*, meaning mouth, and *tome*, meaning cutting. Tracheostomy is a surgical procedure in which an artificial opening, or "mouth" is made in the wall of the trachea. Tracheotomy is a surgical procedure in which an incision is made to open the trachea.

TRACHEOSTOMY

Most medical students trained in first aid procedures are aware of the absolute necessity of maintaining a clear airway between the upper and the lower regions of the respiratory system. They are aware of the need to keep the tongue out of the throat and to clear all debris from the throat so that air can flow freely in and out of the victim's lungs. Many lives have been saved when such measures have been promptly and adequately performed. However, sometimes in clinical practice, for reasons only a clinician can discuss, it is necessary to make a direct entry into the lower respiratory system in order to maintain an adequate airway. Then an incision is made into the wall of the trachea and a curved silver or plastic tube is inserted to provide a new breathing stoma. While the pros and cons of the various methods of tracheostomy need not be discussed, the basic anatomy can be easily reviewed now. Proceed as follows:

ITEM 77-2.   On your cadaver, identify the thyroid cartilage by placing the tip of an index finger on the Adam's apple. Keeping in the midline, slide the finger inferiorly to cross the circothyroid ligament and the cricoid cartilage. Count the number of rings of the trachea between the cricoid cartilage and the isthmus thyroideae. Cross the isthmus and count the rings of trachea between the isthmus and the thoracic inlet.

Now pull the innominate veins inferiorly and somewhat anteriorly to elevate the inferior thyroid veins. Draining into the innominate veins, they lie on the anterior surface of the trachea inferior to the lower aspect of the thyroid gland. Occasionally an additional artery, the thyroidea ima artery (*ima* means lowest), ascends from the brachiocephalic trunk anterior to the trachea to reach the isthmus of the thyroid gland.

The structures mentioned so far are intimately related to the trachea in the neck. In addition, the skin, the platysma, the investing layer of deep cervical fascia, and the jugular arch connecting the two anterior jugular veins lie anterior to the trachea.

No more need be said except to emphasize the significance of the vascular structures anterior to the trachea. Those structures, scarcely visible in an embalmed cadaver, may be engorged tenfold in a patient requiring tracheostomy.

Return now to the lateral lobes of the thyroid gland and examine them as follows:

ITEM 77-3. Examine each lobe and assess its size and shape.

Examine the surface of the lobe. The surface of the lobe is a fibrous capsule, a true capsule from which fibrous septa divide the lobe into lobules. Numerous blood vessels ramify on the capsule and send many tributaries via the septa into the substance of the lobe. Confirm that each lobe is related posterolaterally to the vertebral triangle. The apex of the triangle, the anterior tubercle of the transverse process of C6, is a useful surgical landmark. Identify the tubercle. Observe that it is necessary to displace the carotid sheath and contents and that on the right side the triangle is crossed by the right recurrent laryngeal nerve and on the left by the thoracic duct. The vertebral artery is located in the triangle.

Each lobe is supplied by two arteries and is drained by three veins. The superior, middle, and inferior thyroid veins have already been identified. Identify the arteries now. Locate the inferior thyroid artery at its origin from the thyrocervical trunk and trace the artery in its course toward the apex of the vertebral triangle. At or near the apex, the artery threads its way through the sympathetic trunk anterior to the vertebral column. Trace the artery through the sympathetic trunk; then observe the relationship of the artery to the recurrent laryngeal nerve lying in the groove between the trachea and the esophagus. The relationship is variable and, in general terms, the nerve may pass anterior to, through the branches of, or posterior to the artery.

Trace the superior thyroid artery to the gland. To demonstrate the relationship of the external laryngeal nerve to the superior thyroid artery and to the thyroid gland, cut the isthmus of the gland, and reflect the lobe laterally. Once the cricothyroid muscle is fully exposed it is easy to find the external laryngeal nerve. Find the nerve. How closely is it related to the superior thyroid artery and to the upper pole of the thyroid lobe? Although they are closely related, the nerve is not in immediate peril when the superior pole of the gland and its vessels are mobilized in surgery; the nerve adheres to the musculocartilaginous plane. Read an account of the thyroid gland.

THE PARATHYROID GLANDS

To give an exact location for these glands is to ignore one of the basic problems of parathyroid surgery, namely locating the parathyroid gland that must be removed. The parathyroid glands occupy variable positions, ranging from the level of the thyroid cartilage to the superior mediastinum, and there may be more than or less than four glands.

Usually there are two parathyroid glands located on the posterior surface of each lobe of the thyroid gland, and they may or may not be within the fascial sheath of the gland. Locating the parathyroids in a cadaver is a frustrating experience. Before even an experienced anatomist pronounces that he has located a parathyroid gland, he should first examine microscopically the tissue he has identified. Today modern methods of clinical investigation, such as the use of angiography and radioactive scanning, have resolved some of the difficulty in locating parathyroid tumors.

To safeguard the parathyroid glands during sugical procedures upon the thyroid, a posterior portion of each lobe of the thyroid is left behind. Sometimes, however, it is necessary to remove the entire thyroid gland. Under those circumstances the inferior parathyroids and their blood supply are left intact. This special procedure demands a very careful surgical technique and a dry operative field.

ITEM 77-4. Dissection of the Parathyroids

Examine the posterior surface of each lobe of the thyroid gland. If you can find an anastomosing artery linking the superior and inferior thyroid arteries you may find a parathyroid gland adjacent to it. Do not delay, but, in moving on, do not underestimate the importance of the parathyroid glands.

The parathyroid glands exert an influence on the calcium and phosphorus metabolism of the human frame far out of proportion to their size. It is indeed difficult to conceive how such small structures, measured in millimeters, and weighing approximately 1 g., can have such a profound effect upon the entire body. But this is not the whole story. There is evidence to prove that thyrocalcitonin, a hormone from the thyroid gland itself, also influences calcium levels. The clinical importance of thyrocalcitonin is not yet clear, but there is sufficient evidence to show that the factors controlling the calcium level in the blood have not yet been finally established.

Chapter 78

Regional Dissections of the Head

Introduction

The remaining series of dissections are, to a marked degree, regional in character. In any regional dissection there is always a danger of becoming involved in detail and overlooking the purpose of the dissection. The danger is very real in this series. Accordingly, detail has been reduced to a minimum so that the purpose of the dissection stands forth. Furthermore, in order to simplify the presentation, a complete write-up of the relationship of a region dissected to surrounding regions and to the rest of the head and neck has been omitted. The alert student will observe these relationships in the course of the dissection and, in his own way, he will build up an image of the total anatomy from a series of fragments.

> To grasp this sorry Scheme of Things entire.
> Would not we shatter it to bits — and then
> Re-mould it nearer to the Heart's Desire.
>
> — Omar Khayyam

The nasal cavities, pharynx, larynx, and ear, regarded by some as special regions, are included in the series. The student who wishes to study their anatomy in greater depth is well advised to consult *Fundamentals of Otolaryngology* by L. B. Boies, J. A. Hilger, and R. E. Priest (1964).

The following is the sequence of dissection:
(1) Posterior pharyngeal wall
(2) Atlantoaxial joint
(3) Nasal cavities
(4) Soft palate
(5) Palatine tonsils
(6) Tongue
(7) Three sensory nerves
(8) Submandibular and sublingual glands
(9) Larynx
(10) Ear

405

THE POSTERIOR PHARYNGEAL WALL

ITEM 78-1. To expose the posterior pharyngeal wall, open up the retropharyngeal space and slip a Gigli saw anterior to the disc between vertebra C2 and C3. With the saw divide the column at that level. Tilt the head anteriorly to separate the pharynx and esophagus from the lower cervical vertebra.

The term pharynx is applied mainly to that part of the digestive tract between the oral cavity and the beginning of the esophagus (Fig. 73-6). The part immediately posterior to the oral cavity is described as the oropharynx; the part proximal to the esophagus is described as the laryngopharynx because it is posterior to the larynx. In addition to these two parts, there is an extension of the pharyngeal cavity superiorly beyond the soft palate. This extension has for a long time been named the nasopharynx because it lies posterior to the lower half of the nasal cavities. However, unlike the main part of the pharynx, the nasopharynx does not transmit nourishment and its walls are immobile, so that an alternate term, epipharynx, has been suggested (Cave, 1961). Nasopharynx is the term used here because it is the term used by the majority of clinicians.

At this stage in the dissection it is of great value to review certain levels that help to orient the position of the pharynx in the mind's eye. The roof of the nasopharynx is level with the baseline of the skull (see Figs. 73-1 and 73-6. Thus when one looks at the face from the front, the roof of the pharynx is visualized as level with the inferior margins of the orbits. The roof of the nasal cavities is higher still; it is level with the superior margins of the orbits. The second important level is of considerable diagnostic significance. The oropharynx is immediately anterior to the body of vertebra C2. Thus, when the mouth is opened, the tongue depressed, and the soft palate elevated to expose the internal aspect of the posterior pharyngeal wall (Fig. 78-1), one should know that the body of C2 lies posteriorly. The third level is also of diagnostic significance. The pharynx ends and the esophagus begins at the level of the cricoid cartilage, which is level with C6 vertebra. The cricoid cartilage is not much more than the breadth of a finger superior to the suprasternal notch. It is a surprise to many students to realize the cricoid cartilage and C6 vertebra are, in fact, in the root of the neck.

The lateral aspect of the pharynx, between the level of the cricoid cartilage and the base of the skull, is related first to the carotid arteries and the internal jugular vein, then to the sternomastoid. To reach the lower end of the pharynx for surgical procedures, the sternomastoid and the major blood vessels are retracted laterally on the appropriate side of the neck.

ITEM 78-2. The posterior aspect of the posterior wall of the pharynx is now exposed in your dissection. The three pairs of muscles

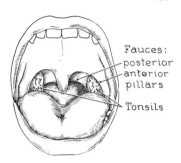

Figure 78-1. Line drawing of a photograph of the tonsils of a male medical student, 20 years old.

that make up the wall, termed the pharyngeal constrictors, are fully illustrated in major anatomic texts. Here we concentrate on the anatomy of the inferior constrictors at the junction of the pharynx and the esophagus, a region commonly called the hypopharynx. Examine an inferior constrictor and observe that it consists of oblique and horizontal fibers. The former are often called thyropharyngeus and the latter cricopharyngeus; both sets of fibers meet their fellows of the opposite side and so create a triangular interval termed a dehiscence. That there are very few muscle fibers covering the dehiscence is one factor in the development, in some persons, of a pouch of mucous membrane whose lumen communicates with the pharynx. The pouch, termed also a pharyngeal diverticulum, may become large enough to extend deep to the sternomastoid to show as a mass in the lower part of the posterior triangle on a level with the cricoid cartilage. The pouch usually increases in size when liquids are swallowed.

Reconstruct the anatomy of the neck as best you can to demonstrate why the sternomastoid and the carotid sheath must be displaced laterally to expose the hypopharynx.

The internal features of the pharynx are seen later.

DIVISION OF THE HEAD

Step 1. At the root of the neck, divide the trachea, esophagus, common carotid arteries, vagus nerves, and internal jugular veins.

Step 2. Make a midline longitudinal slit the length of the posterior pharyngeal wall.

Step 3. With the autopsy saw, divide the mandible at the chin. Do not divide the tongue.

Step 4. Through the pharynx, identify and divide in the midline the soft palate. Then guide a Gigli saw through the wider nasal cavity and out through the oral cavity. Make sure it lies in the cleft you made in the soft palate before you saw through the hard palate.

Step 5. Using a strong saw, divide the rest of the skull and the atlas and the axis. The saw cut must enter the wider nasal cavity.

A good way to divide the head is to use a butcher's bandsaw, if the department of anatomy is equipped with one. The job can be done by the technicians when the students are absent from the laboratory. Using a carefully planned technique, which is obvious when you look at the specimen, it is possible to divide the skull without dividing the tongue.

THE MEDIAN ATLANTOAXIAL JOINT

On the median sagittal section of the head, examine the atlantoaxial joint. Identify first the odontoid, the superior projection of the body of vertebra C2. The odontoid is separated anteriorly from the anterior arch of the atlas vertebra C1 by a synovial cavity, and is separated posteriorly from the transverse ligament by another synovial cavity. Like synovial joints elsewhere in the body, these joints, too, are subject to diseases of synovial joints.

The spinal cord is the most important structure related to the atlantoaxial joint, and the relationship is vital. Life hangs by a thread when the relationship is upset. Nevertheless, fractures of the odontoid are not always fatal.

Exercise

To demonstrate the position of the odontoid in relation to the skull, proceed as follows. Lay a ruler or any straight edge so that it touches the superior margin of the hard palate and the lowermost point in the floor of the posterior cranial fossa. What is the level of the tip of the odontoid in relation to the edge of the ruler? The edge represents one of several lines radiologists draw on a radiograph when displacement of the odontoid is in question. The line is most useful to the beginner in orienting the skull to the column. The tip of the odontoid normally lies below, on, or slightly above the line.

Observe, also, that the odontoid is on the same level as the philtrum, i.e., the central part, of the upper lip. It is possible, therefore, to obtain excellent radiographs of this region through the open mouth (Fig. 78-1).

ITEM 78-3. To expose the transverse ligament, displace the spinal cord, remove the dura, clear away the fat of the extradural space, and expose the membrana tectoria, the expanded and somewhat thickened superior end of the posterior longitudinal ligament. Trace the membrana superiorly to its attachment at the margin of the foramen magnum. Strip off the membrana to expose the transverse ligament. Establish to your own satisfaction that the transverse ligament is attached to the atlas, which is vertebra C1.

At the same time one of the alar ligaments will be exposed. There are two alar ligaments; each one extends superiorly and laterally from the odontoid to the margin of the foramen magnum.

Review

There is a wide range of anomalies common in this region, some of them congenital and others associated with bone-softening disease such as rickets. They may or may not affect the C.N.S. The congenital anomalies range from total fusion of the three skeletal parts, namely the occiput, the atlas and the axis, to persistence of one or more of the embryologic components of one or both these vertebrae. For example, the odontoid may not fuse; on a radiograph, then, it will be seen separated from the body of the second cervical vertebra, the axis.

This small region brings together many disciplines, embryology, anatomy, biochemistry, pathology, preventive medicine, neurology, radiology, and neurosurgery. It is therefore a region that can be studied in depth.

THE NASAL CAVITIES

The two cavities are separated by the nasal septum. The septum is usually deflected to one side so that one nasal cavity is wider than the other. This difference was taken advantage of when the head was sectioned. If all went according to plan, when that was done, an intact nasal septum and an exposed lateral nasal wall are available for examination.

ITEM 78-4. Examine first the "nasal septum" specimen. The nasal cavity opens anteriorly at the nostril. Slit the nostril, pull apart the flaps, and look at the septum. Without slitting the nostril but by using a nasal speculum to spread apart its walls, a doctor can easily examine the anteroinferior region of the septum. One type of recurrent nose bleeding is from a vessel in this region. The vessel can be seen and cauterized.

Examine the choana, which is the posterior nasal aperture. The posterior ends of the inferior and middle conchae (also known as turbinates) can be seen. They can also be seen clinically in a laryngeal mirror skillfully manipulated to reflect their image (see Gardner, Gray, and O'Rahilly, 1963, plate 65B, p. 954).

Then examine the roof of the nasopharynx for the adenoids, a collection of lymphoid tissue known also as the nasopharyngeal tonsil. You will not find them in an elderly cadaver, but the examination will remind you of the existence and the position of the adenoids present in children.

The nasopharynx lies immediately posterior to the nasal cavities, and the dominant feature of the side wall of the nasopharynx is the opening of the pharyngotympanic tube. Bartolomeus Eustachius, an

Italian professor of anatomy, described the tube and its connection with the ear in 1563; today the need to open the eustachian tube by forceful swallowing or yawning is well known to scuba divers.

Next slide a probe posteriorly on the floor of the nasal cavity. Observe how the tip of the probe reaches the pharyngeal orifice of the eustachian tube without your altering the general direction of the probe. Measure the distance between the margin of the nostril and the orifice. What is it in your specimen? By inserting a eustachian catheter in much the same way as you have inserted a probe, a clinician can blow air into the pharyngotympanic tube, thence to the middle ear, for diagnostic or therapeutic purposes.

The next exercise is locating the site of the sphenopalatine foramen, an important landmark in the posterior region of the nasal cavity. The foramen is a focal point for several nerves, which are composed of both sensory and autonomic nerve fibers to the major part of the mucous membrane of the nasal cavity. Like focal points elsewhere in the body, this one is a site for anesthesia. The sphenopalatine foramen, however, cannot be seen because it is deep to mucous membrane and the nerves and vessels passing through the foramen proceed in the submucosa to their destinations. The anesthetic, therefore, is applied to the mucous membrane and reaches the nerves by absorption. This is an example of topical anesthesia.

Identify the posterior end of the middle concha. Posterosuperior to the end, and deep to the mucous membrane, the sphenopalatine foramen is located. Strip off sufficient mucous membrane to expose the foramen. Insert a probe through the nostril and direct the tip to the foramen. Measure the distance between it and the margin of the nostril. Clinically, when necessary, a pledget of wool soaked in an anesthetic agent and a small amount of adrenalin is applied to this location; the success of the procedure depends to a large extent on an accurate visualization of the distance involved. Why use adrenalin?

What is meant by a submucous resection is easily demonstrated on the exposed aspect of the nasal septum of your specimen. Make an incision into the mucous membrane of the septum. Insert the end of curved scissors into the plane between the mucous membrane and the skeleton of the septum, and by blunt dissection elevate the mucous membrane. Similarly, an otolaryngologist can separate mucous membrane from both sides of the septum in order to resect all or part of its skeleton.

ITEM 78-5. Examine the lateral wall of the nasal cavity as seen on the other half of the head, Identify the superior, middle, and inferior conchae; inferior to each concha identify the corresponding cleft or meatus. Confirm the position of the orifice of the pharyngotympanic tube and the location of the sphenopalatine foramen in relation to the inferior meatus and the middle concha.

The Paranasal Air Sinuses

The nasal cavities lie in the shelter of an extensive irregularly formed arch of air sinuses of varying size and shape (Fig. 69-1). Each pillar of the arch is made up of the solitary maxillary sinus inferiorly and a cluster of ethmoidal air sinuses superiorly. The sphenoidal air sinuses complete the arch superiorly. From each curve of the arch a frontal sinus extends superiorly and laterally. The sinuses separate the nasal cavities from regions of major importance such as the orbits, the anterior cranial fossa, and the sella turcica. All the air sinuses open into the nasal cavities, as you will now see. Begin with the sphenoidal air sinuses.

ITEM 78-6. Dissection of the Paranasal Air Sinuses

Inspect the sphenoidal air sinuses and confirm that they are separated from each other by a septum and that each sinus opens into a part of the nasal cavity, superior to the superior concha, known as the sphenoethmoidal recess.

The ethmoidal air sinuses are lateral to the superior concha, the middle concha, and the intervening superior meatus. These sinuses usually have three openings into the nasal cavity in the location just described, but the openings are not always easily located in a cadaver.

The frontal air sinus opens into a narrow funnel, the infundibulum. To find the infundibulum trace the free border of the middle concha superiorly to its termination. At that point slip the tip of a probe lateral to the concha and into the infundibulum. In a cadaver it is usually possible to demonstrate that the frontal air sinus and the infundibulum are continuous through a fairly narrow opening. Establish the size of each frontal sinus.

Cut off the middle concha at its root to expose fully the middle meatus. Observe the ethmoidal bulla, a bulge very characteristic of the middle meatus. The bulla is merely one of the ethmoidal air cells larger than the others and projecting toward the nasal cavity. To establish the level of the ethmoidal air cells in relation to the orbit, place the tip of a finger or a probe on the ethmoid bulla, then look at the orbit from the front.

The gutter anteroinferior to the ethmoid bulla is termed the hiatus semilunaris. The sharp edge forming the anteroinferior boundary of the hiatus is termed the uncinate process. Observe how the floor of the infundibulum continues into the hiatus.

The opening of the maxillary sinus is located in the hiatus. It is important to know that the opening of the maxillary sinus is at a higher level than the floor. Accordingly, with the aid of bone forceps, break through the external wall of the maxillary sinus sufficiently to be able to compare the level of the floor of the sinus with the level of the opening. At the same time observe the proximity of the roots of the teeth of the upper jaw to the sinus. The mucous membrane of the sinus is delicate and may be overlooked in the dissection.

Finally cut off the inferior concha to uncover the inferior meatus. At the anterior end of the meatus look for the nasal end of the nasolacrimal duct. The importance of the nasolacrimal duct, especially in infants, was described on p. 347.

Then, at the level of the floor of the nasal cavity thrust a probe into the maxillary sinus. Clinically the same maneuver, with more careful technique, is used to admit a cannula into the sinus for a therapeutic measure termed antral washout (antrum is another name for the maxillary sinus).

Mucous Membrane

The mucous membrane of the paranasal sinuses is quite delicate, in marked contrast to the thick membrane upon the conchae (also known as the turbinates). The latter membrane has a substantial submucous layer as well as well-developed vascularity—it includes venous sinuses of considerable size. Between these two varieties of mucous membrane is an intermediate variety, found upon the nasal septum and the walls of the meatuses. All three varieties are parts of one continuous surface, coated, in life, with a blanket of mucus. The mucus has special bacteriocidal properties and is constantly on the move because of the action of the cilia, which are so characteristic of respiratory epithelium.

The exquisite sensitivity of the normal nasal mucosa is well known and its profuse vascularity is often demonstrated.

THE SOFT PALATE

When the mouth is closed and the teeth are together, the soft palate and the tongue are in apposition, closing off the nasal airway from the oral cavity. As a result of the closure one can chew food and breathe at the same time. Then, during swallowing, the soft palate is elevated to close off the nasopharyngeal isthmus and open up the oropharyngeal isthmus. At the same time the posterior pharyngeal wall moves forward as peristalsis begins (Calnan, 1957).

During speech, however, there is little or no movement of the pharyngeal wall while the soft palate is elevated to a higher level to completely close the nasopharyngeal isthmus, but not for all sounds. For example, the sound "ng" as in "kissing" is nasal and is effected by an escape of air into the nasal cavities.

The two muscles solely responsible for elevation of the soft palate are the right and left levator palati. They are to be examined now.

ITEM 78-7. Dissection of the Soft Palate

Examine the orifice of the pharyngotympanic tube. In the floor of the orifice there is usually an elongated bulge to be seen. Without digging deep, strip off the mucous membrane from the bulge to expose the underlying levator palati muscle. Continue to strip off the mucous membrane and expose as much of the muscle as possible.

To demonstrate the action of the muscle pull it laterally, posteriorly, and superiorly, i.e., in the direction of its fibers; it is certain that you will observe the muscle elevating, first, the intermediate third of the palate, and second, the anterior third, while the posterior third, including the uvula, remains suspended (Fig. 78-2). To demonstrate what happens during swallowing, push the entire posterior pharyngeal wall anteriorly while you pull the levator palati in the direction specified. Remember that during speech, in contrast to what happens in swallowing, there is little or no anterior movement of the pharyngeal wall.

It is appropriate now to stress the importance of the adenoid pad in the normal closing of the nasopharyngeal isthmus during speech. Figure 78-2, adapted from Calnan (1957), shows the adenoid pad in a normal female, aged six. Calnan discussed (in 1959) the occurrence of nasal speech following removal of the adenoids. It is clear that the removal of the adenoids in children is a serious decision governed by the health of the child on the one hand and the possibility of nasal speech on the other. As the years advance the adenoids shrink; nasal speech develops if the depth of the pharynx becomes greater than the length of the soft palate.

ITEM 78-8. Dissection of the Tensor Palati Muscle

The soft palate is also controlled by the right and left tensor palati. It is easier to understand this fascinating little muscle by seeing it in a dissection than by reading a description.

Use the infratemporal fossa that has been dissected and, with a sharp tap with a mallet and chisel, crack the lateral pterygoid plate. Remove the plate and with it the superior half of the medial pterygoid

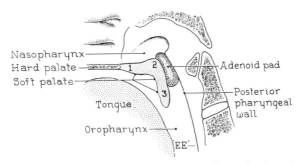

Figure 78-2. This is a reproduction of an actual radiograph taken when the sound ("EE") was being uttered. It shows that during oral speech, in contrast to nasal speech, the intermediate third of the soft palate is hoisted by the right and left levator palati muscles to meet the adenoid pad. (Courtesy of Professor Calnan.)

muscle. The lateral aspect of the tensor palati is exposed. Its muscle fibers taper rapidly to form a very small tendon that turns medially inferior to the hamulus and into the palate, where it joins the palatine aponeurosis. It is most helpful to make sure the tendon is slack as it passes inferior to the hamulus. Then pull the tendon laterally and observe the result. Together the tensor palati muscles tighten the soft palate but only when the soft palate is intact. When the palate is cleft each muscle pulls its half of the palate to its own side. Sometimes in the surgical treatment of cleft palate, both pterygoid hamuli are fractured to reduce the effectiveness of the tensor palati.

THE PALATINE TONSILS

Each palatine tonsil (Fig. 78-1) is a mass of lymphoid tissue located between the palatoglossal fold anteriorly and the palatopharyngeal fold posteriorly. Because the palatoglossal fold serves as the boundary between the oral cavity and the oropharynx, the palatine tonsil, in theory, lies in the sidewall of the oropharynx. The tonsil extends superiorly to the soft palate and inferiorly to lie lateral to the pharyngeal part of the tongue. In the age group to which the majority of cadavers belong, the tonsils are usually absent or atrophied. Therefore study Figure 78-1 with care. The arches referred to are often spoken of as the pillars of the fauces (fauces means throat), and the site of the tonsil as the tonsil bed or tonsillar sinus.

The pharyngeal surface, i.e., the medial surface, of the tonsil is uneven and is studded with several orifices, each orifice leading into a tonsillar crypt. An additional feature is the intratonsillar cleft, which extends quite deeply into the substance of the tonsil.

The lateral surface of the tonsil is related to a sheet of fascia termed the capsule of the tonsil, an erroneous term because the capsule does not completely surround the tonsil. The other deep relations of the tonsil, the exact anatomy of the arteries and veins of the tonsil, and the precise attachments of the tonsil are extremely important to the surgeon but they need not be reviewed here. All clinicians, however, must be familiar with the lymph drainage of the tonsil because acute tonsillitis is such a common ailment. It is accompanied by swollen lymph nodes in the deep cervical chain. The jugulodigastric node is the one most commonly affected; the node is palpable just posterior to the angle of the jaw.

Exercise

Use the half of the head in which the infratemporal fossa is undissected. Locate the bed of the tonsil and establish its position with reference to the angle of the jaw. Then replace the internal jugular vein and the posterior belly of the digastric muscle so that you can establish the position of the jugulodigastric lymph node.

At some convenient time, with the aid of a good light and a mirror examine your own fauces and palatine tonsils, if the tonsils are still present. Identify the tonsillar cleft.

THE TONGUE

The position of the tongue is easily misconceived by examining the tongue in a cadaver, by browsing over anatomic illustrations drawn from a cadaver, and by reading that the tongue lies in the floor of the mouth. Therefore, first of all, establish the position of the tongue in yourself by observing where the tip of the tongue lies when the mouth is closed and the teeth together. You will agree that the tip rests against the posterior surface of the upper incisor teeth and that the forepart of the tongue abuts the forepart of the hard palate. In the living, then, the tongue rises from the floor to reach the roof of the oral cavity and lies, really, in the attic. The close relationship of the tongue to the upper incisor teeth is revealed in its worst form in tongue thrust, a childhood orthodontic problem in which the upper incisor teeth become displaced by repeated powerful forward movements of the tongue during growth.

Posteriorly the tongue and the uvula of the soft palate are in contact. Indeed, in some individuals, the uvula may be long enough to touch the epiglottis. It is only when the mouth is opened and "ah" is said that the uvula and the tongue are apart. Even then it may be necessary to push the tongue down with a tongue depressor to see the oropharyngeal isthmus and the oropharynx properly.

The proximity of the tongue to the hard and soft palates is in keeping with the embryologic development of the tongue. The tongue begins to develop in a region destined to separate into the two nasal cavities and, as development proceeds, the tongue descends into the oral cavity, which is then separated from the nasal cavities by the development of the hard and soft palates. In severe forms of cleft palate the tongue intrudes into the nasal region.

For descriptive purposes the surface of the tongue, also known as the dorsum, is divided into thirds. The anterior two-thirds are horizontal; directed toward the hard palate, this portion is usually called the palatine surface. It is the part seen when the mouth is open. The posterior third is oblique; directed posterosuperiorly toward the pharynx it is usually called the pharyngeal surface. The sulcus terminalis indicates the junction of the anterior two-thirds and the posterior third.

ITEM 78-9. Dissection of the Tongue

Examine the tongue of the cadaver. Notice how it is poised over the larynx. Then identify the anterior two-thirds and the posterior one-third of the dorsum of the tongue. Examine particularly carefully the posterior third because it is out of sight in most people, even when the mouth is wide open and the tongue well forward. Identify the glossoepiglottic fold, a median fold of mucous membrane between the tongue and the epiglottis, separating the right and left valleculae. Then observe how this region of the tongue is studded with irregular masses of lymphoid tissue, known collectively as the lingual tonsil. Sometimes, as a result of an error in development, thyroid tissue may also be found in this location. Finally, at the sulcus terminalis identify the 10 or 12 vallate papillae, and the foramen cecum, a tiny pit indicative of the site at which the thyroid gland originally developed.

To examine the mucous membrane of the anterior two-thirds of the dorsum of the tongue, use a mirror and inspect your own tongue. The roughness that can be seen and felt is due to the presence of many thousands of filiform papillae (*filum* means thread) partially embedded in a layer of white desquamated cells. Scattered sparsely throughout the filiform papillae are very small red spots, fungiform papillae, red because they are vascular and fungiform because they are shaped rather like mushrooms. Thrust the tongue out and direct the tip toward the nose. This maneuver throws the frenulum into relief and shows clearly the fold of mucous membrane between the undersurface of the tongue and the floor of the mouth.

Observe the dark blue vein on each side of the frenulum. This vein ultimately joins with other veins to form the lingual vein you have already identified. To feel the pulsations of the right lingual artery grasp the right side of your tongue between the left index finger and thumb. Nip the tongue until you feel the pulsations of the lingual artery.

ITEM 78-10.   On the cadaver, in the carotid triangle identify the lingual vein and the lingual artery. Identify also the hypoglossal nerve going to the muscles, not the mucous membrane, of one half of the tongue. The sensory innervation of the tongue is dealt with in the next section.

The Lymphatic Drainage of the Tongue

It is not generally realized by junior medical students that muscles have lymphatic drainage and that the volume of lymph is related to muscular activity. Experimentally, in dogs, it has been shown that the flow of lymph from a hind limb is very slight when the limb is at rest and considerable in amount when the limb is exercised. The human heart has a rich lymphatic drainage and so does the human tongue.

Read an account of the lymphatic drainage of the tongue, for it is very significant in the assessment and therapy of a cancer of the mucous membrane of the tongue.

The Tongue and the Airway

Although the tongue is firm in life, it is also very flexible, so in most people the tip of the tongue can examine the exposed surfaces of each tooth. The contortions the tongue can perform are possible because of its substance, entirely muscle. Although this has obvious advantages, it is a marked disadvantage, indeed a hazard, in an unconscious person, for the tongue is transformed into a mass of relaxed muscle that can so easily flop into the oropharynx and block the airway.

The tongue is moored to the mandible. Pulling the mandible forward brings the tongue forward, but this maneuver may not necessarily clear the airway because the relaxed tongue can adopt some very unusual positions. In every unconscious person, therefore, it is vital to establish where the tongue is before resuscitation is begun.

THE LINGUAL, GLOSSOPHARYNGEAL, AND INTERNAL LARYNGEAL NERVES

ITEM 78-11. On the half of the head in which the infratemporal fossa has *not* been dissected, peel off the mucous membrane at the junction of the alveolar margin and the ramus of the mandible. Careful blunt dissection posteroinferiorly will bring the lingual nerve to light. In the living, the nerve can actually be felt as a linear bulge deep to the mucous membrane, 1 to 2 cm. posteroinferior to the site of the last molar tooth.

Then, on the other half of the head identify the lingual nerve in the same location and in the infratemporal fossa. Observe that the nerve is external to the pharyngeal wall in the infratemporal fossa. Thus the nerve penetrates the pharyngeal wall to reach the oral cavity.

Carefully incise the mucous membrane of the floor of the mouth parallel to the mandible. Reflect the mucous membrane to expose the lingual nerve. Trace the nerve under the submandibular duct (Fig. 78-3) as far as the tongue.

The lingual nerves supply the mucous membrane of the anterior two-thirds of the dorsum of the tongue, the floor of the mouth, and the gums. Both the chorda tympani—in the oral cavity the fibers of the chorda tympani are incorporated in the lingual nerves—are the nerves of taste to the anterior two-thirds of tongue.

ITEM 78-12. To expose the glossopharyngeal nerve, expose fully the external aspect of the sidewall of the pharynx in order to see the stylopharyngeus muscle, upon which the glossopharyngeal nerve descends to the level of the tonsil bed. Elevate and free the nerve by gentle dissection and trace it to where it disappears through the pharyngeal wall.

From the pharyngeal aspect of the tonsil bed, strip away mucous membrane and fascia to expose the glossopharyngeal nerve. By now the nerve is dividing into branches to the tonsil bed, the mucous membrane of the fauces, and the pharynx as well as to the posterior third of the tongue.

The glossopharyngeal nerves are essentially somatic sensory nerves subserving the sensations pain, temperature, and touch, but they also transmit fibers concerned with taste, not only from the taste buds of the vallate papillae but from taste buds scattered throughout the region of the oropharyngeal isthmus.

ITEM 78-13. The internal laryngeal nerve has already been identified passing through the thyrohyoid membrane. Examine now the piriform fossa, an anterior extension of the pharynx on each side of the inlet of the larynx. Reflect the mucous membrane of the fossa to expose the internal laryngeal nerve. The nerve is dividing into its terminal branches and has quite an extensive distribution to the epiglottis and the vestibule of the larynx as far as the vocal cords.

Both internal laryngeal nerves are sensory to a particularly sensitive region, namely the entrance to the airway. Each nerve may be anesthetized before it pierces the thyrohyoid membrane or by an anesthetic agent introduced into the piriform fossa.

THE SUBMANDIBULAR SALIVARY GLANDS AND LYMPH NODES

Each submandibular salivary gland has a deep part lying deep to the mucous membrane forming the floor of the mouth and a superficial part covered by skin, platysma, and deep fascia between the angle and tip of the jaw. Both parts join at the posterior border of the mylohyoid muscle (Fig. 78-3).

ITEM 78-14. Reflect the mucous membrane from one side of the floor of the mouth to expose the submandibular duct. Trace the duct posteriorly to the deep part of the gland. Identify the posterior border of the mylohyoid muscle.

To expose the superficial part of the submandibular gland and associated lymph nodes in a surgical procedure, it is necessary to incise the skin, platysma, and deep fascia. In your present dissection these layers have been removed. If not, remove what remains to expose the inferolateral surface of the submandibular gland and look for lymph nodes embedded in its substance.

Establish the continuity of the deep and superficial parts of the gland at the posterior border of the mylohyoid muscle.

Now trace the submandibular duct anteriorly and locate its orifice lateral to the frenulum.

The sublingual gland is another salivary gland lying between the

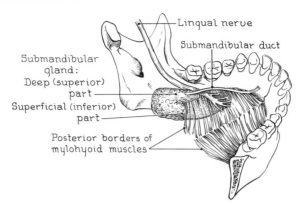

Figure 78-3. The two mylohyoid muscles form a muscular diaphragm, as shown here. Very little of each mylohyoid muscle is attached to the hyoid bone. Each submandibular gland is cleft by the posterior border of the mylohyoid muscle.

submandibular duct and the internal aspect of the mandible. The gland is immediately deep to a feature of the mucous membrane of the mouth, the sublingual fold, on which the numerous small sublingual ducts have their openings.

Finally, on your specimen, "examine" the floor of the mouth by placing the tip of the index finger of the right hand in the oral cavity (Fig. 78-4) and support the soft tissues from below with the fingers of your other hand.

Press your hands gently together and palpate the sublingual gland, the submandibular duct, and the deep and superficial parts of the submandibular gland.

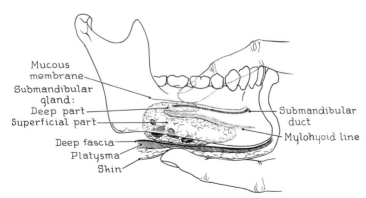

Figure 78-4. Clinically, the floor of the mouth, including the submandibular gland, is examined bimanually. In this way the soft tissues can be "held" so that the site, size, shape, substance, surface, and other features of a tumor can be established.

Exercise

At some convenient time, inspect the floor of the mouth of your colleague and identify the frenulum, orifice, and duct of both submandibular glands and, in addition, both sublingual glands and sublingual folds. Also palpate those structures bimanually, as described above.

THE VOICE

Introduction

Mankind is so accustomed to the sound of the human voice that it is not surprising that many junior medical students are completely unaware of the significance of the voice in medicine. They have yet to see how the astute clinician gleans considerable information about his patient by listening to the voice. From now on, therefore, the student must regard the voice, invisible though it is, as an integral part of clinical anatomy.

In listening to a patient the student must distinguish between the voice and speech. Is there a distinction? Yes, there is. The voice is sound produced by a movement of air through the larynx, pharynx, and oral and nasal cavities. Speech, on the other hand, puts thoughts into words and is, therefore, a function of the brain. In speech, sounds are marshalled to make sense. Without certain parts of the brain, speech becomes garbled or is lost altogether, yet the larynx is perfectly normal. Furthermore, at birth the larynx may be perfectly normal while hearing is imperfect or absent. Thereafter speech will not develop without special training.

The distinction between speech and sound explains why surgical removal of the larynx does not rob the individual of the power of speech; the power remains and speech can be restored with proper training. This type of speech is termed esophageal speech because air is "swallowed" and regurgitated across the tissues at the superior end of the esophagus; once the surgeon has removed the larynx he refashions these tissues to substitute, to some extent, for the larynx. Although this is a subject of great interest and deserving further commentary, sufficient has been said to show why the clinician who has detected an abnormality as he listens to his patient must distinguish between the function of the brain and the function of the larynx as he seeks the cause of the disorder.

The anatomy of the larynx is basically the same as anatomy elsewhere in the body. The larynx has a skeleton consisting of supporting parts, linked at joints and moved by muscles. Fascia, both well-defined and ill-defined, is present in the larynx, but the larynx is covered by mucous membrane instead of skin. Nerves, lymphatic vessels, and blood vessels are present also, and the first two groups are of considerable significance in the larynx. To understand the shape of the mucous membrane it is necessary to know the shape of the skeleton (Fig. 78-5).

The cricoid cartilage is the key cartilage (Fig. 78-5*A*), for it supports the two arytenoid cartilages and the thyroid cartilage (Fig. 78-5*B*, *C*, *E*). The cricoarytenoid and the cricothyroid articulations are synovial; thus it is possible for the arytenoid cartilages to swivel and slide on the summit of the lamina of the cricoid and for the thyroid cartilage to do likewise where its inferior cornu meet the cricoid.

On each side there is a cricothyroid ligament, also known as the cricovocal membrane (Fig. 78-5*G*) attached to the cricoid, thyroid, and arytenoid cartilages. The free edge of the membrane is the core of the

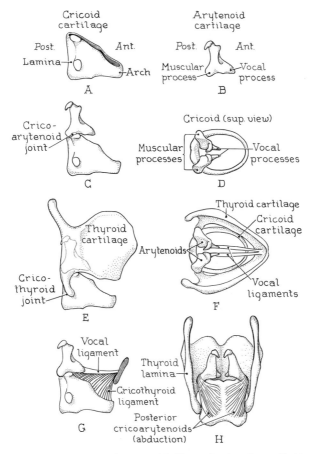

Figure 78-5. Structure of the larynx. This illustration is to be studied in conjunction with the text.

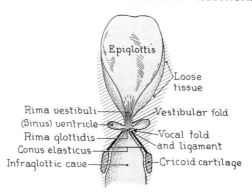

Figure 78-6. A coronal section of the larynx.

vocal cord (Fig. 78-5*F*). Thus adjustments in the relative positions of the three cartilages alter the position and tension of the vocal cord. For example, while the other muscles of the larynx stabilize the cartilages, the posterior cricoarytenoid muscles swivel the arytenoids (Fig. 78-5*H*) to separate the vocal cords. This action is discussed in more detail later.

The right and left cricovocal ligaments form a cone as they slant superiorly and medially (Fig. 78-6). Hence they form the conus elasticus.

Clinical Examination of the Larynx

Direct laryngoscopy, in which the laryngologist looks directly at the larynx with the aid of an instrument, is employed when it is necessary to scrutinize the larynx. Because of the powerful reflexes of the pharynx and larynx, some form of anesthesia is necessary to give the laryngologist optimal conditions to examine with care the distal as well as the proximal parts of the larynx.

Indirect laryngoscopy, in which the doctor looks at the reflection of the larynx in a mirror (see Gardner, Gray, and O'Rahilly, 1963, plate 65) is a technique easily acquired with practice. With it the doctor obtains a brief but sufficient view of the larynx to establish the presence or absence of an obvious abnormality as well as the range of movement in each vocal cord.

Examination of the Cadaveric Larynx

ITEM 78-15. The fossae around the inlet to the larynx, namely the piriform fossae and the valleculae, have already been identified. Proceed now to examine the inlet to the larynx. Identify the epiglottis. Then, on each side of the inlet, identify and grasp the aryepiglottic fold. Grasp the fold between finger and thumb, and observe that it is quite soft and slack, for it contains mostly muscle, some supporting fascia, and a tiny piece of cartilage, the cuneiform cartilage. Slide the finger and thumb posteriorly until they grasp the arytenoid cartilage (for accuracy one should explain that the apex of the arytenoid is a separate little cartilage, the corniculate cartilage, but this cartilage is rarely named). Grasp each arytenoid and gently pull each one laterally to reveal the interarytenoid fold. Thus the inlet of the larynx is bounded by the aryepiglottic folds, which incorporate the corniculate and cuneiform cartilages, the superior margin of the epiglottis, and the interarytenoid fold.

ITEM 78-16.   The vestibule of the larynx is the cavity between the inlet and the vestibular folds (Fig. 78-6). Explore the cavity with the tip of an index finger. Peer down through the vestibule and identify the vestibular folds.

Inferior to the vestibular folds identify the vocal folds. They may be hidden from view if they are widely separated.

The larynx is also known as the glottis, which explains why the gap between the vocal cords is often called the rima glottidis. In adults, the rima is the narrowest part between the laryngeal inlet and the beginning of the bronchi. The student may not appreciate the practical significance of "narrowest" parts: the size of an instrument to be passed through a hollow system is determined by the caliber of the narrowest part of the system.

However in children and especially in infants, the narrowest part of the larynx may be at the level of the cricoid cartilage, which is inferior to the vocal cords. Thus an endotracheal tube that passes through the gap between the vocal cords may fail to pass through the cricoid, so a smaller tube must be used. In addition to this major difference, the child's larynx is more superior than the adult's, and the epiglottis is longer and more prominent.

The anterior region of the rima glottidis where the vocal cords come together is termed the anterior commissure. On each side of the larynx there is a cavity called the sinus of the larynx, which is inferior to the vestibular fold and superior to the vocal fold (Fig. 78-6). The sinus is also called the ventricle.

The saccule of the larynx is a blind-ended narrow tube that opens into the anterior end of the sinus. It is rarely found in a cadaver. It becomes significant, clinically, if it increases in size and bulges into the neck when the air pressure in the glottis is raised. Then it is known as a laryngocele.

All these features of the larynx can be examined more closely when the larynx is divided.

The Musculature of the Larynx

There are numerous muscles in the larynx, named according to the cartilages they link together, e.g., the cricoarytenoid muscle and the cri-

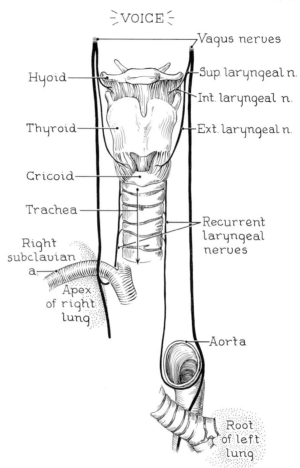

Figure 78-7.   A scheme of the nerve supply of the larynx.

cothyroid muscle. The novice, inclined to spend time learning the names of all of the muscles of the larynx and their precise attachments, may overlook a general principle that serves as a basis for clinical decisions. Accordingly the principle alone is emphasized here. The student who wishes to study the muscles in greater detail must consult a larger text.

The muscles of the larynx form three functional groups. The first group includes muscles with a sphincteric action to shut down the entrance to the airway as a protective measure. This group includes the muscle fibers within the aryepiglottic folds. They bring together the arytenoids and the epiglottis. The second group includes muscles bringing the vocal cords closer to each other with precision in the production of sound. Each vocal cord is brought toward the midline, therefore this group is referred to as the adductor group. The third group is an abductor group and refers especially to the paired posterior cricoarytenoid muscles. It must be stressed that the paired posterior cricoarytenoid muscles are the only muscles responsible for abduction of the vocal cords. Accordingly, paralysis of one cricoarytenoid muscle is serious and paralysis of both is grave.

It is a curious fact that each recurrent laryngeal nerve supplies both the adductors and the sole abductor of one vocal cord. It is even more curious that when the recurrent laryngeal nerve is becoming involved in the growth of a cancer the first muscle to weaken is usually the abductor, the posterior cricoarytenoid.

The nerve supply of the larynx is illustrated in Figure 78-7.

The Submucous Tissue of the Larynx

ITEM 78-17. Make a median sagittal section through the tongue, hyoid bone, thyroid, epiglottis, cricoid cartilages, and trachea. Now that the internal aspect of the larynx is fully exposed, identify the inlet, the vestibule, the vestibular fold, the sinus, and the vocal fold. Observe how the rima glottidis may be divided into a large anterior part between the anatomic cords and a much smaller part between the medial borders of the bases of the arytenoids. Identify now the vocal process. Observe the shape of the infraglottic space.

On one side make a longitudinal incision the length of the vestibular fold and reflect the edges sufficiently to expose the underlying sub-mucous layer. This layer is demonstrable throughout the vestibule, but at the level of the vocal cords the submucous layer disappears and the mucous layer becomes firmly adherent to the cricovocal ligament and the cricoid and tracheal cartilages.

In the larynx the existence of a loosely woven submucous layer down to the level of the vocal cords determines the extent of edema, which is the accumulation of excessive fluid in tissues. Edema of the larynx is usually due to infection of the mucous membrane, to irritation by obnoxious fumes, or even to trauma, and may be severe enough to close the vestibule. Under those circumstances the doctor faces a grave medical emergency. Briefly, how would you deal with the emergency?

Continue to strip off mucous membrane to expose the abductor, the posterior cricoarytenoid muscle, an adductor, the lateral cricoarytenoid muscle, and a sphincter, the aryepiglotticus.

Review

Read an account of the laryngeal nerves (Fig. 78-7) and of the lymphatic drainage of the larynx. Also, this is an appropriate time to review the anatomy of the entire respiratory system, including its upper and lower parts.

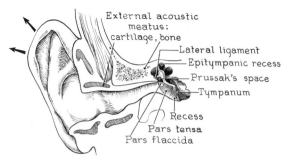

Figure 78-8. The anterior wall of the external ear and of the middle ear were removed in this dissection to show the position of the tympanic membrane in the adult. The arrows indicate the direction to pull the auricle to straighten the meatus.

THE EAR

The ear has three parts, external, middle, and internal. The external ear consists of the auricle (the part called the ear by the layman) and a tunnel called the external acoustic meatus (Fig. 78-8) that ends at the tympanic membrane. Both the membrane and the meatus are so frequently examined by the doctor that they warrant first consideration by the student. However, to understand easily certain very important features of the membrane it is advisable to look at the middle ear first. In doing so a brief explanation of certain relevant aspects of the anatomy of the internal ear will be included.

Dissection of the Middle Ear

The middle ear is also called the tympanum (adjective, tympanic). Unlike the timpano of a symphony orchestra, the human tympanum has

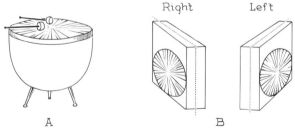

Figure 78-9. Tympanum is another name for the middle ear. Unlike *A*, the timpano of an orchestra, the human tympanum has six sides and is irregular in shape, and its tympanic membrane is off center. Furthermore the human tympanum lies on its side.

For descriptive purposes, however, it is useful to conceive the middle ear as a six-sided box. The dotted lines in *B* indicate the second saw cut in the dissection dividing the box into two parts.

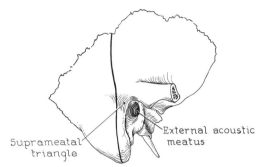

Figure 78-10. The black line indicates the saw cut to expose the tympanic antrum deep to the suprameatal triangle.

six sides (Fig. 78-9). Accordingly it is frequently described as box-shaped, but the shape is not regular, the sides are not parallel, and some of the sides have openings.

There are two stages to the dissection of the middle ear: the first exposes the tympanic antrum; the second divides the tympanum in half.

Stage One. The tympanic antrum is a mastoid air cell, usually larger than the others; it communicates by an opening called the aditus ad antrum (opening to the antrum) with the superior region of the middle ear, a region called the epitympanic recess (*epi* means above) or the attic.

ITEM 78-18. In the adult the antrum is 15 mm. medial to the suprameatal triangle, which is a depression on the skull posterosuperior to the attachment of the cartilaginous part of the external acoustic meatus to the skull. The depression is easily felt in the living and easily identified on a skull (Fig. 78-10). Identify it on the cadaver. Incise the soft tissues along the line shown in Figure 78-10; make sure the tissues

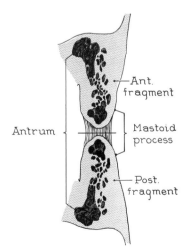

Figure 78-11. The two fragments obtained after the saw cut referred to in Figure 78-10.

are cut to the bone, otherwise the autopsy saw will not work well. Then cut medially into the skull at the line (Fig. 78-10) until the bone separates into an anterior and posterior fragment (Fig. 78-11).

Examine the specimen carefully, then proceed cautiously with the next instruction if the antrum is not revealed; sometimes the antrum is absent from birth or it becomes obliterated by disease. If the antrum is not immediately exposed another sawcut, a millimeter or so anterior to the first cut, is required. Examine the antrum.

The aditus ad antrum can be observed by peering anteriorly from the antrum.

In the infant the antrum is only 2 mm. from the external surface of the skull. The suprameatal triangle is poorly defined. Furthermore, the antrum is superior to the external acoustic meatus.

Stage Two. Under a good overhead light, peer forward through the aditus ad antrum. By placing the tip of an index finger on and off the roof of the aditus, observe how translucent the floor of the middle cranial fossa is in this region. This translucent portion, which is the roof of the middle ear and of the antrum, is called the tegmen tympani (tegmen means roof). Be sure you identify the tegmen correctly before you proceed. It is only 15 to 20 mm. long and a few millimeters wide. The novice must realize that the translucent tegmen is all that separates the mucous membrane of the middle ear from the dura mater, the arachnoid, the cerebrospinal fluid in the subarachnoid space, and the temporal lobe of the brain, in which the optic radiation is located; middle ear infections sometimes spread into these adjacent structures.

ITEM 78-19. With forceps, carefully nibble away the tegmen until first the aditus ad antrum, then the middle ear is exposed. Examine the middle ear (with a dissecting microscope if possible) and identify the head of the malleus (Fig. 78-12) articulating with the body of the incus. With fine pointed forceps remove the incus. It is into the narrow space between the malleus and the stapes that the blade of the autopsy saw descends for the next cut.

In making the next cut, the blade of the saw must be tilted to lie parallel to the tympanic membrane, which cannot be seen clearly at the present stage of the dissection, but the malleus, attached to the internal

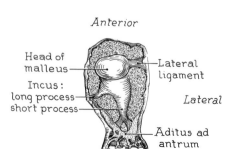

Anterior

Head of malleus
Incus:
long process
short process

Lateral ligament

Lateral

Aditus ad antrum

Figure 78-12. Looking down on the middle ear after the tegmen, or roof, of the middle ear has been nibbled away. The long process of the incus articulates with the stapes. The illustration is greatly magnified; the length of the body of the incus is normally 3 mm.

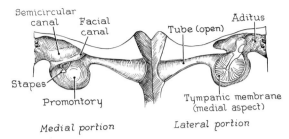

Semicircular canal Facial canal Tube (open) Aditus

Stapes

Promontory Tympanic membrane (medial aspect)

Medial portion Lateral portion

Figure 78-13. The two fragments obtained after the second saw cut. The technique is precise. The blade of the saw must lie parallel to the slant of the membrane. The results vary from specimen to specimen. In this instance, the eustachian tube was cut perfectly lengthwise.

surface of the membrane, provides a clue to the location and slant of the membrane. The membrane lies at an angle of 55° so that its external surface faces laterally inferiorly and anteriorly. With this information in mind, study the orientation of the specimen carefully. Then, with the autopsy saw blade immediately medial to the malleus and tilted to lie parallel to the malleus, make an oblique anteroposterior cut through the middle ear. Continue the cut until there are two loose portions, a lateral one with the tympanic membrane and a medial one with the internal ear (Fig. 78-13). Wash away all bone dust and debris. The findings in each middle ear opened in this way are a little different, depending on the precise direction of the cut. Figure 78-13 shows some of the structures to be examined on the medial surface of the tympanic membrane and the lateral aspect of the internal ear.

The Internal Ear

In order to understand the features of the medial wall of the middle ear it is necessary to digress for a moment to consider certain gross features of the internal ear.

The internal ear includes two organs, the organ of balance and the organ of hearing. The latter is located in the cochlea, the former in the semicircular canals; the cochlea is anteromedial to the canals in the petrous part of the temporal bone (Fig. 78-14).

Each organ consists of sensitive structures supported in a membranous tube called a labyrinth because of its complicated shape. The exact anatomy of the membranous labyrinth (*Grant's Atlas of Anatomy,* Fig. 650) is established by building a model using tracings of enlargements of a series of histologic slides of the petrous part of the temporal bone.

The membranous labyrinth is housed in a bony labyrinth that does not fit closely around the membranous labyrinth (Fig. 78-15). The bony

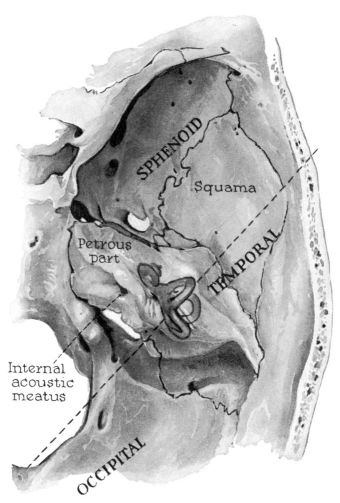

Figure 78-14.   Right bony labyrinth; position in the skull. The labyrinth, drawn from a reconstruction, is shown as if the surrounding part of the temporal bone were transparent.

The bony labyrinth is 20 mm. in length. It lies approximately parallel to the posterior surface of the petrous part of the temporal bone.

The base of the cochlea adjoins the internal acoustic meatus; it lies parallel to the plane of the posterior semicircular canal. Both form an angle of approximately 45 degrees with the median plane, as does also the plane of the superior semicircular canal (in the course of the broken line). (From B. J. Anson: Atlas of Human Anatomy. 2nd ed. Philadelphia, W. B. Saunders Co., 1963.)

labyrinth is usually illustrated as a separate structure (see *Grant's Atlas of Anatomy*, Fig. 649) but it is important for the student to realize that the bony labyrinth is not a separate structure. The bony labyrinth is tightly embedded (Figs. 78-14 and 78-15) in the petrous part of the temporal bone, but not entirely, as you will see.

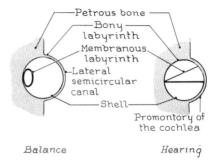

Figure 78-15. Scheme to show the principal difference between the membranous and the bony labyrinth.

What is said now is very important in the teaching of practical anatomy. It is possible to free the bony labyrinth by delicate dissection with fine dental drills. More easily, a cast of the bony labyrinth can be made by injecting latex or metal to fill the labyrinth; in doing so the membranous labyrinth is destroyed. Then the petrous part of the temporal bone is dissolved in acid. In most anatomic models used for teaching purposes, the bony labyrinth has been created from casts of this kind, and lies free in the rest of the model. Therefore, it must be reemphasized that in reality the bony labyrinth is totally embedded in bone, except for two aspects exposed in the middle ear. The exposed part of the organ of hearing is called the promontory (Fig. 78-15); the exposed part of the organ of balance is the lateral semicircular canal (Fig. 78-15).

The Fenestra Vestibuli and the Fenestra Cochleae (Fig. 78-16). The vestibule of the bony labyrinth is a cavern between the semicircular canals and the cochlea. *Fenestra vestibuli* is Latin for window of the vestibule; *fenestra cochleae* means window of the cochlea. The footplate of the stapes is held in the fenestra vestibuli by pliant ligamentous tissue; when this tissue is normal the foot plate of the stapes is free to move

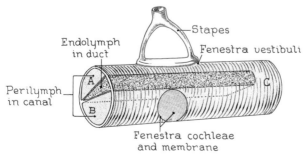

Figure 78-16. A diagram to illustrate the mechanism of the internal ear. The perilymph apparently isolated in A and B meet at C, for the duct is shorter than the canal. Thus when movement of the stapes sets up a disturbance in the perilymph in A, the disturbance proceeds through the perilymph at C into the perilymph in B.

slightly, in and out of the fenestra vestibuli. The fenestra cochleae, on the other hand, is closed completely by a membrane, but it is a membrane that is slack enough to quiver. A simple explanation of the function of these structures follows next.

Study Figure 78-16 and visualize how movements transmitted from the tympanic membrane by the malleus and incus ultimately end at the stapes. Movement of the stapes at the fenestra vestibuli sends a disturbance through the perilymph to stir the duct. Thus a stimulus reaches the nerve endings of the organ of hearing located in the duct. The existence of a second window, the fenestra cochleae, is believed to be necessary because otherwise movement of the stapes would merely raise the.pressure of the perilymph and not necessarily set up a disturbance. This is far too simple a concept, no doubt, but it serves to draw attention to the accepted functional relationship of the foot plate of the stapes in the fenestra vestibuli and the membrane closing the fenestra cochleae.

In conclusion, there are many causes of deafness; one cause involves the stapes—any pathologic condition that diminishes movement of the stapes diminishes hearing.

ITEM 78-20. Examination of the Walls of the Middle Ear

Through a dissecting microscope focused on the medial wall of the middle ear, identify the promontory, the stapes, the stapedius muscle, the fenestra cochleae, the lateral semicircular canal, and the canal for the facial nerve. The facial canal here lies between the organs of hearing and balance. Examine with particular care how the stapes fits into the fenestra vestibuli (Fig. 78-16).

The significant feature of the anterior wall of the middle ear is the opening of the pharyngotympanic (eustachian) tube. Obtain a firm piece of nylon thread or a slender stick and push it into the nasopharyngeal end of the tube. Provided the tip of the stick stays in the lumen of the tube, the tip will emerge at the tympanic end, which is located in the superior half of the anterior wall. By reconstructing the anatomy, establish the direction of the pharyngotympanic tube from the nasopharynx to the middle ear. The direction is medial, inferior, and somewhat anterior. What is the length of the tube?

In the infant the pharyngotympanic tube is more horizontal, has a larger lumen, and its pharyngeal opening is nearer the oropharynx. It is generally agreed that these are major factors in the incidence of middle ear infections in childhood, and it is certainly true that the risk of middle ear infections decreases as childhood slips by.

The significant feature of the posterior wall is the aditus ad antrum. Observe how it leads off the superior part of the middle ear cavity, a part named the epitympanic recess, often called simply the attic. Establish also the position of the lateral semicircular canal and the facial canal with reference to the aditus.

The Lateral Wall of the Middle Ear

Introduction

There can be little doubt that the lateral wall is by far the most important part of the middle ear to the practicing physician. The lateral wall is partly bone, but mainly membrane. It is the membrane the doctor examines with the aid of a speculum inserted into the external acoustic meatus. The student will have the opportunity to examine the external aspect of the tympanic membrane at a later stage in the dissection.

ITEM 78-21. Inspect the malleus lying deep to the mucous membrane of the middle ear (Fig. 78-13). Observe how its handle, also known as the manubrium, has an intimate relationship with the membrane and how the center of the membrane is pulled medially. Very gently maneuver the malleus to demonstrate its lateral process projecting into the membrane. From the process anterior and posterior malleolar folds extend and isolate a segment of the membrane called the pars flaccida from the rest of the membrane, the pars tensa (Fig. 78-8). The pars flaccida is frequently called Shrapnell's membrane after an English anatomist. Microscopically it can be shown that the pars tensa has three layers, an outer layer of modified skin, an inner layer of mucous membrane, and an intermediate fibrous layer. The intermediate layer is absent in the pars flaccida.

The interval between the pars flaccida and the neck of the malleus is known clinically as Prussak's space (Fig. 78-8) after Prussak, who was a nineteenth century Russian otologist. A serious complication of a middle ear infection is perforation of the pars flaccida; the complication may go further and obliterate Prussak's space, but the details of these interesting aspects come later in your training. Carefully identify Prussak's space.

The tympanic membrane responds to changes of pressure in the middle ear. To demonstrate this, gently pull the malleus medially to increase the convexity of the membrane. Such an increase occurs when the eustachian tube is blocked and the air in the middle ear is absorbed; the increase is particularly obvious in the pars flaccida. Next, gently push the malleus laterally to demonstrate how fluid in the middle ear can cause the tympanic membrane to bulge toward the external acoustic meatus.

Now observe how the head of the malleus is in the epitympanic recess, higher than the superior margin of the tympanic membrane. Examine the lateral aspect of the head and the adjacent bone for an example of one of the tiny ligaments mooring the ossicles to the side walls. This one is the lateral ligament of the malleus.

Finally, the tendons of the two small muscles may be identified most easily with magnification. The tendon of the tensor tympani is usually cut in the second stage of the dissection. The tendon of the stapedius is usually intact.

Although the floor of the middle ear can be quickly examined, its relationships are nevertheless important. Establish the relationship of the bulb of the jugular vein to the floor of the middle ear and, at the same time, establish the relationship of the sigmoid sinus to the antrum. Also trace the internal carotid artery through the carotid canal and note its relationship to the ear.

The Mucous Membrane of the Middle Ear

To begin with it is important to stress the size of the middle ear cavity. The cavity is usually likened to a box (Fig. 78-9), but the simile conveys an impression of great size unless it is stressed that the anterior to posterior length is only 15 mm. and the height is the same. Furthermore, the width varies because of the presence of the promontory; the width at the level of the promontory is only 2 mm., so the depth of an incision into the membrane from the external acoustic meatus must be controlled to an extreme degree.

Superior to the promontory the width increases to 6 mm. and below the promontory to 4 mm. These measurements alone decree that the tympanum is a very small space but the space is even further reduced by the presence of the ossicles, the several ligaments that support the ossicles, the chorda tympani, two slender muscle tendons, and several little bony projections that have not been named in this description. In addition these structures are "coated" with a mucous membrane.

When the student first examines the middle ear he does not appreciate immediately that the ossicles and other structures are covered by a delicate mucous membrane. To visualize the extent of the membrane some students find it useful to imagine that the middle ear and its contained structures has been dipped into molten wax; the surplus wax is then shaken out, leaving a thin continuous coating of wax, i.e., mucous membrane, over all the internal structures, projections, and recesses of the cavity, with some surplus here and there to form folds.

The small size of the actual void in the middle ear and the presence of a continuous sheet of mucous membrane are significant factors in the effects of inflammation of the middle ear. Unfortunately, further discussion requires a knowledge of bacteriology and pathology, but it can be explained now that the inflammation is usually referred to as otitis from the Greek word *otos*, which means ear.

The External Acoustic Meatus

All that has been done so far concerning the ear brings us to the most important part, the external aspect of the tympanic membrane.

ITEM 78-22. Examination of the Tympanic Membrane

Examine Figure 78-8; then cut away a strip from the anterior aspect of the cartilaginous meatus. Complete the opening of the bony meatus with the narrow blade of the autopsy saw. Proceed carefully until the tympanic membrane can be seen.

Wash away all cerumen and debris before you examine the membrane. The membrane is nearly circular, measuring 8 to 9 mm. in diameter; it is 0.1 mm. thick. Note the direction of the surface of the membrane, anterior, inferior, and lateral. Identify the position of the malleus embedded in the membrane and observe the *umbo*, which is Latin for the boss on a shield; in this instance the umbo is the tiny white bulge at the inferior end of the handle of the malleus and at the center of the membrane. Identify the lateral process of the malleus and distinguish between the pars flaccida and the pars tensa. There may be some evidence that the membrane is, indeed, a vascular structure. Study Figure 78-8 carefully, then reexamine your specimen for abnormal findings such as a perforation.

Finally examine the external acoustic meatus. In the adult it measures 2.5 to 3.5 cm. Observe how the long axis of the meatus ascends gradually and then descends gradually. The meatus, therefore, at the junction of the floor and the membrane is wedge-shaped. Demonstrate that pulling the auricle superiorly, laterally, and posteriorly is necessary to straighten the canal.

Anyone who has had a furuncle (boil) of the external auditory meatus will testify to the pain it causes. This is because the skin lining the meatus is firmly adherent to the perichondrium and the periosteum, so the furuncle cannot enlarge with ease.

The secretions of the modified sebaceous glands found in the skin of the meatus form the cerumen or wax.

The External Acoustic Meatus in the Child

Nowhere else in the body is it more important to know that the anatomy of the child is different from that of the adult. Examination of the ear is always required in the physical examination of a child. It is therefore absolutely essential to know that the tympanic membrane is much more superficial in the child than in the adult (Fig. 78-8) and that the membrane faces much more inferiorly. Therefore to prepare the external acoustic meatus for the insertion of the speculum the child's auricle must be pulled inferiorly and laterally. And the doctor's eye must look through the speculum as he inserts it into the very short meatus.

Exercise

Examine the skull of an infant and that of a full term fetus. Observe the length of the bony external acoustic meatus and the size of the mastoid process.

Review

Read an account of the nerve supply of the external acoustic meatus. Place some emphasis on the auricular branch of the vagus nerve; it is recognized that clinical procedures in the external ear may precipitate reflex coughing, nausea, or even vomiting; hard wax in the external ear is one cause of a persistent, dry unproductive cough.

REFERENCES

Boies, L. B., Hilger, J. A., and Priest, R. E.: Fundamentals of Otolaryngology. Philadelphia, W. B. Saunders Co., 1964.

Calnan, J.: Modern views on Passavant's ridge. British Journal of Plastic Surgery, *10*:89, 1957.

Calnan, J.: The surgical treatment of nasal speech disorders. Annals of the Royal College of Surgeons of England, *25*:119, 1959.

Cave, A. J. E.: Epipharynx (nomen novum). Journal of Anatomy, *95*:281, 1961.

Fulton, J. F.: Horner and the syndrome of paralysis of the cervical sympathetic. Archives of Surgery, Chicago, *18*:2025, 1929.

Gardner, E., Gray, D. J., and O'Rahilly, R.: Anatomy. Philadelphia, W. B. Saunders Co., 1963.

Gordon-Taylor, Sir Gordon, and Walls, E. W.: Sir Charles Bell. Edinburgh, E. & S. Livingstone Ltd., 1958.

Grant, J. C. B., and Basmajian, J. V.: Method of Anatomy. Baltimore, Williams & Wilkins Co., 1965.

Patey, D. H., and Ranger, I.: Some points in the surgical anatomy of the parotid gland. British Journal of Surgery, *45*:250, 1957.

Sicher, H.: Oral Anatomy, 4th ed. St. Louis, C. V. Mosby Co., 1965.

Wolff, E.: The Anatomy of the Eye and Orbit. London, H. K. Lewis & Co. Ltd., 1946.

PART 7

THE UPPER LIMB
The Organ of Manual Activity

by R. D. LAURENSON
and B. J. GREENHILL

Introduction

The upper limb is also known as the upper extremity. It should be noted that the upper limb includes the arm, forearm, and hand. The arm, then, is only part of the upper limb.

"To make a body of a limb" should be the intent of every student dissecting a limb. In other words, he must view the limb in its entirety, not in a series of parts. Moreover, he must not view the limb as remote from the rest of the human frame for:

> The head is not more native to the heart,
> The hand more instrumental to the mouth
> Than is the throne of Denmark to thy father.
>
> Hamlet.

In the following dissection, therefore, emphasis is laid upon a systemic and total approach and the horizons of dissection are: skin, superficial venous system, superficial lymphatics, the deep fascia, the deltoid region, the extensor and flexor aspects of the limb, the hand, and, last, the joints of the upper limb. In the process of dissection the student's attention will be drawn to the regions of clinical importance.

If you have not yet read the chapter on skin and fascia (p. 1), you are advised to do so now.

Separation of the Upper Limbs

If the order of dissection presented here has been followed the vertebral column should now be completely divided down the midline to separate the limbs. It is an advantage to have the technicians do this when the students are absent from the laboratory. A butcher's bandsaw is ideal, but a strong carpenter's saw is satisfactory for the purpose.

Chapter 79

Skin, Superficial Veins, Lymphatics, Deep Fascia, and Muscle Groups

Examine the skin of the entire limb. In addition to the general features of skin (Chapter 1), look especially at the tips of the fingers and the fingernails. Changes in the fingernails are found in many diseases. Thus your clinical tutors will expect you to report on the condition of the patient's fingernails. Furthermore, when the endocrine system is under review, a report on the presence or absence of axillary hair is essential. As your experience grows you will realize how much indeed can be learned about a patient's health by a methodical inspection of his skin and its appendages. Finally, look for scars that may be the result of a previous injury or a surgical procedure. (You must rewrap the hands of the cadaver very carefully to prevent their mummifying.)

ITEM 79-1. To remove the skin from the upper limb begin at the wrist. (Do not remove skin from the hand at this stage. Experience has taught us that the hand of an embalmed cadaver dries out more quickly than any other part.) Proceed as follows:

About 5 cm. from the base of the thumb on the lateral aspect of the forearm, make a transverse incision 2 or 3 cm. long and expose the cephalic vein (Fig. 79-1). It is a common clinical procedure to "cut down" in this manner to expose the cephalic vein, or some other vein of the upper limb, for the administration of blood, plasma expanders, and electrolytes. Of course, there is a precise technique for this procedure, but for the moment you are only concerned with the anatomy.

Then, by means of the closed-open scissors technique (Fig. 46-2), make a longitudinal cut in the skin and fat superficial to the vein while you trace the vein toward the shoulder. About the middle of the arm, i.e., halfway between the shoulder and the elbow, the vein slips under the deep fascia. From that point on, therefore, the vein is obscured from view by a thin, gray membranous sheet. Without disturbing that sheet follow the cephalic vein into the groove between the deltoid and pectoralis major. Then slit the sheet to mobilize the vein and trace it to where it passes posterior to the pectoralis major, penetrates the clavipectoral fascia (see Thorax, p. 12), and joins the subclavian vein.

Now that you have identified the depth of the superficial venous plane, strip back each long flap of skin to expose the rest of the super-

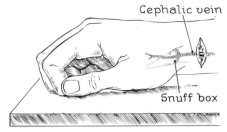

Cephalic vein

Snuff box

Figure 79-1. Incision to expose the cephalic vein.

ficial veins. On the medial aspect of the forearm identify the basilic vein and trace it to where it penetrates the deep fascia. Ultimately it joins the axillary vein, as you will see more easily at a later stage of the dissection. Skin the entire limb, including the deltoid region and the axilla. In removing skin from the region of the olecranon a bursa between the tendon of triceps and skin is usually found.

BURSAE

A bursa is a membranous sac, usually empty except for a little fluid that makes the internal surface of the sac slippery. Accordingly, a bursa is a means of reducing friction between moving parts. There are many bursae throughout the body but only a few of them are recognized. They are the bursae prone to distend with fluid or to become hot, red, and painful (bursitis) as a result of persistent repetitive movements, pressure, or infection. Bursitis is an occupational hazard; some of the bursa involved are commonly identified by occupation: student's elbow (olecranon bursa); housemaid's knee (prepatellar bursa).

Baker's cyst is named not after an occupation but after William Baker, an English surgeon. The term Baker's cyst is loosely applied to any cystic swelling of the popliteal fossa. The commonest swelling there is enlargement of a bursa related to the medial head of the gastrocnemius; this bursa usually communicates with the knee joint.

ITEM 79-2. Examine the veins in front of the elbow joint, a region called the cubitus. The antecubital veins are the commonest site for intravenous injections or for obtaining a sample of blood. These veins must be studied with care not just on the cadaver but also on your own arm and on the arms of your colleagues.

Exercise

On your own arm, compress the tissues superior to the elbow joint to obstruct the venous return. Observe the pattern of the superficial veins of the hand and forearm. The proximity of the major artery and nerve of the forearm and the possibility of an anomalous superficial artery in the cubital fossa are borne in mind by the anesthetist who uses the antecubital veins for intravenous anesthesia.

THE LYMPHATIC DRAINAGE OF THE UPPER LIMB

The drainage is superficial and deep. Superficial drainage is mainly from the skin; deep drainage is from muscle. The principal group of lymph nodes, located in the axilla deep to deep fascia, is termed the axillary nodes. They will be exposed when the axillary fascia is removed.

It is difficult, at first, to conceive that lymph from the skin of the fingers finally filters through the lymph nodes in the axilla, yet that is so. Long and normally inconspicuous lymph vessels accompany the major superficial veins and terminate in the axilla. Thus, when the axillary lymph nodes are tender and swollen, obviously reacting to an infection somewhere in their field of drainage, the skin of the entire limb must be examined. The skin of the trunk, the mammary glands, and the umbilicus must also be included in the examination.

The deep lymphatic vessels, accompanying the deep veins, also drain into the axillary nodes.

From the axillary nodes an efferent vessel finally emerges. It is the subclavian trunk, and it joins the venous system in the root of the neck. The subclavian lymph trunk may have been seen when the neck was dissected, but it is rarely found.

DEEP FASCIA

ITEM 79-3.   Removal of the Superficial Fascia

To expose the deep fascia remove the superficial fascia, which may be abundant (see Fat, p. 6). To remove the superficial fascia from an obese cadaver, incise the fascia until you expose the deep fascia, gray in color. Then peel off the superficial fascia in one layer. If you proceed with reasonable caution you will note cutaneous nerves piercing the deep fascia. Even though you do not have time to demonstrate these nerves by dissection, it is useful to know something about their distribution, which is usually adequately illustrated in anatomy texts. The sensory innervation of the hands, which is particularly important and deserves careful attention, will be dealt with later.

Inspection of the Deep Fascia.   The deep fascia of the palm of the hand, the palmar aponeurosis, and the flexor retinaculum have clinical importance that will be mentioned when the hand is dissected. The extensor retinaculum, which is a thickening of deep fascia superior to the wrist on the extensor (posterior) aspect, is similar in structure and function to the retinacula of the leg (see Retinaculum, p. 257).

The deep fascia of the forearm forms an investment of the muscles of the forearm. In the living the deep fascia is tense, not slack, and the muscles are full, not shrunken. Sometimes, therefore, as in the management of swelling in the anterior tibial compartment (p. 257), the deep fascia of the forearm is incised (fasciotomy) to safeguard the underlying muscles from the effects of increased pressure. If fasciotomy is not done the pressure may increase to a degree that the muscles perish. To understand how serious that is the student should consult an orthopedic textbook for an account of Volkmann's ischemic contracture.

ITEM 79-4.   On the anterior aspect of the forearm, inferior to the cubital fossa, carefully make a slit 2 to 3 cm. long into the deep fascia. Slip the tip of the scissors deep to the fascia and, by pressing the tip of the scissors toward you, test the strength of the fascia.

Examine particularly the deep fascia over the cubital fossa, i.e., the anterior aspect of the elbow, where the bicipital aponeurosis spreads out from the medial aspect of the tendon of biceps to blend with the deep fascia of the superomedial aspect of the forearm. The superficial veins lie superficial to the aponeurosis and must be displaced or removed. The brachial artery and the median nerve lie deep to it. This regional zone of fascia may serve to protect those significant deep structures during venipuncture. On the other hand, the toughness of the fascia enhances any increase in pressure that may occur deep to it.

The axillary fascia, a regional part of the deep fascia, can be demonstrated in an embalmed cadaver although it is adherent to the superficial fat and to the fat within the axilla. Laterally the axillary fascia is continuous with the deep fascia of the arm, medially with fascia on the chest wall and, anteriorly and posteriorly with the fascia on the muscles that form the anterior and posterior axillary walls. Because of these periph-

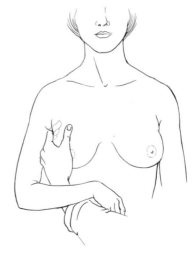

Figure 79-2.   Palpation of the axilla.

eral connections the axillary fascia is slack only when the upper limb is close to the side of the body and the boundary muscles completely relaxed. Thus the axilla is examined with the patient's arm at the side and supported (Fig. 79-2).

Chapter 80

Muscle Groups of the Upper Limb

The key to an understanding of the upper limb is a knowledge of the location and nomenclature of the muscle groups.

The deltoid is a solitary muscle and is therefore included in the descriptive term, deltoid region. The pectoralis major is another solitary muscle forming the anterior axillary fold. The latissimus dorsi and teres major form the posterior axillary fold.

The muscles of the arm form two groups, anterior and posterior. The anterior group flexes the elbow, so it is frequently described as the flexor group; the posterior group is described as the extensor group. The muscles of the forearm also form an anterior (flexor) and a posterior (extensor) group.

The muscles of the posterior axillary fold, the deltoid muscle, and the extensor muscles of the arm and forearm have one thing in common—they are all supplied by nerves derived from the posterior divisions of the brachial plexus. The muscle forming the anterior axillary fold and the flexor muscles of the arm and forearm are supplied by nerves derived from the anterior divisions of the brachial plexus. How this happens is discussed with the brachial plexus.

Exercise

At a convenient time, demonstrate on the living body, the major muscle groups just referred to. They are seen best of all when they contract against resistance, such as gravity, the weight of a book, or the resistance of a colleague (Fig. 53-1).

It is an oblique upward and outward flinging of the upper limb that brings into action the extensor muscles, i.e., those muscles supplied through the posterior divisions of the brachial plexus. The opposite movement, bringing the limb down across the front of the body, brings into action the flexor muscles, i.e., those muscles supplied through the anterior divisions of the brachial plexus.

Meantime, in the gross anatomy laboratory, locate the deltoid, pectoralis major, teres major, and latissimus dorsi, then the flexor and extensor muscle groups of the arm and forearm.

Removal of Deep Fascia

In the region of the elbow the distal parts of the muscles of the arm are related intimately with proximal parts of the muscles of the forearm.

ITEM 80-1. The deep fascia of the flexor compartment of the arm is thin and may have been torn or removed in the removal of the superficial fascia. If the fascia is intact, make a midline longitudinal incision into it from shoulder to elbow and reflect the flaps laterally and medially as far as the intermuscular septa (p. 6). If the fascia is damaged proceed to reflect it as best you can. Do not delay, but as you approach the medial septum look out for the brachial artery and median nerve.

Then make a similar midline longitudinal incision into the fascia over the posterior aspect of the arm and reflect the flaps as far as the intermuscular septa. As you approach the medial septum look out for the ulnar nerve proceeding to the posterior aspect of the medial epicondyle of the humerus.

Before you remove the fascia from the forearm, reexamine the bicipital aponeurosis and extensor retinaculum and read Synovial Sheaths (p. 258). Then, from elbow to wrist make a midline longitudinal incision into the deep fascia. Reflect the flaps medially and laterally. It will be necessary to detach by sharp dissection the investing layer of deep fascia from several well-marked intermuscular septa between individual muscle bellies close to the elbow. The major attachment of the investing layer of deep fascia is to the posterior border of the ulna. Continue to reflect the layer until the attachment is demonstrated. It is usually necessary to make transverse incisions into the fascia to create flaps that can be reflected more easily.

Exercise

Demonstrate that the posterior border of the ulna is subcutaneous from end to end and separates the anterior and the posterior muscles of the forearm. In contrast to this exposed position of the ulna, you will find that the radius is "buried" in muscles except at both ends, which are easily palpated.

ITEM 80-2. Finally, use the inferior border of the pectoralis major (which may have been mobilized already, p. 12) as a guide to the correct plane of separation in the removal of the axillary fascia. Continue to reflect the fascia posteriorly until the posterior axillary fold is exposed. Be careful not to cut deep and to keep the edge of your scalpel directed

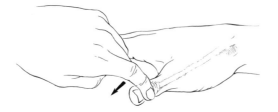

Figure 80-1. Testing the muscle belly and tendon of the extensor pollicis longus. Try it on yourself.

toward the fascia to avoid lacerating muscles. Nonetheless, the more extensive and adequate the removal of the deep fascia, the easier the remainder of the dissection.

Now that the major muscle groups have been located and the deep fascia reflected, the limb is ready for further dissection to identify the muscles in each group, principal vessels, and nerves. In reflecting muscles, nerves and vessels will come into view. Each muscle is connected to at least one nerve, artery, and vein (collectively known as a neurovascular bundle). Individual bundles will not be earmarked for identification. In general, as each muscle is identified its neurovascular bundle becomes obvious.

It is a practical necessity for the student to know how to test the action not only of a muscle group but also of many significant individual muscles. The method is illustrated in Figure 53-1, where it is obvious that the patient is keeping his foot in a position of dorsiflexion while the clinician pulls in the opposite direction. All muscle groups or individual muscles of the upper limb are tested in this way, and the required position of the patient and the most suitable grip for the clinician are fully illustrated in Aids to the Investigation of Peripheral Nerve Injuries, M.R.C. War Memorandum No. 7, from which Figure 80-1 has been adapted.

It is recommended that the student reflect the deltoid first. The deltoid lies on the superolateral aspect of the upper limb; anteriorly and posteriorly it overlaps the muscle groups of the arm. Then the student should reflect the pectoralis major and minor if this has not already been done (p. 12).

Chapter 81

The Deltoid Region

The strength or weakness of an individual is often judged by the size of his deltoid muscles. "He has a powerful pair of shoulders" is a common expression, but what is not generally realized is the part played by the underlying skeleton in the characteristic shape of the shoulder. The skeleton, therefore, of the deltoid region must be examined in some detail.

Examine a skeleton and observe how the lateral extremity of the clavicle articulates with the medial margin of the acromion (Fig. 81-1). Then observe how the greater and lesser tuberosities protrude anteriorly and laterally beyond the lateral margin of the acromion. The scapulohumeral articulation of the skeleton you are examining may be hinged so that the protrusion is greater than normal, but you can confirm by palpation of your own shoulder the relationship of the upper end of the humerus to the acromion.

The protrusion of the humeral tuberosities bolsters the deltoid. Take away the bolster and the shoulder loses its plump shape, the hallmark of a good physique. It must be made clear, however, that deltoid paralysis, accompanied by marked wasting of the muscle, produces a similar effect. In summary, then, both the deltoid and the underlying skeleton are responsible for the rounded shape of the deltoid region.

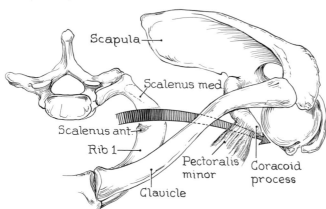

Figure 81-1. The arrow indicates the route taken by the brachial plexus and accompanying artery through the cervicoaxillary canal. The vein travels in the opposite direction to pass anterior to the scalenus anterior.

445

Next, observe that the head of the humerus, in particular its articular surface, is greater than the glenoid fossa of the scapula. Clearly skeletal stability is not a characteristic of the scapulohumeral articulation. Indeed, the articulation is notorious for its instability, and dislocation is common. The head of the humerus usually dislocates anteromedially so that the deltoid is deprived of the underlying skeletal support and, thus, the deltoid region becomes flattened or "square" shaped because of the prominent acromion.

Palpate on yourself the deltoid region and identify the bony landmarks you have just observed on the skeleton. Then expose the structures deep to deltoid as follows.

ITEM 81-1. Identify the anterior border of the deltoid. The border forms the superolateral boundary of the groove occupied by the cephalic vein. Mobilize that border by blunt dissection, removing fascia until the entire anterior border of the deltoid is free. Then cut the clavicular attachment of the deltoid close to the clavicle and peel the deltoid posteriorly to expose the head of the humerus and related structures. Continue to detach the deltoid from its clavicular and acromial attachments until the underlying structures are fully exposed. Expect to find the circumflex nerve entering the deep surface of the deltoid posteriorly when you detach the muscle from the spine of the scapula. The nerve is accompanied by the posterior circumflex humeral vessels. It is important to realize that this neurovascular bundle passes immediately inferior to the shoulder joint before it reaches the deltoid muscle.

The coracoacromial arch, consisting of the coracoid, the coracoacromial ligament, and the acromion, is now exposed. The immediate inferior relationship of the arch is a bursa. The nomenclature of this bursa is confusing probably because there may be two bursa in this region. When there are two, one is subacromial and the other is subdeltoid, but the terms subacromial and subdeltoid are often regarded as synonymous.

Identify the coracoid, the coracoacromial ligament, and the acromion, all forming the coracoacromial arch. Probe gently the extent of the remainder of the subacromial bursa inferior to the arch. Remove the bursa. Then identify, from anterior to posterior, the following structures: the pectoralis minor, the coracobrachialis, and the short head of the biceps, all attached to the coracoid process; the humeral attachment of the subscapularis; the proximal tendon of the long head of the biceps (hidden in a tunnel); the humeral attachment of the supraspinatus, infraspinatus, and teres minor.

To see the subscapularis tendon more clearly it may be necessary to cut the attachments of the coracobrachialis and the short head of the biceps close to the coracoid process.

The tendons of the subscapularis, supraspinatus, infraspinatus and teres minor, blending with the superior aspect of the shoulder joint capsule, are termed clinically the rotator cuff (p. 501). The rotator cuff is separated from the coracoacromial arch only by the subacromial bursa. The interval between the coracoacromial arch and the upper end of the humerus is minimal and will be mentioned later under the heading Rotator Cuff Syndrome.

Chapter 82

The Muscles of the Scapula

For descriptive purposes these muscles may be grouped as the muscles of the shoulder girdle, the subdeltoid muscles, and the posterior axillary fold muscles. The first group includes the trapezius, levator scapulae, rhomboids, serratus anterior, and pectoralis minor; the second includes the subscapularis, supraspinatus, infraspinatus, and teres minor; the third includes the teres major and latissimus dorsi. Begin with the first group.

ITEM 82-1.   Dissection of the Muscles of the Scapula

The trapezius has already been detached from the skull and the ligamentum nuchae. It may have also been detached from the lower thoracic spines. If these steps have not been taken, take them now and detach the trapezius entirely from the vertebral column and skull. Reflect the trapezius laterally and demonstrate how it is attached to the spine of the scapula, to the acromion, and to the clavicle. Confirm that the accessory nerve enters its deep surface.

Observe how the superior muscle fibers of the trapezius slope inferiorly and laterally and that the superior portion, i.e., the portion with cranial and cervical attachments, is more bulky. It is easy to visualize how paralysis of the trapezius allows the lateral aspect of the shoulder girdle to drop to a lower level. Under those circumstances, the medial border of the scapula is held at a normal, or nearly normal, level by the levator scapulae and the rhomboids. The normal action of the trapezius is referred to under Arm and Trunk Mechanism (p. 502).

Examine the levator scapulae and the rhomboids. Their position and shape is illustrated in *Grant's Atlas of Anatomy*, Figure 477.

Examine the digitations of the serratus anterior on the chestwall and identify its nerve descending from the neck vertically across the digitations. Observe how the lower four digitations crowd on to the inferior angle of the scapula, whereas the fibers of the upper four digitations have a linear attachment to the medial border of the scapula. To see these attachments to better advantage, cut the rhomboids and elevate the scapula from the chest wall. The normal action of the serratus anterior is referred to under Arm and Trunk Mechanism (p. 502).

Now examine the second group of muscles, the subdeltoid muscles, particularly their scapular attachments, for their attachments to the humerus have already been seen. Begin with the teres minor and infraspinatus. The distinction between the two muscles is not easy to see. It is the contribution of their tendons to the rotator cuff rather than their muscle bellies that is important.

The next muscle is the supraspinatus. Its muscle belly, occupying the supraspinous fossa, is deep to the part of the trapezius attached to the spine of the scapula. Thus, to expose the muscle belly of supraspinatus, it may be necessary to make a prudent cut through the trapezius. Expose the supraspinatus and demonstrate how its fibers proceed laterally, inferior to the acromion, to a tendinous insertion into the humerus. The tendon of the supraspinatus is the one most commonly torn in injuries of the rotator cuff. The normal action of this muscle is referred to on p. 503.

The subscapularis is attached medially to almost the entire anterior surface of the scapula and narrows considerably as it proceeds laterally to pass anterior to the shoulder joint to the lesser tuberosity of the humerus. Examination of the scapular attachment must be postponed until the axilla is opened up or until the shoulder joint is dissected. The humeral attachment has already been examined.

Finally, examine the third group of muscles, namely the teres major and latissimus dorsi. To avoid confusion it must be stated immediately that the latissimus dorsi has scarcely any attachment to the scapula. However, the latissimus has an intimate relationship with the teres major in the posterior axillary fold and that is why it is included here. The latissimus dorsi was reflected from the vertebral column and pelvis (p. 160). With care, so as not to damage the neurovascular bundle of the upper limb, clean the muscle sufficiently to show how it narrows rapidly to a broad strap that passes anterior to the teres major to be inserted into the humerus. Also clean the teres major sufficiently to be able to recognize its attachments. What is the likely action of these two muscles?

The step-by-step dissection and examination of the scapular muscles you have now completed is necessary to see individual muscles, but it must not leave an impression of erratic movement in your mind. The harmony of the action of the scapular muscles is seen to perfection in "the man on the flying trapeze," and is described in more detail under the heading Arm and Trunk Mechanism.

Chapter 83

How the Major Artery, Nerves, and Vein Enter or Leave the Upper Limb

If you have dissected the lower limb first you will be aware that the sciatic nerve, the femoral nerve, and the obturator nerve each have different points of entry into the limb. Only the femoral nerve accompanies the femoral vessels, which are the principal vessels of the lower limb. In the upper limb, however, the arrangement is different, for all the major nerves as well as the principal artery and vein of the limb have a common point of entry into the limb. They pass through the cervicoaxillary canal (see Fig. 82-1) where they lie side by side, crowded together.

For descriptive purposes the cervicoaxillary canal begins at the scalenus anterior and medius muscles and ends at the base of the axilla. Figure 82-1 shows how the intermediate part of the canal is bounded by the first rib, the clavicle, and the upper border of the scapula and coracoid process. It is this intermediate part of the canal that forms the apex of the axilla. Read an account of the location, extent, and boundaries of the axilla.

Exercise

Identify the intermediate part of the cervicoaxillary canal on a skeleton.

ITEM 83-1. Opening the Cervicoaxillary Canal

Four items of dissection are necessary to open the canal.

(1) Reflection or retraction of the sternomastoid muscle to expose the scalenus anterior and medius. This was done when the neck was dissected.

(2) Removal of the intermediate third of the clavicle.

(3) Reflection of the omohyoid. This was done when the neck was dissected.

(4) Reflection of the pectoralis major and minor. This was done when the thorax was opened.

Reflect the sternomastoid to expose the scalene muscles. Then, on one side only, with an autopsy saw remove the intermediate third of the clavicle—one side only because the shoulder girdle has yet to be examined. Finally peel the pectoralis major and minor laterally toward

449

their humeral and scapular attachments. As the pectoralis major is reflected laterally, it is necessary to detach it from the axillary fascia if this has not already been done adequately.

The pectoralis minor is a significant landmark because all the major vessels and nerves proceeding to and from the limb lie deep to it (see Fig. 83-1). A sheet of fascia, the clavipectoral fascia, extends between the muscle and the clavicle. The cephalic vein pierces this fascia to enter the subclavian vein. One of the nerves to the pectoralis major also pierces the fascia and may have been ruptured when the pectoralis major was reflected. The other nerve to the pectoralis major pierces the pectoralis minor. Remove the clavipectoral fascia by blunt dissection and see to it that the pectoralis minor is reflected as far as possible toward the coracoid process. The cervicoaxillary canal is now wide open on its anterior aspect, but not all its contents are in clear view because of the presence of the axillary sheath.

Axillary Lymph Nodes

In the cadaver, during the dissection of the axilla, groups of lymph nodes are often found lying parallel to the axillary vein. They extend from the base, i.e., the axillary fascia, to the apex of the axilla.

The axillary lymph nodes receive lymph from the forequarter, which includes the upper limb and the breast. The student must reread the account of the lymphatic drainage of the breast (p. 15).

One method of examining the axillary lymph nodes is illustrated (Fig. 79-2).

Specific instructions to remove axillary nodes and fat will not be given here. The dissector must use his initiative to maintain a clear field of view as his dissection proceeds.

The Axillary Sheath

There is on the anterior surface of the scalenus anterior a sheet of fascia that is part of a more extensive sheet called the prevertebral fascia. As the subclavian artery and its close relation, the brachial plexus, proceed beyond the scalenus anterior toward the axilla they obtain a sleeve of fascia termed the axillary sheath. It should be noted that the accompanying axillary vein and its continuation, the subclavian vein, lie outside the sheath although loose fascia around the veins and attached to the sheath may give a different impression. The axillary sheath extends along the axillary artery and adjacent nerves into the upper arm.

ITEM 83-2. With care because of the proximity of the phrenic nerve, incise the prevertebral fascia on the anterior surface of the

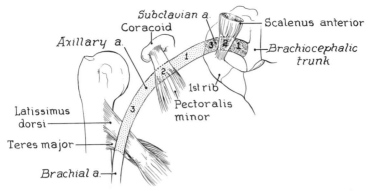

Figure 83-1. The subclavian and axillary arteries are each divided into three parts, but only for descriptive purposes. The numbers show the approximate location of these divisions. The third part of the axillary artery becomes the brachial artery at the lower border of the teres major.

scalenus anterior. Reflect the fascia to deliberately expose the phrenic nerve. Once the nerve and muscle fibers are seen deep to the fascia the correct plane of cleavage can be established.

Next extend the incision to open the axillary sheath and expose the main artery and accompanying nerves. Do not become concerned about identifying the nerves while you open the sheath throughout the length of the axilla.

The Principal Nerves and Vessels of the Cervicoaxillary Canal

The axillary vein, which may be obscured from view by axillary lymph nodes, is the most conspicuous vessel in the cervicoaxillary canal. In a cadaver the vein is usually distended, rigid, and adherent to adjacent structures; little can be seen until it is removed. Accordingly it is advantageous to first review the venous drainage of the upper limb, then to deal with the axillary vein.

THE VENOUS DRAINAGE FROM THE UPPER LIMBS

Read the section on the difference in the location of the superficial and deep veins (p. 7). Then proceed with this brief introduction to, and dissection of, the venous drainage of the upper limb.

The superficial venous system of each upper limb begins in the dorsal venous arch (or plexus) on the dorsal aspect of the hand. The plexus is readily seen in the living and therefore needs no further description. Two principal veins arise from the plexus, the cephalic and basilic veins, both of which have already been dissected to where they terminate by joining the deep venous system.

The deep venous system of each upper limb consists primarily of venae comitantes, veins accompanying the arteries of the limb. Thus the venae comitantes are located in the hand, forearm, and arm. In the axilla the venae comitantes of the brachial artery, the artery of the arm, and the basilic vein join the axillary vein. The axillary vein is a massive vein that is renamed the subclavian vein superior to the first rib, where it lies anterior to the scalenus anterior. The subclavian vein then joins the internal jugular vein to form the innominate vein. The junction of the two innominate veins to form the superior vena cava has already been seen in the thorax.

Exercise

To establish a concept of the continuity of the venous system, trace the pathway of the tip of a cardiac catheter from the right and then the left basilic vein to the cavity of the right ventricle. What is the difference between the right and left innominate veins?

ITEM 83-3.   Venous Drainage of the Upper Limb

Veins obscure the field of view and should be removed even though it may take a little time. Begin at the cubital fossa. The subsequent dissection in that region is much easier if the fossa is cleared of veins. The brachial veins may be left undisturbed if they are not obstructing the field of view.

Usually the axillary vein is huge and must be removed. Tie the vein proximally close to the first rib and distally in the arm. Tying the vein prevents debris within the vein from trickling into the field of view. Cut out the part of the vein between the ties.

As you deal with the axillary vein, consider what would be the effect in the living upon the venous return from the upper limb if the blood in the vein were to clot. Axillary vein obstruction and thrombosis occur for reasons that are not clearly understood. It ought not to be difficult to visualize the appearance of the upper limb when axillary vein obstruction or thrombosis occurs.

Now that the veins have been removed from the cervicoaxillary canal, the student has a choice, to dissect the artery or to dissect the nerves next. Both lie so close together. The artery, however, is the landmark on which the nomenclature of some of the nerves is based, so it is probably advantageous to deal with it first.

THE ARTERIAL SUPPLY OF THE UPPER LIMBS

The supply line of blood to each upper limb is a subclavian artery, which is soon renamed axillary. Renaming the artery, however, is not the only source of confusion to the junior student. In addition each artery is divided into three parts for descriptive purposes. Accordingly, the changes of name and the subdivisions of the proximal part of the main artery to the upper limb are illustrated in Figure 83-1. Observe that the subclavian artery and the axillary artery each have three subdivisions, and that the intermediate part, the second part of each artery, is posterior to a muscle. It is worth clarifying that the short distance of the artery exposed between the outer border of the scalenus anterior and the outer border of the first rib is indeed the third part of the subclavian artery.

Exercise

Measure the width of the scalenus anterior and of the pectoralis minor to get some idea of the lengths of the intermediate subdivisions of the two arteries. Then on the cadaver identify the subdivisions of the subclavian and axillary arteries on each side of the body. The small portion of teres major shown so clearly on Figure 83-1 is usually obscured from view by heavy fascia, so you may not be able to establish precisely where the axillary artery ends and the brachial artery begins.

The Origins of the Subclavian Arteries

ITEM 83-4.   Confirm that the left subclavian artery arises directly from the arch of the aorta and that the right subclavian artery is a branch of the brachiocephalic (previously known as the innominate) artery.

In 1 per cent of the population the right subclavian artery arises directly from the arch of the aorta and, to reach the root of the neck, passes posterior to the esophagus. For an explanation of how this alternate course is possible a textbook of embryology should be consulted. The anomaly is mentioned here because it is an excellent example to make the student aware that anatomic structures do vary and that anatomic descriptions are not absolute. Furthermore, it is of practical significance in many surgical procedures on the neck.

Branches of the Arterial Tree

From each subclavian artery trace the arterial tree distally. Identify the following major branches as you go. Clean each artery sufficiently to be able to identify it accurately. Remember, arterial anomalies are common. Therefore do not become unduly alarmed if your specimen does not match an illustration or text. Use those aids as a guide to the interpretation of your actual findings.

Subclavian Artery
    Vertebral artery
    Internal thoracic artery
    Thyrocervical trunk
    Costocervical trunk
Axillary Artery
    Subscapular artery
    Circumflex humeral arteries
    Numerous branches to adjacent muscles
Brachial Artery
    Profunda brachii artery
    Terminal branches, the radial and ulnar arteries

THE NERVE SUPPLY TO THE UPPER LIMB

To prevent the student of gross anatomy from jumping to the conclusion that the nerve supply of the upper limb begins and ends in the brachial plexus, a concept is described briefly now that will be developed in much greater detail in neuroanatomy.

The predominant control of voluntary activities of the upper and lower limbs of the same side of the body is from the motor cortex of the opposite cerebral hemisphere. Similarly the sensory representation of the limbs is contained predominantly in the opposite cerebral hemisphere. However, present knowledge of the functional activity of the central nervous system shows clearly that to consider the motor control and sensory representation of any limb to be confined entirely to the opposite cerebral hemisphere is far too simple a concept. Much integrated activity of widely separated parts of the entire central nervous system (C.N.S.) is involved in both voluntary and reflex movement. Also, sensory input affects more than those areas in which conscious impressions are generated. Any single sensory stimulus evokes widespread activity in many parts of the C.N.S. These facts, as well as the concept of contralateral motor control or of contralateral sensory representation, must be borne in mind in the interpretation of the signs and symptoms of injury or disease of the C.N.S.

Now that you have been reminded of the part the C.N.S. plays in the function of the limbs, proceed to examine the proximal part of the peripheral nervous system of the upper limb beginning with the spinal cord and its ventral and dorsal roots.

ITEM 83-5. After the vertebral column was sectioned (p. 437) perhaps a portion of the spinal cord was left. If not, at least some of the dorsal and ventral root should still be present. The roots attached to the superior segments of the cord lie transversely in the subarachnoid space. The lower cervical and then the thoracic roots become more and more oblique in direction, until finally the lumbar and sacral roots are vertical and form the cauda equina.

ITEM 83-6. Observe that the ventral root, which is motor, and the dorsal root, which is sensory, leave the subarachnoid space in separate sleeves of the arachnoid and dura mater. That the sleeves remain separate as far as the posterior root ganglion is not obvious, but it can be demonstrated once the intervertebral foramen is opened (Fig. 83-2).

ITEM 83-7. Pull the dura and arachnoid medially to see the dural sheath that encloses the dorsal and ventral roots. The sheath is surrounded by the fat and veins of the extradural space. Clinicians refer to the sheath and its contents as the "nerve root." The relationship of the proximal part of the nerve root to an intervertebral disc is important, and is examined next.

ITEM 83-8. Identify the cut surface of the disc between cervical vertebra 7 and thoracic vertebra 1. Observe its relationship to the eighth cervical nerve root.

A protrusion of the disc between C7 and T1 vertebrae, impinging on the root of C8, produces signs and symptoms in the motor and sensory distribution of that root in regions remote from the actual protrusion. Similar signs and symptoms occur in other regions of the upper limb, depending on the nerve root involved. However, the interpretation of signs and symptoms indicative of nerve root pressure somewhere in the cervical region is far from easy and really requires considerable clinical instruction. The reference to nerve root disorders is

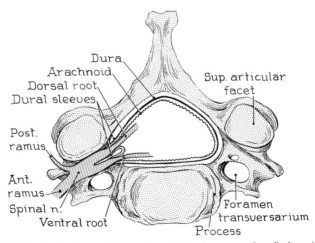

Figure 83-2. A spinal nerve is very short. What is commonly called a spinal nerve is really the anterior ramus. The process indicated forms part of the joint of Luschka. The superior articular facet and the inferior facet of the vertebra above form the zygapophyseal joint. Between these two joints lie the nerve components.

introduced here merely to indicate the breadth of vision that is necessary in the successful diagnosis of the cause of a peripheral disorder.

ITEM 83-9. After drawing attention to the significant relationship of the C7 and T1 disc and eighth cervical nerve root it would be logical to expose that particular nerve root in its intervertebral foramen. From a practical point of view, however, it is much easier to expose a root at a higher level, close to where the column was sectioned when the head was removed. Therefore, making sure you gain as wide exposure as possible, but with minimal destruction, use bone forceps and an autopsy saw to remove bone and trace the second or third cervical root into its intervertebral foramen. Observe how the root lies inferior to the pedicle above.

The posterior root ganglion is soon exposed. It is an obvious swelling and serves as an ideal landmark. Beyond the ganglion, identify the cervical spinal nerve and its division into an anterior and posterior ramus. Note the following facts:

(1) The posterior root ganglion is located in the intervertebral foramen. This is true of all posterior root ganglia except in the sacral region, where the ganglia are located in the sacral canal.

(2) The actual spinal nerve is short (Fig. 83-2), for it quickly divides into an anterior and posterior ramus. This is true of all spinal nerves. Each spinal nerve is only slightly longer than an intervertebral foramen.

ITEM 83-10. Examine first a skeleton and then your specimen, and note that the intervertebral foramen in which a spinal nerve lies is bounded posterolaterally by a zygapophyseal joint and anteromedially by a joint of Luschka. The joints of Luschka are small joints between the lateral margins of adjacent cervical vertebrae. The process labeled in Figure 83-2 indicates the site of the joint of Luschka. For an interesting and instructive account of these small joints that have provoked much debate as to their exact origin and function, the student should read *Luschka's Joints* (Hall, 1965).

Clinically, it is of practical significance that the intervertebral foramina of the neck become narrower when the neck is extended. In mild flexion, the foramina are at their widest.

The Brachial Plexus

Between the anterior rami of nerves C5, C6, C7, C8, and T1 and the actual nerves of the upper limb, the nerve fibers of each ramus pass through what appears at first to be an unrelated series of short interconnections termed upper, middle, and lower trunks, anterior and posterior divisions, and posterior, medial, and lateral cords. The rami, trunks, divisions, and cords together are named the brachial plexus. Within the plexus, a stage by stage redistribution of nerve fibers occurs until the nerve fibers that pass through all the posterior divisions of the plexus proceed to form the posterior cord. The fibers that pass through all the anterior divisions proceed to form the medial and lateral cords.

This redistribution has little or no significance until it is added that the extensor muscles of the upper limb are innervated by nerves that arise entirely from the posterior cord, and the muscles of the flexor aspect of the limb by nerves from the medial and lateral cords. In simpler terms, the posterior divisions of the brachial plexus serve the extensor muscles of the limb, while the anterior divisions serve the flexor muscles (p. 442). Therefore it may be said that the function of the brachial plexus is a redistribution of the nerve fibers to the flexor and extensor muscles of the upper limb. There is no ready explanation of why such a complicated method of redistribution is necessary. Knowledge of the pattern of distribution that finally emerges, however, is useful in the interpretation of physical signs that appear in certain neurologic disorders. Therefore, one of the aims in dissecting the brachial plexus is the demonstration of the formation of the anterior and posterior divisions as well as of the posterior, medial, and lateral cords.

The anterior rami of spinal nerves C5, C6, C7, C8, and T1, which combine to form the brachial plexus, are known as the roots of the brachial plexus. In this region of the body the word root means several things. To avoid the confusion that can arise, the student must make sure that he understands how the roots of the brachial plexus differ from the dorsal and ventral roots of the spinal cord and from the nerve roots of clinical significance. To add to the confusion, the median nerve, a branch of the brachial plexus, has medial and lateral roots.

ITEM 83-11.   To expose the superior roots of the brachial plexus, separate the scalenus anterior and medius muscles. To get the anterior ramus of T1, which is the inferior root of the plexus, examine the region of the neck of the first rib from within the thorax. This ramus forms a conspicuous bundle ascending to cross the rib in association with the subclavian artery.

ITEM 83-12.   Usually rami C5 and C6 join to form an upper trunk, ramus C7 remains as a middle trunk, and rami C8 and T1 join to form the lower trunk of the brachial plexus. This regrouping occurs between the scalenus anterior and scalenus medius. Identify the trunks of the brachial plexus.

ITEM 83-13.   Each of the three trunks divides into an anterior and posterior division. Identify the anterior divisions first, as follows. Identify the upper trunk of the brachial plexus. Trace the trunk distally beyond the origin of the suprascapular nerve to the point where the anterior divisions of the upper and middle trunks meet to form the lateral cord of the brachial plexus. The musculocutaneous nerve arises from the lateral cord and enters the coracobrachialis.

Next trace the lateral root of the median nerve from the lateral cord to the median nerve. From the median nerve, trace proximally the medial root of the nerve to reach the medial cord and then the anterior division of the lower trunk of the brachial plexus.

Slide a probe posterior to all three anterior divisions. Elevate them and the corresponding posterior divisions are obvious. They join to form the posterior cord of the brachial plexus.

ITEM 83-14. Identify the three cords of the brachial plexus as they are related to the second part of the axillary artery (Fig. 83-1).

The clue usually used to identify the medial and lateral cords accurately is the M formation, which has already been examined to some extent. The medial and lateral roots of the median nerve are the oblique strokes of the M. The musculocutaneous nerve forms the lateral upright stroke and the ulnar nerve the medial upright stroke.

Identify the radial nerve and the circumflex nerve arising from the posterior cord.

The Direction of the Brachial Plexus

Diagrams of the brachial plexus are useful in outlining the components of the plexus that have just been examined, but they may leave the student with the impression that the plexus is a horixontal formation like a group of streamers in a breeze. The brachial plexus is, in fact, an oblique structure in the root of the neck, as Figure 83-3 shows, and the components of the plexus are not spread out but crowded together. From a clinical and practical point of view, knowledge of the exact position of the plexus is most important. It can be seen in Figure 83-3 that if one shoulder is held down and the head bent forcibly to the opposite side that the upper "margin" of the plexus will be stretched and perhaps torn. Similarly, if the body is fixed and the upper limb pulled upward with force, then the lower part of the plexus will be stretched or torn. Thus there are two distinct types of injury to the brachial plexus in the root of the neck, both of which are related to the slant of the brachial plexus.

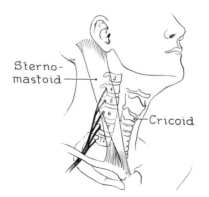

Figure 83-3. The brachial plexus is an oblique, not a horizontal, structure.

The Position of the Brachial Plexus

Often the student has no idea of the level of the brachial plexus in relation to the clavicle. Let us, therefore, consider the position of the roots first. The levels of the roots of the brachial plexus may be determined as follows: The cricoid cartilage is at the level of vertebra C6. The anterior ramus of nerve C7 (note C7 especially well), which is the middle root of the brachial plexus and forms the middle trunk, emerges inferior to vertebra C6. Thus, normally, two roots of the plexus will lie above and two below the level of the cricoid cartilage.

The trunks of the plexus lie between the scalene muscles (Fig. 81-1). The position of the muscles may be visualized by studying the position of the first rib. The long axis of the body of the first rib is essentially at right angles to the clavicle, and the most lateral point of the lateral border of that rib is directly posterior to the midpoint of the clavicle. The scalene muscles descend almost vertically from the cervical column to the rib. Clearly, the muscles do not lie lateral to the midpoint of the clavicle, and the same may be said of the trunks of the brachial plexus.

The divisions of the plexus lie adjacent to the third part of the subclavian artery. A finger pressed in behind the midpoint of the clavicle can palpate the pulsation of that artery. Thus, in the living, the position of the divisions of the plexus may be located.

The cords of the plexus extend from the midpoint of the clavicle to the inferomedial aspect of the coracoid process. The tip of the coracoid is readily palpable inferior to the lateral third of the clavicle. A mnemonic for the position of the brachial plexus is "the three C's," that is, clavicle-cords-coracoid.

Exercise

Examine a skeleton and confirm the position of the brachial plexus in relation to the first rib and the clavicle.

The Branches of the Brachial Plexus

Branches of the plexus are designated as supraclavicular and infraclavicular.

The supraclavicular branches include the following nerves to muscles concerned with activity of the upper limb: the nerve to the rhomboids and levator scapulae, the nerve to the serratus anterior, the nerve to the subclavius, and the suprascapular nerve, to the supra- and infraspinatus. The branches mentioned are quite easily found if you have the time to look for them. From a clinical point of view, however, there is little to be gained by searching for and dissecting out the supraclavicular branches of the brachial plexus.

The infraclavicular branches are best dealt with cord by cord. The posterior cord gives rise to the radial nerve and the circumflex nerve; in addition the cord gives branches to the latissimus dorsi, subscapularis, and teres major. The lateral cord gives rise to the musculocutaneous nerve and the lateral root of the median nerve. The medial cord gives rise to the ulnar nerve and the medial root of the median nerve. The pectoralis major is supplied from the lateral and medial cords.

ITEM 83-15. Identify the infraclavicular branches of the brachial plexus. They contain fibers conveying impulses from skin and from joints as well as to muscle. However in addition to cutaneous, articular, and motor fibers, they also contain sympathetic fibers destined to innervate the musculature of blood vessels. The origin of those vascular fibers is dealt with next.

The Sympathetic Innervation of the Upper Limb

On p. 3, in the chapter on skin, brief mention was made of the sympathetic innervation of arteries. Figure 1-2 shows diagrammatically what is meant by vasoconstriction and vasodilation. The sympathetic supply to the upper limb reaches the limb mainly through connections from the stellate ganglion to the roots of the brachial plexus. More precisely, these connections, called rami communicantes, join the anterior rami of C8 and T1, the lowermost roots of the brachial plexus, which form the lowermost trunk.

ITEM 83-16. Trace the sympathetic trunk out of the thorax, and at the neck of the first rib you will find the stellate ganglion lying posterior to the vertebral artery. Sometimes the ganglion is in two parts, recognized as the inferior cervical ganglion and the first thoracic ganglion. Those two ganglia are usually fused into one ganglion, the stellate ganglion. Identify some of the rami communicantes between the stellate ganglion and the roots of the brachial plexus.

The nerve fibers in the rami communicantes are eventually distributed through the peripheral nerves to the arteries of the limb. An easily found example of a vascular branch of a peripheral nerve is the slender branch from the ulnar nerve to the proximal part of the ulnar artery.

A good, brief account of the components of the autonomic nervous system is included in *The Essentials of Neuro-anatomy*, by Mitchell (1966).

REVIEW

The student is well advised to ignore the classical concept of the well-defined separate regions, upper limb, thorax, and neck, and to look upon the root of the upper limb, the root of the neck, and the superior mediastinum as one region. If he has a clear understanding of the major vessels and nerves of the upper limb as they lie in that region, he will be well set to tackle the diagnosis of a vascular or neurologic peripheral disorder manifest in the hand while the cause nestles unseen somewhere in the root of the neck.

Accordingly, take the structures that have been exposed piece by piece. Put them together to establish their continuity as they proceed to the upper limb from the superior mediastinum and the neck, through what has been aptly described as an anatomic no mans land.

Dissection of the upper limb continues in two stages. In the first stage the muscles of the arm and forearm are mobilized; the purpose of this stage is orientation with minimal dissection. In the second stage there is maximal dissection in order to obtain the widest exposure of nerves and vessels. In the first stage, therefore, when the muscles are mobilized nerves and vessels will be mentioned only briefly, but because this is so, do not underestimate the significance of the nerves and vessels. Mobilize the muscles with reasonable care (see Fig. 50-1) and be alert for their neurovascular bundles.

The first series of muscles to be mobilized are those on the extensor aspect of the limb. They are muscles whose nerve supply passes through the posterior divisions and then the posterior cord of the brachial plexus. The second series of muscles are those on the flexor aspect of the arm and forearm. Their nerve supply passes through the anterior divisions and then the medial and lateral cords of the brachial plexus.

In advance of the dissection the terms pronation and supination must be explained. The forearm is supinated when you turn the palm up to receive loose change; it is pronated when you turn the palm down to spill the change into a box. The movements of supination and pronation occur at the radiohumeral and radioulnar joints. The forearm of an embalmed cadaver is usually pronated.

The anatomist describes the structures of the forearm as they are in the position of supination. In that position the forearm is "untwisted," so to speak, and the longitudinal structures are more parallel. The student dissecting a cadaveric forearm for the first time must note carefully the position of the forearm so that he may correlate his findings with standard anatomic descriptions. The descriptions and instructions in this text are based on the position of full supination. Once the forearm structures are mobilized it is possible to twist the forearm into supination and keep it there tied by string to an arm board.

Chapter 84

The Extensor Muscles of the Arm and Forearm

In the arm the extensor group consists entirely of the three heads of triceps. Except for anconeus, a very small muscle close to the elbow joint, triceps alone extends the elbow joint. Descriptions of triceps are confusing until you appreciate its three parts lie in two layers. Figure 84-1 shows how the *l*ong and *l*ateral heads (the two "l's") lie side by side on the same superficial plane while the medial head lies alone on a deeper plane. When this arrangement is appreciated it is quite easy to under-

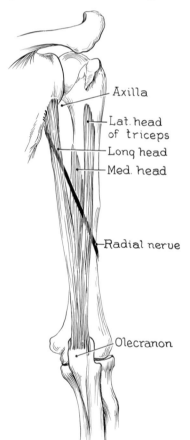

Axilla

Lat. head
of triceps

Long head

Med. head

Radial nerve

Olecranon

Figure 84-1. A schematic illustration to show how the long and lateral heads of triceps (the two "l's") lie on one plane and the medial head on another. The radial nerve travels inferolaterally between the two planes.

stand detailed descriptions that read: "The radial nerve and profunda vessels lie first between the long and medial head of triceps, then between the lateral and medial head." In simpler terms, the radial nerve and profunda vessels proceed inferolaterally between the two planes of triceps.

ITEM 84-1.   Dissection of the Extensor Muscles of the Arm

Identify the V-shaped junction of the long and lateral heads of triceps. Slip the tip of an index finger deep to the V and make a vertical incision to separate the long and lateral heads (Fig. 84-1) as far distally as the olecranon. The medial head of triceps is now exposed but, in addition, the radial nerve and the profunda vessels are seen crossing the muscle superiorly.

Investigate the thick aponeurosis of the triceps attached to the olecranon. The thickness is in keeping with the function of the muscle, powerful extension of the elbow.

Trace the branches of the radial nerve into the muscle.

Follow the radial nerve inferolaterally to where it leaves the extensor compartment to enter the flexor compartment of the arm, where the next stage of exposing the nerve will begin.

Extensor Muscles of the Forearm

In the forearm, on the extensor aspect, three groups of muscles can be identified (Fig. 84-2). Group I consists of the brachioradialis, extensor carpi radialis longus, and extensor carpi radialis brevis. These three muscles form the fleshy, mobile mass on the superolateral aspect of the forearm. A. K. Henry (1957) describes them as the "mobile wad of three." The brachioradialis is more obvious on the flexor aspect (Fig. 84-3).

Group II (Fig. 84-2) consists of the anconeus, extensor carpi ulnaris, and extensor digitorum (the extensor digiti minimi is an offshoot from the medial side of extensor digitorum). They lie on the same plane within an imaginary triangle, the base of which is the posterior border of the ulna and the apex the lateral epicondyle.

Group III (Fig. 84-2) includes the abductor pollicis longus, extensor pollicis brevis, extensor pollicis longus, and extensor indicis. The supinator is on the same plane as this group.

ITEM 84-2.   Dissection of Forearm

Specific instructions to slit open the separate compartments of the extensor retinaculum will not be given. The compartments are to be slit open as the tendons are completely mobilized.

Begin with Group I. Mobilize the brachioradialis and establish where its tendon is attached distally. The radial artery lies close to the tendon. Establish the humeral attachment close to the previously identified radial nerve.

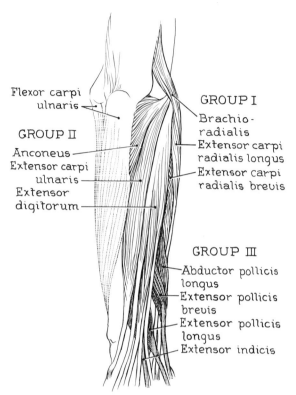

Flexor carpi
ulnaris

GROUP I
Brachio-
radialis
Extensor carpi
radialis longus
Extensor carpi
radialis brevis

GROUP II
Anconeus
Extensor carpi
ulnaris
Extensor
digitorum

GROUP III
Abductor pollicis
longus
Extensor pollicis
brevis
Extensor pollicis
longus
Extensor indicis

Figure 84-2.   Scheme to show how the extensor muscles of the forearm may be considered in three groups according to their location.

The muscle bellies of the extensor carpi radialis longus and brevis are adjacent to the brachioradialis, but their tendons run deep to the muscles of Group III. Leave these muscles undisturbed meantime.

Proceed to Group II and mobilize the extensor digitorum as far as the wrist. The lateral tendon of this muscle is joined by the tendon of the extensor indicis. An offshoot of the digitorum, the extensor digiti minimi, proceeds independently through the extensor retinaculum. How these tendons terminate will be reviewed when the hand is dissected.

The next muscle in Group II is the extensor carpi ulnaris. Mobilize the muscle and trace its tendon distally. Peel skin off the dorsum of the hand to expose the attachment of the tendon to the base of the fifth metacarpal bone.

Now cut across the belly of the extensor digitorum at the junction of its middle and distal thirds. Leave enough muscle distally so that the tendons may be reidentified when the hand is dissected.

Group III muscles are exposed by reflecting the extensor digi-

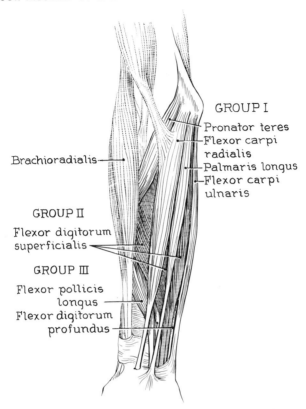

GROUP I
Pronator teres
Flexor carpi radialis
Palmaris longus
Flexor carpi ulnaris

Brachioradialis

GROUP II
Flexor digitorum superficialis

GROUP III
Flexor pollicis longus
Flexor digitorum profundus

Figure 84-3. Scheme to show how the flexor muscles of the forearm form three planes. Group I is superficial, group II is intermediate, and group III is deep. Brachioradialis and the extensor carpi muscles (Fig. 84-2) are considered as group I of the extensor aspect.

torum. Deep to this muscle find three muscles of the thumb, the extensor pollicis longus, extensor pollicis brevis, and abductor pollicis longus, in addition to the extensor indicis. Mobilize the tendons of the first two muscles of the thumb and extensor indicis just as far as the wrist. Mobilize the tendon of the abductor pollicis longus to its attachment to the base of the metacarpal bone of the thumb. Peel off skin from the base of the thumb if this is necessary.

Return now to the extensors carpi radialis longus and brevis. Mobilize their muscle bellies and trace their tendons distally. Peel skin off the dorsum of the hand to expose their distal attachments at the bases of the second and third metacarpal bones. Avoid cutting the tendon of the extensor pollicis longus.

Identify the Λ shaped interval between the extensor carpi radialis brevis and extensor digitorum. Along the line from the apex of the Λ to the lateral epicondyle, use your thumbs to separate the two muscle bellies. Begin at the apex, which is distal, and proceed to the epicondyle, which is proximal. The supinator is now in view, as are the terminal branches of the posterior interosseous nerve and vessels, which emerge from the supinator to reach the extensor muscles of the forearm.

The Radial Nerve

Experience reveals that it is opportune to complete dissection of the radial nerve at this time.

ITEM 84-3. Return to the point where the radial nerve left the extensor compartment of the arm to enter the flexor compartment. Using the thumbs, separate brachioradialis from the brachialis, a muscle on the anterior aspect of the humerus and the elbow joint. In the cleft between these muscles, the radial nerve descends to give off a major branch, the posterior interosseous nerve, and then continues deep to the brachioradialis.

Trace the posterior interosseous nerve into the supinator. To complete the dissection, return to the extensor aspect to the Λ shaped interval between extensor carpi radialis brevis and digitorum and reexamine supinator. Slide the tip of the scissors along the path of the posterior interosseous nerve and cut the supinator to expose the nerve.

A complete review of the radial nerve is given on p. 470.

Chapter 85

The Flexor Muscles of the Arm and Forearm

In the arm the flexor group includes the coracobrachialis, biceps brachii, and brachialis. The coracobrachialis (which may have been detached) is a flexor of the shoulder joint, lying in the superomedial region of the arm. The biceps, on the other hand, is a muscle with a long span; it stretches from its proximal attachments proximal to the shoulder joint to its distal attachment distal to the elbow joint and relative to the radioulnar joint. The biceps is primarily a supinator of the forearm, but acts also as a flexor of the elbow joint when the forearm is supinated (Basmajian and Latif, 1957). The brachialis is a flat muscle immediately related to the anterior aspect of the elbow joint. All three muscles are innervated by the musculocutaneous nerve, which usually passes through the substance of the coracobrachialis muscle.

ITEM 85-1. Dissection of the Flexor Muscles of the Arm and Forearm

One cannot mobilize the muscles of the flexor aspect of the arm and forearm without encountering major vessels and nerves. Proceed, therefore, with caution. Deal with the coracobrachialis first. Gently, because the musculocutaneous nerve is not robust, mobilize the muscle between its attachment proximally to the coracoid process and distally to the midshaft of the humerus.

Then mobilize the muscle belly of the biceps. Leave the tendon of its long head undisturbed until the shoulder joint is dissected, but mobilize the attachments of its short head to the coracoid process. Deep to the medial border of the biceps muscle belly lie the brachial artery and the median nerve. Therefore remain on the lateral aspect. Elevate the muscle belly from its bed and, by careful blunt dissection, release the musculocutaneous nerve; then proceed to the distal attachment of the muscle on the posteromedial aspect of the radial tuberosity. Be alert and avoid lacerating the important neurovascular structures you are bound to encounter.

Between the biceps and brachialis lies the musculocutaneous nerve. Avoiding the nerve, define the brachialis muscle. Observe the extent of its proximal attachment to the humerus and to the lateral intermuscular septum. Slide a finger distally on the anterior surface of the muscle to determine the muscle's distal attachment to the coronoid process of the ulna. Lying in the cleft between the brachialis and brachioradialis is the radial nerve. The anatomy of the flexor aspect of the arm is reviewed when the musculocutaneous nerve is considered in more detail (p. 471).

In the forearm three layers of muscles, superficial, intermediate, and deep, are readily identified. The superficial group is overlapped laterally by three muscles A. K. Henry describes as "the mobile wad of three" (Figs. 84-2 and 84-3), the brachioradialis and the long and short radial extensors of the wrist. Those three muscles have been dealt with fully in the dissection of the extensor aspect of the limb.

The superficial layer includes pronator teres, flexor carpi radialis, palmaris longus (sometimes absent), and flexor carpi ulnaris, in that order from lateral to medial.

The intermediate layer consists of one muscle, the flexor digitorum superficialis.

The deep layer consists of two muscles concerned with the fingers, namely, the flexor pollicis longus and the flexor digitorum profundus. In addition, a small muscle, pronator quadratus, will be found deep to the tendons of those two muscles as they proceed through the distal half of the flexor aspect of the forearm.

ITEM 85-2. The Superficial Muscle Layer

Bearing in mind that the neurovascular bundle to each muscle will not be specially named, mobilize the muscle bellies of the superficial group. Their proximal attachment is essentially to the medial epicondyle.

Pull the muscle belly of the brachioradialis laterally to expose the radial attachment of pronator teres. The radial artery and the radial nerve are also seen when the brachioradialis is pulled laterally.

The pronator teres is related posteriorly first to the median nerve and second to the ulnar artery.

Clean the muscle carefully and trace it proximally to its humeral attachment. The pronator teres is one muscle that must be cleaned completely to assure success in the further stages of dissection. Make sure its superior and inferior borders are distinct. At this time it is worth cleaning the median nerve and the short length of the ulnar artery between the bifurcation of the brachial artery and the pronator teres.

Next, identify the muscle belly of the flexor carpi radialis. The tendon of the flexor carpi radialis proceeds into the hand and cannot be exposed fully at present.

The palmaris longus may be absent. Although it seems to be a muscle of little consequence, it has an important relationship to the median nerve. When the muscle is present, its tendon lies anterior and medial to the median nerve at the wrist. Both structures may be cut when the wrist is slashed. In the consequent repair the doctor must be careful to identify the structures correctly so that he does not inadvertently suture the proximal cut end of the nerve to the distal cut end of the tendon. Such a mishap may seem impossible on inspection of a wrist laid bare in the dissecting laboratory. In the emergency room of a hospital, however, under vastly different circumstances, the mishap is a real possibility.

Confirm that the flexor carpi ulnaris is attached not only to the medial humeral epicondyle but also to the olecranon and the posterior border of the ulna. Its flat muscle belly swathes the medial aspect of the forearm and so covers the flexor profundus digitorum. It is the bulky muscle belly of the profundus that gives the characteristic shape to the medial aspect of the forearm. Pull the flexor carpi ulnaris medially to expose the ulnar artery and ulnar nerve lying superficial to profundus in the distal third of the forearm. Trace the tendon of the flexor carpi ulnaris to its distal attachment, the pisiform bone.

Mark and cut the tendons of flexor carpi radialis and palmaris longus. This is done so that their muscle bellies may be displaced more easily to expose the intermediate muscle, the flexor digitorum superficialis.

ITEM 85-3. The Intermediate Muscle Layer
The flexor digitorum superficialis has a flat muscle belly giving rise

to two pairs of tendons, one pair for the ring and middle fingers, the other pair for the little and index fingers. The tendons for the ring and middle fingers are the more superficial. Identify all four tendons of this muscle, and then, by pulling on the fingers, establish to which finger they belong.

The median nerve passes deep, first of all, to the pronator teres then to the proximal border of the flexor superficialis digitorum, which lies under the so-called sublimis bridge (sublimis is equivalent to superficialis). The nerve proceeds distally, adhering to the deep surface of the muscle. At the wrist the nerve appears from under the lateral border of the muscle. Identify the nerve at the wrist.

ITEM 85-4.   The Deep Muscle Layer

Pull the flexor carpi ulnaris medially and the flexor digitorum superficialis laterally, while the wrist is flexed, to improve access to the deep layer. The flexor digitorum profundus is now seen. Manipulate the fingers to demonstrate the tendons of the muscle.

Lateral to the muscle belly of the profundus lies the muscle belly of the flexor pollicis longus. By manipulating the thumb confirm that you have correctly identified the tendon and muscle belly of that muscle.

Deep to the tendons of the flexor digitorum profundus you can see the pronator quadratus.

Chapter 86

The Vessels and Nerves of the Upper Limb

The second stage of the dissection is to trace the vessels and nerves from the axilla to the wrist.

THE MAJOR ARTERIES

Axillary artery
Brachial artery

Radial artery
Ulnar artery

ITEM 86-1.   Identify the axillary artery. It continues under a different name, the brachial artery (see Fig. 83-1), into the upper limb. The brachial artery is accompanied at first by the median and ulnar nerves, but the ulnar nerve soon departs, leaving the median nerve and brachial artery to travel together, first in the shelter of the biceps muscle, then deep to the bicipital aponeurosis. Confirm those facts.

Having entered the forearm, the brachial artery divides into the radial and ulnar arteries. Trace the radial artery to the wrist, where it becomes subcutaneous and may be compressed against the radius. On both your wrists identify the pulsations of the radial artery and compress the artery against the radius. Trace the ulnar artery deep to pronator teres, and then distally as far as the lateral aspect of the pisiform bone of the carpus. In its course through the forearm the artery meets and accompanies the ulnar nerve.

To appreciate the full importance of these three arteries, brachial, ulnar, and radial, read the commentary Arterial Distribution on p. 255.

NERVES

The Nerves to the Extensor Muscles of the Upper Limb

Circumflex nerve
Radial nerve

The Circumflex Nerve

This nerve has already been identified entering the deltoid and at its origin from the posterior cord. Now, as a review, trace the nerve from the cord and note that it passes close to the shoulder joint, where it is vulnerable to pressure from the head of the humerus if the bone has been dislocated from its socket. After reduction of a dislocation of the shoulder the integrity of the nerve must be checked. How?

The Radial Nerve

From the posterior cord, trace the radial nerve inferolaterally and observe that, of the major nerves in the axilla, it is the one most obviously slung across the cavity of the axilla. In this position it is vulnerable to pressure from the crosspiece of the upper end of a crutch. Thus, a patient obliged to use crutches is advised not to lean on the crutches but to use his "arms" to support his weight. Once you have reviewed the posterior interosseous nerve, a branch of the radial nerve, determine the form of "crutch" paralysis.

Trace the radial nerve into the plane of cleavage between the medial head of triceps anteriorly and the long and lateral head of triceps on the same plane posteriorly. The nerve supplies the three heads of the triceps. Trace the nerve distally to the point where it pierces the lateral intermuscular septum. Observe its relationship to the shaft of the humerus.

Now turn to the anterolateral aspect of the lower humeral region. Identify the muscle bellies of the brachioradialis and brachialis. Separate them and, in the cleft between them, find the radial nerve. Trace the nerve distally until it is beyond the elbow joint.

The muscular branches arising from the radial nerve before the nerve passes the elbow joint are branches to the triceps, anconeus, brachioradialis, and extensor carpi radialis longus.

Find the posterior interosseous branch of the radial nerve. Then trace the posterior interosseous branch into and out of the supinator muscle. Pronate and supinate the forearm, establish the relationship of the nerve to the head and neck of the radius, and appreciate that the nerve is easily injured by ill-advised surgical exposures about the radial neck, which may result in paralysis of the long extensors to the fingers and the thumb (Turek, 1959). Here, then, is an excellent region to illustrate why a knowledge of anatomy, attention to detail, and common sense are essential for first class orthopedic surgery.

The posterior interosseous nerve supplies the following muscles in order: the extensor carpi radialis brevis, supinator, extensor carpi ulnaris, extensor pollicis brevis, extensor indicis, extensor pollicis longus, extensor digiti minimi, extensor digitorum, abductor pollicis longus. In brief, apart from the extensor carpi radialis longus and brachioradialis, supplied by the radial nerve, the posterior interosseous nerve supplies the extensors of the wrist, the extensors of the fingers, and the extensors and the long abductor of the thumb. The result of paralysis of the nerve is termed dropped wrist. Why?

The Nerves to the Flexor Muscles of the Upper Limb

Musculocutaneous Nerve

Median nerve

Ulnar nerve

ITEM 86-2. Identify the musculocutaneous nerve arising from the lateral cord and piercing the coracobrachialis. Trace the nerve from the coracobrachialis into the plane of cleavage between the biceps and brachialis. The nerve supplies those muscles and terminates as a cutaneous nerve to the lateral aspect of the forearm.

At this time it is opportune to introduce a simple principle applicable to all nerve lesions (injury to a nerve is spoken of clinically as a nerve lesion). The principle can best be expounded by the question, "If the musculocutaneous nerve is severed after it leaves the shelter of biceps, will the victim have paralysis of the coracobrachialis, biceps, and brachialis?" In other words, the extent of motor or sensory loss after a nerve lesion depends precisely upon where the lesion is located.

ITEM 86-3. Identify the median nerve arising by two roots, one from the lateral cord and one from the medial. The nerve passes through the arm closely related to the brachial artery in the shelter of the biceps muscle. Note how the nerve and artery are separated from the supracondylar part of the shaft of the humerus and from the elbow joint by the brachialis. The nerve and vessel are vulnerable in supracondylar fractures of the humerus and in dislocations of the elbow joint. Recall that the nerve and vessel lie deep to the bicipital aponeurosis.

In the arm, i.e., between the shoulder and elbow, the median nerve has no branches although it may have one or more connections with the ulnar nerve. These connections are said to explain variations in the nerve supply of the small muscles of the hand.

The median nerve enters the forearm and passes deep to the pronator teres. To expose the nerve slide the tip of a pair of curved scissors into position on the anterior aspect of the nerve, and with a scalpel cut through the pronator teres to expose the scissors, and the nerve.

After passing the pronator teres, the median nerve passes deep to the flexor digitorum superficialis. To expose the nerve slide the scissors into position deep to the radial attachment of the muscle. Cut the radial attachment to expose the scissors. Turn the muscle medially and the entire course of the median nerve in the forearm comes into view.

The anterior interosseous branch of the median nerve can now be found going to supply the flexor pollicis longus and the lateral half of the flexor digitorum profundus.

Complete this stage of the dissection by tracing the median nerve as far as the carpal tunnel. The palmar cutaneous brach of the nerve may be found. The close relationship of the median nerve to the tendon of the palmaris longus has already been referred to (p. 468).

Finally, if you have time, confirm that the median nerve supplies all the flexor muscles of the forearm except the flexor carpi ulnaris and the medial half of the flexor digitorum profundus.

ITEM 86-4. The ulnar nerve should be identified leaving the medial cord of the brachial plexus. The nerve travels for a short distance with the brachial artery and median nerve; then it leaves them to proceed posteroinferiorly toward the medial epicondyle. Confirm that that is so.

At the elbow joint the nerve becomes subcutaneous. Furthermore, it is an immediate medial relation of the elbow joint. Thus the nerve can easily be involved in fractures of the medial epicondyle and in fracture-dislocations of the elbow joint.

Passing beyond the elbow joint, the nerve passes deep to the flexor carpi ulnaris bridge to enter the forearm. Using the closed-open scissors technique, trace the ulnar nerve posterior to the medial epicondyle and under the flexor carpi ulnaris bridge. Cut the bridge and expose fully the ulnar nerve.

Before proceeding further, observe how it is feasible to transplant the ulnar nerve to the anterior aspect of the medial epicondyle. The transplant is employed for the following reason. Flexion of the elbow is normally accompanied by gliding of the ulnar nerve posterior to the medial epicondyle. Sometimes, however, after an injury the alignment of the skeleton may be altered sufficiently to cause stretching of the ulnar nerve in flexing the elbow, a state of affairs that cannot be allowed to persist because of the eventual deleterious effect upon the nerve. It is under those circumstances that ulnar nerve transplantation is undertaken. Transplantation is also used to "lengthen" the nerve when the nerve has been cut and it is not possible to bring the cut ends easily together to be sutured. It is always interesting how significant anatomy becomes when its application is understood.

In the forearm, pull the flexor carpi ulnaris medially and observe how the ulnar nerve and artery meet and journey together on the flexor profundus digitorum toward the lateral aspect of the pisiform bone. If you have time, identify the branches of the ulnar nerve to the flexor carpi ulnaris and the medial half of the flexor profundus digitorum. Occasionally, in dissecting a cadaver one finds a vascular branch from the ulnar nerve to the ulnar artery to illustrate by example how the sympathetic part of the autonomic nervous system controls the caliber of the entire arterial system.

All the pertinent structures relative to the anatomy of the hand have now been revealed as far as the wrist.

Chapter 87

The Hands

The selection of a key from a bunch of keys, the choice of a coin from a handful of coins, the buttoning of a garment, the signing of your name, the twist of a door handle—these are a very few of the effortless activities of a normal pair of hands taken for granted. Behind these effortless activities, however, lies the infinite control of the human brain. Realizing the bond between the hands and the brain, Wood Jones, a distinguished anatomist, wrote thus: "What we are admiring in the multitude of actions of the useful human hand is the human cerebral perfection, not the bones, the muscles, and joints which carry out complex volitions" (Wood Jones, 1944). The same idea was expressed by Michelangelo in quaint but impressive language: "It is necessary to keep one's compass in one's eyes, and not in the hand, for the hands execute, but the eye judges." When one appreciates the bond between the activity of the brain and the action of the hands, it is easy to understand why the disabling effect of an injury to the hand is far out of proportion to the extent of the injury. Clearly, once the hand is maimed, restoration of its functions is imperative.

The student of anatomy must realize, however, that restoration of function does not necessarily mean complete restoration of structure. Of course sensory and motor nerves and blood supply must be reestablished, but the function of the hand is to grip. Accordingly, it may well be necessary to remove, displace, refashion, or replace skin, muscles, tendons, bones, and joints of the hand in order to restore the grip. Sometimes, indeed, after extensive surgical procedures, the restored hand looks like a lobster claw, but it can grip.

Clinically three grades of grip are recognized, namely the pinch grip, the grip, and the power grip. In the pinch grip the object is held between the pulps of the fingers and the pulp of the thumb; in the grip it is held firmly but not tightly within the hand; in the power grip it is held tightly. That all three grades of grip may be restored almost completely to a mutilated hand is testimony to the skill of modern reconstructive surgery.

The student of the anatomy of the hand cannot ignore its function. Indeed, in the hand, function and structure go hand in hand.

Chapter 88

The Skin, Sensation, and Movements of the Hand

The Skin of the Hand

To demonstrate the remarkable texture of the skin of the hand, first stretch and spread the fingers of your own hand, and then make a tight fist. Observe how the skin of both the palmar and dorsal surfaces of the hand, especially of the fingers, accommodates with ease and with a mark of elegance to the movements of the hand. Then identify the special features illustrated in Figure 88-1. Once you have seen a patient whose hands are hidebound following severe burns and inadequate medical care, you will realize how much the use of the normal hand depends upon the plasticity of the skin. So called redundant skin over the knuckles and skin creases, illustrated to some extent in Figure 88-1, are of more than passing interest, for they are mainly responsible for the plasticity of the skin of the hand and therefore must be taken into account in surgical procedures on the hand. For example, incisions that cross skin creases are not recommended because residual scar tissue may reduce the range of movement normally allowed for by the creases.

The skin and underlying layers are not easily separated on the hand of an embalmed cadaver, for the skin is, usually, hard and unyielding. Appreciate, therefore, that in life the epidermis (see Fig. 1-1) of the palmar surface of the hand may be soft, lily-white, and easily blistered, or it may be studded with calluses as tough as horn. The dermis (see Fig. 1-1) is dense but it is also mobile. The subcutaneous fat lies in pads; numerous strong fibrous septa binding the dermis to the deep fascia divide the fat into lobules; the pads resemble sponge rubber, with fat instead of air. The deep fascia is thin where it covers the muscles of the thenar and hypothenar eminences, but it is dense in the midpalm, where the fascia, the palmar aponeurosis, covers the long tendons to the index, middle, ring, and little fingers and many vessels and nerves. Together these four layers, the epidermis, the dermis, the subcutaneous fat, and the deep fascia, provide for the palmar surface of the hand a covering that, in life, is tough and yet exquisitely sensitive. Furthermore the fat

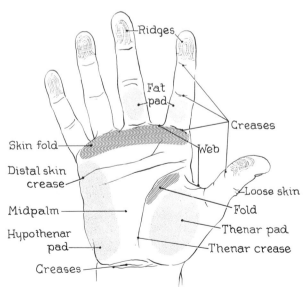

Figure 88-1. The palmar aspect of the hand. Identify the features illustrated on your own hand.

pads strengthen the grip while they mold themselves to the object held. The mobility of the layers of the palm allows a quick release when the grip goes slack. Similar fat pads are present on the sole of the foot and on the heel, where they function as cushions to soften the impact of the tread.

On the dorsum of the hand the epidermis, dermis, subcutaneous fascia, and deep fascia are much thinner and much more mobile than on the palm. Compare the skin on the back of your own hand with that on the palm. Having done so you will appreciate why the abnormal amount of fluid (edema) that may appear in response to an infection of the palm of the hand makes its appearance on the dorsum of the hand rather than in the palm.

Sensation in the Hand

The exquisite sensibility of the hands, especially of the tips of the fingers while they caress an objet d'art, is well known to all students and needs no further description. Nevertheless, surgeons experienced in the restoration of function to the injured hand stress the importance of restoring sensory nerves as well as motor nerves. "Without sensation in the hand, a manual worker is greatly crippled. . ." (Bunnell, 1948).

Clearly the sensibility of the hands requires further discussion, but it involves a knowledge of special nerve endings, central pathways, and modalities of sensation beyond the scope of this text. The anatomy, however, of the cutaneous nerves of the hand is within the scope of this text. Their distribution is of considerable clinical importance, so the student should locate as best he can the cutaneous nerves of the hand, especially those of the fingers, while he skins the hand of a cadaver.

The distribution of the cutaneous nerves of the hand is beautifully illustrated in Grant's Atlas, Figures 83, 84, and 85. It should be noted,

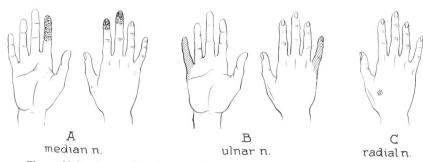

| A | B | C |
| median n. | ulnar n. | radial n. |

Figure 88-2. Areas of total sensory loss after each of the three main nerves to the hand have been cut. (Adapted from S. Bunnell: Surgery of the Hand. Philadelphia. J. B. Lippincott Co., 1948.)

however, that the area of total anesthesia when a nerve is severed is much smaller than the distribution of the nerve (Fig. 88-2).

Exercise

On the hand of the cadaver scratch a line to indicate the boundaries of the areas of skin innervated by the median, ulnar, and radial nerves. Also trace the boundaries of those areas on your own hand.

Movements of the Hand

Many of the muscles of the hand are named according to the movements they control, and some of these movements are not in the same direction as movements with the same name elsewhere in the body. Accordingly, to prevent the student's jumping to erroneous conclusions, the movements of the hand are dealt with now (Fig. 88-3). In the following description "fingers" refers only to the index, middle, ring, and little fingers, and does not include the thumb. To demonstrate the movements on your own hand proceed as follows:

Fingers

Flexion Clench the fingers to make a fist.

Extension Stretch the fingers as in pointing with the index finger.

Abduction Keep the fingers straight and spread them away from each other. The middle finger is unusual; it can abduct to one or other side of the center line (Fig. 88-3).

Adduction Keep the fingers straight and press them together. The middle finger can adduct to the center line from one side or the other (Fig. 88-3).

Thumb

Flexion Clench the fist and the thumb flexes.

Extension Spread the fingers and thumb. Note that the axis for flexion and extension of the thumb is at right angles to the axis for flexion and extension of the fingers.

Abduction Hold the hand palm uppermost and point the thumb to the ceiling.

Adduction Hold the hand palm uppermost. Keep the thumb straight and place it alongside the index finger. The plane of

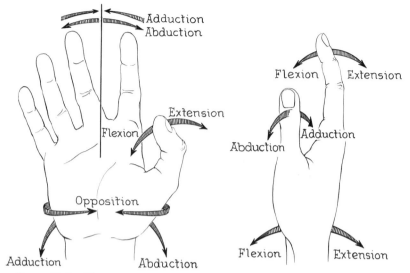

Figure 88-3. The movements of the wrist, palm of the hand, fingers, and thumb.

abduction and adduction of the thumb is at right angles to the plane of abduction and adduction of the fingers.

Opposition   Bring the borders of the palm toward each other to cup the palm. Observe that there is opposition of both the hypothenar and thenar eminences as each eminence moves toward the midpalm. As a result of opposition, the thumb is rotated so that its tip faces and can easily touch the tips of the fingers. In opposition, however, it is the cupping of the palm and the rotation of the thumb that are significant.

Chapter 89

The Muscles and Tendons of the Index Finger

Rather than remove skin from every finger it is recommended that the student concentrate on a careful dissection of the index finger and thumb, both of which are the essential parts of the grip.

In removing skin from the hand of a corpse it is customary to begin with the palm. Experience, however, has shown that the significant structures to the index finger are not so frequently lacerated when the following approach is adopted.

REMOVAL OF SKIN FROM THE FINGER AND THUMB

ITEM 89-1. On the dorsal aspects of both the finger and thumb, make shallow longitudinal incisions (Fig. 89-1). Elevate the apex of the triangular flap bounded by the incisions and proceed to reflect the flap toward the web of the thumb. Where it is necessary, make judicious cuts in the skin you are reflecting to create extra flaps rather than struggle to remove the skin in one piece. At all times, keep the blade of the knife directed toward the skin and not toward the underlying tissues.

ITEM 89-2. The extensor tendons to the index finger and to the thumb are visible and should be used constantly as a guide to depth. With care so that you do not go deeper than the extensor tendon and the dorsal expansion, reflect the flaps to each side of the index finger. Reflect the flaps far enough to expose the dorsal expansion as well as the attachments of the extensor tendon itself. A similar procedure will be adopted for the palmar surface of the finger. Do likewise for the thumb.

ITEM 89-3. In this next step proceed with caution because of the presence of cutaneous nerves and arteries. Continue to remove skin

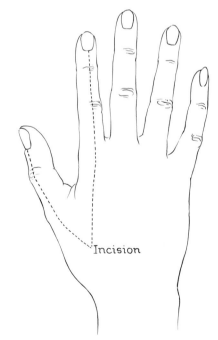

Figure 89-1. The incision recommended for skinning the index finger and thumb.

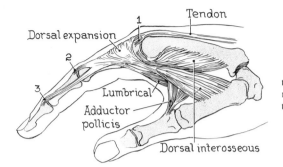

Figure 89-2. Muscles and tendons exposed as skin is removed from the dorsal aspect of the index finger and thumb.

from between the thumb and index finger. The first dorsal interosseous muscle will appear and its attachment to the dorsal expansion can be recognized (Fig. 89-2). In order to expose the muscle adequately you may have to remove areolar tissue by blunt dissection until the muscle belly is clearly seen. Then locate the first lumbrical muscle. Each lumbrical muscle lies in a sheath of fascia termed a lumbrical canal. Parallel to its lateral border of the first lumbrical muscle lies the digital nerve to the lateral aspect of the index finger.

ITEM 89-4. Expose (do not incise) the fibrous flexor sheath by means of a longitudinal incision the length of the palmar aspect of the index finger. Carefully reflect the flaps to each side and expect to reveal the cutaneous nerves and digital vessels to the index finger. If the hand is very "fleshy" there may be a considerable amount of fat between the skin and the fibrous sheath.

ITEM 89-5. With the dorsal expansion and its attached muscles, cutaneous nerves and digital arteries now in view, judiciously remove all skin from the index finger.

If you have been successful you should have exposed a perfect example of the dorsal expansion (Fig. 89-2). Completion of the dissection of the palm, however, is essential before you study the function of the expansion.

REMOVAL OF SKIN FROM THE PALM

ITEM 89-6. The palmar aponeurosis is fixed to the skin by numerous septa, especially numerous at the skin creases. In an embalmed hand the septa are particularly tough, so separation of the skin from the aponeurosis is difficult even with a sharp scalpel. Thus in removing skin it is usual to remove some of the aponeurosis too. Furthermore, the digital vessels and nerves, which appear at the distal margin of the aponeurosis, are liable to be lacerated. However, it is important to see the nature of the aponeurosis, if not its extent.

ITEM 89-7. Identify the ulnar artery and nerve. Thrust closed, blunt-ended curved scissors along their route into the palm. Open the scissors as you withdraw them. Cut the skin parallel to the vessel and nerve as you proceed. Proceed only a few centimeters, until you see the vessel and nerve divide. As the ulnar artery and nerve enter the palm they are superficial to the flexor retinaculum with which the apex of the palmar aponeurosis blends. Reflect the lateral (radial) margin of the incision across the midpalm to expose the palmar aponeurosis.

Now continue to remove skin from the midpalm to the bases of the fingers. This is hard work, especially with a blunt scalpel, but persevere until you see the aponeurosis dividing into four slips, one for each finger. Accordingly three intervals, or archways, will appear, through which three sets of digital vessels and nerves emerge.

Finally, using the digital nerve and artery to the medial (ulnar) side of the little finger as a guide to the correct depth, skin the hypothenar eminence. Then—but proceed cautiously, for the motor branch of the median nerve is superficial, in fact subcutaneous—skin the thenar eminence.

THE PALMAR APONEUROSIS

Even in a crude dissection the palmar aponeurosis is easily recognized because it is strong and in possession of fairly well defined medial and lateral edges. The aponeurosis is triangular in shape; its apex gains attachment to the flexor retinaculum as well as receives the tendon of the palmaris longus when the palmaris longus is present. The base of the aponeurosis lies at the bases of the fingers, and from the aponeurosis a fibrous prolongation extends distally into each finger to blend with the fibrous flexor sheath. For several reasons the palmar aponeurosis is clinically significant, but the reason selected to illuminate the anatomy of the aponeurosis is Dupuytren's contracture.

Dupuytren's contracture affects the deep fascia of the hand, particularly the prolongations of the palmar aponeurosis to the little and ring fingers. The fascia becomes thickened and, losing its resilience, contracts, pulling the fingers into a permanently flexed position. The treatment is expert surgical removal of the deep fascia, including the palmar aponeurosis. There is no doubt that such surgery requires skill and patience, not only because of the extent and the intricacies of the deep fascia but also because of its vulnerable neurovascular relationships. The following rough summary of a method for removing the palmar aponeurosis is adapted from *Surgery of the Hand*, (Bunnell, 1948). In this way the significant anatomy of the aponeurosis is quickly demonstrated.

ITEM 89-8. Removal of the Palmar Aponeurosis

Return to the ulnar artery as it enters the palm. Trace it distally to where it divides into a deep branch proceeding into the depths of the palm and a superficial branch. Using the closed-open scissors technique, mobilize the superficial branch as it proceeds deep to the palmar aponeurosis. Snip the aponeurosis until the superficial palmar arch (the continuation of the superficial ulnar branch) is fully exposed. It may be joined by a palmar branch from the radial artery. Then, with strong toothed forceps, or, preferably, a pair of hemostats, seize the aponeurosis, elevate it, and demonstrate the fibrous septa that leave its deep surface to enter the depths of the palm. Pull the aponeurosis toward the fingers and snip, close to the aponeurosis, the various septa. Continue until the tendons of the index, middle, ring, and little fingers and accompanying structures lie exposed.

THE FLEXOR RETINACULUM

Examine the carpus of an articulated skeleton and observe that it is "hollowed out." Its anterior surface is concave and somewhat quadrangular in shape. At each corner there is a bony landmark; these are the tubercle of the scaphoid, the ridge of the trapezium, the hook of the hamate, and the pisiform on the triquetrum. Identify those landmarks on the cadaver and on your own hand. Between them the flexor retinaculum extends. Now examine your specimen. The retinaculum is a tough band of tissue continuous proximally with the deep fascia of the forearm and distally with the palmar aponeurosis. The retinaculum converts the anterior concave surface of the carpus into the carpal tunnel for the long flexor tendons and the median nerve. Clinically it happens that the median nerve may be "compressed" as it advances into the tunnel for reasons not fully established. The sensory and motor signs that result are known as the carpal tunnel syndrome.

ITEM 89-9.   Keeping toward the ulnar side, open the carpal tunnel by using the closed-open scissors technique along the flexor tendons. Snip the retinaculum as you proceed. Once the retinaculum is completely divided the median nerve is fully exposed. The motor branch of the median nerve, also known as its recurrent branch or its thenar branch, should be clearly visible curving acutely toward the thenar eminence. Identify it and the several digital cutaneous branches of the median nerve itself. With care it should be possible to demonstrate the tiny, but nevertheless important, branch to the first lumbrical muscle. It is a branch of the digital nerve to the lateral (radial) side of the index finger.

ITEM 89-10.   Having passed through the carpal tunnel and then deep to the palmar aponeurosis, the long flexor tendons to each finger enter a fibrous flexor sheath. Trace the flexor tendons of the index finger into their fibrous sheath; then slit the sheath as far as the tip of the finger. Observe how the sheath thins out on the palmar aspect of the joints. In disturbing the fibrous sheath and tendons you have also disturbed the synovial sheath. The surface of the tendons is slimy with synovia.

Read the account of synovial sheaths (p. 258) and then a more detailed account of the synovial sheaths of the hand.

ITEM 89-11. The relationship of the tendon of the flexor digitorum superficialis to the flexor digitorum profundus should be studied next. Review their arrangement in the forearm. Then observe how the profundus tendon penetrates the superficialis and how the tendon of the superficialis is molded at all times to the profundus tendon. The superficialis tendon is inserted into the palmar surface of the middle phalanx, the profundus tendon into the base of the distal phalanx.

ITEM 89-12. Of the various muscles acting on the index finger, the last one to be demonstrated is the first palmar interosseous muscle. To do so, remove the skin from the web between the index and middle fingers. By blunt dissection clear away areolar tissue to reveal the deep transverse ligament between the adjacent heads of the metacarpal bones. Slit the ligament to demonstrate the palmar interosseous muscle that lies posterior to it. Trace the muscle to its insertion. It is a slender muscle, not well seen from this angle, but it will be seen to better advantage in the voyage through the depths of the palm. It is worth drawing your attention to the obvious dorsal interosseous muscle to the lateral (radial) side of the middle finger, which is much more obvious than the palmar interosseous muscle to the index finger. All the dorsal interosseous muscles are more bulky than their palmar counterparts.

ITEM 89-13. The Dorsal Expansion

The attachments to the dorsal expansion have now all been exposed. By moving the finger and by pulling the attachments demonstrate how the expansion glides proximally and distally. The demonstration is never very convincing in a cadaver because of the artificial adherence of the expansion to the underlying proximal phalanx. You are seeking only to demonstrate a long-established principle, more easily seen on autopsy specimens and in the course of operative procedures.

Review

The muscles acting on the index finger are divided into two groups for descriptive purposes, an extrinsic and an intrinsic group. The extrinsic group includes the extensor digitorum and indicis and the flexor digitorum superficialis and profundus. The intrinsic group is composed of the first lumbrical muscle and a dorsal and a palmar interosseous muscle. Review the attachments of these muscles before proceeding to the next section.

MUSCLE ACTION ON THE INDEX FINGER

There is a marvelous balance of muscle power in the hand, not only between the extrinsic muscles and the intrinsic muscles, but also between the flexors and extensors. "The whole arrangement in the finger shows perfect synchronism, each muscle and tendon doing its part, conserving its limited amplitude of motion and so relaying its action that by co-ordination with each other the complete motion is carried out" (Bunnell, 1948). The outcome in the normal hand is movement so smooth and effortless that the change from one muscle to the other goes on unseen.

When it is difficult to comprehend the various joint movements and muscle actions that are involved in a synchronized activity of the limbs, it is best to select a key structure and study its function in certain basic static positions. This has been done here. The dorsal expansion is considered to be a key structure and the two basic static positions are moderate flexion of the finger and full extension.

Finger Flexion

In Figure 89-3 the lower finger is in moderate flexion. The dorsal expansion is distal relative to the metacarpophalangeal joint (often abbreviated to m/p), and the tendons of the lumbrical and the interosseous muscles lie anterior to the axis of the joint. Another important fact (not illustrated) must now be taken into consideration. The proximal attachment of the lumbricals is to the tendons of the flexor profundus digitorum. Thus, in flexion, as the flexor profundus tendons withdraw from the palm the lumbrical muscles accompany them. In other words, the lumbrical muscles are maintained at an optimal length for contraction throughout flexion of the fingers. The two factors mentioned, that is, the relationship of lumbrical tendon to the axis of the metacarpophalangeal joint and the maintenance of an optimal length of its muscle belly, allow the lumbrical to flex the metacarpophalangeal joint.

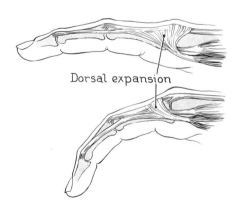

Dorsal expansion

Figure 89-3. The two basic locations of the dorsal expansion with reference to the metacarpophalangeal joint (for further discussion return to the text). The dorsal expansion is also known as the extensor expansion and as the extensor hood.

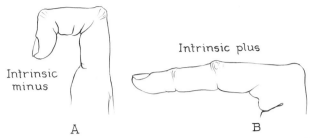

Figure 89-4. In *A*, the intrinsic muscles to the finger are paralyzed, so full flexion of the metacarpophalangeal joint is absent. In *B*, only the long flexor muscles of the finger are paralyzed, so it is flexion of the interphalangeal joints that is absent. Clinically, these two positions, demonstrated on flexion of the finger, are referred to as the intrinsic minus and the intrinsic plus positions.

To be more precise, clinical experience reveals that the lumbrical muscles, assisted by the interossei, are in fact responsible for the final degrees of flexion of the metacarpophalangeal joints. When the intrinsic muscles are paralyzed the fingers, on flexion, adopt the so-called intrinsic-minus position (Fig. 89-4). And when the extrinsic flexors are paralyzed the fingers, on flexion, adopt the intrinsic-plus position (Fig. 89-4).

The main points concerning flexion of a finger are summarized as follows:

(1) The flexor digitorum profundus flexes the distal and proximal interphalangeal joints.

(2) The flexor digitorum superficialis flexes the proximal interphalangeal joint.

(3) Both muscles just listed flex the metacarpophalangeal joint, but not completely (see 4).

(4) The lumbrical muscle and the interossei flex the metacarpophalangeal joint completely. Thus, when the intrinsic muscles are paralyzed the finger cannot be flexed into the palm, as in making a fist.

Finger Extension

In Figure 89-3 the upper finger is extended and the dorsal expansion is proximal relative to the metacarpophalangeal joint. The tendons of the lumbrical muscle and the interossei are now on the same plane as the axis of the metacarpophalangeal joint. Thus, when the lumbrical contracts, that joint remains immobile while the pull is transmitted distally to extend the intermediate and distal interphalangeal joints.

Extension of the interphalangeal joints when the metacarpophalangeal joint is flexed is an important movement that must now be considered. When the metacarpophalangeal joint is fully flexed, extension of the interphalangeal joints is achieved by the slips of the extensor tendon to the intermediate and distal phalanges (2 and 3, Fig. 89-2), and not by the lumbrical and interosseous muscles. Thus, the summary of the action of the lumbrical muscle that is usually given in anatomical texts, namely, "it flexes the metacarpophalangeal joint and extends the interphalangeal joints" is not accurate. The two events do not occur at the same time. The lumbrical and interosseous muscles only extend the interphalangeal joints when the metacarpophalangeal joint itself is extended.

The main points concerning extension of the index finger are summarized as follows:

(1) extensor digitorum extends the metacarpophalangeal joint.

(2) when the metacarpophalangeal joint is flexed the interphalangeal joints are extended by extensor digitorum.

(3) when the metacarpophalangeal joint is extended the interphalangeal joints are extended by the lumbrical.

The interossei abduct or adduct the finger as indicated in Figure 88-3. Abduction and adduction are most powerful when the fingers are fully extended.

Exercise

Flex and extend your index finger and analyze the muscle actions responsible for the movements.

Chapter 90

The Muscles and Tendons of the Thumb

The extrinsic muscles are the abductor pollicis longus, extensor pollicis longus and brevis, and flexor pollicis longus.

The intrinsic muscles are the abductor pollicis brevis, flexor pollicis brevis, opponens pollicis, and adductor pollicis.

ITEM 90-1. The tendons of the extrinsic muscles are to be mobilized now and their distal attachments should be established. In doing so synovial sheaths are to be taken into consideration. Read the account of synovial sheaths (p. 258).

The extensor pollicis longus and brevis were exposed when skin was removed from the dorsum of the thumb. Mobilize those tendons to their distal attachments, and in doing so review their attachments in the forearm.

The tendon of the abductor pollicis longus has already been mobilized to its insertion into the base of the metacarpal bone to the thumb.

ITEM 90-2. To reach the flexor pollicis longus proceed thus. Remove all skin from the thumb. Mobilize the median nerve proximal to the carpal tunnel. Place two ligatures about 1 cm. apart on the nerve. Cut the nerve between the ligatures and "peel" the distal part out of the carpal tunnel. Elevate the nerve and by blunt dissection isolate its peripheral branches, including the branch to the muscles of the thenar eminence. The way is now clear to trace the tendon of the flexor pollicis longus through the carpal tunnel into its fibrous sheath. Do so and slit the sheath to expose the tendon as far as its distal attachment.

ITEM 90-3. To examine the intrinsic muscles of the thumb proceed as follows: Mobilize by blunt dissection the flexor pollicis brevis and the abductor pollicis brevis. Both lie on the same plane superficial to opponens pollicis. The opponens must be clearly seen. Therefore divide the two superficial muscles and reflect them clear to bring opponens into full view.

To see adductor pollicis clearly it is necessary to divide between ligatures the long flexor tendons at the level of the carpal tunnel. Then "peel" the tendons distally. By finger dissection clear away areolar tissue to expose adductor pollicis.

Muscle Action on the Thumb

The comments on the synchronization of the activity of the extrinsic and intrinsic muscles of the index finger (p. 484) apply also to the thumb. The following are the facts.

(1) The abductor pollicis longus may be likened to an instant guy rope for it steadies the metacarpal bone of the thumb in whatever position the thumb adopts. "Without it the thumb is useless" (Bunnell, 1948).

(2) The action of the extensor pollicis longus is demonstrated by stretching the thumb away from the index finger in a dorsal direction (Fig. 80-1). The tendon of extensor pollicis longus is readily identified. Ventral to the tendon is a hollow termed the anatomic snuffbox, the other boundary of which is formed by the tendons of extensor pollicis brevis and abductor pollicis longus .

(3) The flexor pollicis longus flexes the interphalangeal joint.

(4) The adductor pollicis serves to pull the thumb toward the hand. Furthermore it is responsible for stabilizing the metacarpophalangeal joint of the thumb when the tips of the index finger and thumb are pressed together.

(5) The opponens pollicis rotates the thumb so that the pulp of the thumb faces the tips of the fingers.

The Anatomic Snuffbox

The tendons forming the boundaries of the snuffbox have already been identified. The radial artery crosses the snuffbox. Press the tip of your index finger lightly into the snuffbox and you will feel the artery pulsating. The floor of the snuffbox is mainly the lateral aspect of the scaphoid.

Opposition

To experience a feeling of utter helplessness, try holding scissors, scalpel, or forceps without using the thumb. As the instruments slip through the fingers one is convinced that the strength of the hand lies in the strength of the thumb. The movement that is basic to the thumb is opposition; demonstrate it by holding your hand out palm uppermost. If the hand is relaxed, the thumbnail faces laterally. Now, keeping the palm uppermost, bring the pulps of the fingers and thumb together. The thumb rotates. The thumbnail faces the ceiling. It is rotation of the thumb through 90° or more that is the chief characteristic of opposition.

Clinical experience with nerve injuries reveals that the opponens pollicis is the chief muscle of opposition. Experience also reveals, however, that in the pinch grip, in which the pulps of the thumb and index finger are pressed firmly together, all the muscles of the thumb, both intrinsic and extrinsic, contribute to stabilize the thumb. Thus clinicians, who are more concerned about the patient's grip and less concerned about simple anatomic movements, describe the adductor, flexor, and extensor components in opposition of the thumb as well as the rotation component. Clinicians recognize that weakness of any one of those components weakens opposition of the thumb.

With these facts in mind review the muscles and movements of the pinch grip.

Identify the muscles of the hypothenar eminence. Their control over abduction and opposition of the little finger needs no further discussion.

Chapter 91

Arteries and Nerves
Entering the Hand

Arteries

Radial and ulnar arteries alone convey blood to the hand. Within the hand arteries are numerous and their anastomoses abundant. Thus when a vessel is cut in a laceration of the hand, bleeding is profuse; usually both ends of a bleeding artery must be tied in order to stop the hemorrhage. It is because of the profuse blood supply that surgical procedures on the hand are done with a tourniquet on the arm. In this way small but significant structures, nerves for example, are not obscured from view by blood oozing from cut surfaces. Naturally, when the tourniquet is released at the end of the surgical procedure steps are taken to ensure that bleeding will not resume.

In view of the significance of hemorrhage in the hand it is curious how little detail concerning the arteries of the hand appears in surgical texts, in contrast to the extensive detail in standard anatomic texts. Therefore it is considered unnecessary, from the clinical point of view, for the undergraduate to do an elaborate dissection of the arteries of the hand.

ITEM 91-1. Location of Arteries

The ulnar artery has already been traced to some extent, and the superficial palmar arch has been demonstrated by reflecting the palmar aponeurosis. The superficial palmar arch is beautifully illustrated in *Grant's Atlas of Anatomy*, Figure 67. The other division of the ulnar artery is its deep branch, which proceeds into the depths of the palm. The deep branch joins the deep arch, but it is not easily traced to its junction with the deep arch, so proceed to trace the radial artery into the palm.

ITEM 91-2. Identify the radial artery at the wrist. Trace it across the anatomic snuffbox to where it disappears into the palm at the proximal end of the first interosseous space. With careful use of the closed-open scissors technique the artery can be mobilized in its course through the dorsal interosseous muscle and the adductor pollicis muscle until its connection with the deep palmar arch is established. Grant's Atlas of Anatomy, Figure 71 shows the radial artery emerging from the adductor pollicis and the size and length of the deep arch. It is from both the superficial palmar arch and the deep palmar arch that the vessels to the hand emanate.

Read an account of the arterial supply of a digit. The two volar (palmar) digital arteries convey most of the blood required by the digit, so they must be preserved by the surgeon if gangrene of the digit is to be avoided.

ITEM 91-3. If the arteries of your cadaver have been successfully injected with latex or a similar substance it should be easy to define the digital arteries of the index finger you have already dissected. Identify the proximal parts of the palmar digital arteries of the index finger.

The Nerves to the Muscles of the Hand

ITEM 91-4. The ulnar nerve should be reidentified where it enters the forearm deep to flexor carpi ulnaris, which it supplies. Trace the nerve distally. Take heed of its innervation of the ulnar half of the flexor digitorum profundus. This half gives rise to the deep tendons to the ring and little fingers. The two lumbricals arising from those particular tendons are also supplied by the ulnar nerve.

ITEM 91-5. Accompanied by the ulnar artery, the ulnar nerve remains superficial to the flexor retinaculum. Then, close to the hook of the hamate, the nerve divides into a superficial and deep branch. This division has already been found. If not, find it now. Then read an account of the cutaneous branches of the ulnar nerve.

ITEM 91-6. The motor branches of the deep branch of the ulnar nerve are to the three muscles of the hypothenar eminence, the medial (ulnar) two lumbricals, the interossei, and the adductor pollicis. The deep branch of the ulnar nerve is important, but spend little time looking for its branches except the branch to the adductor pollicis. The student is so often in error on the nerve supply of that muscle that it is worth tracing the deep branch of the ulnar nerve into the hand until it reaches the adductor pollicis. Very occasionally, however, the adductor pollicis is supplied by the median nerve. This may just be so in your specimen. Did you observe the close relationship of the deep branch of the ulnar nerve to the hook of the hamate?

ITEM 91-7. You have already seen how the median nerve enters the forearm deep to pronator teres and then travels distally on the undersurface of the flexor digitorum superficialis. Reidentify the nerve. In its course through the forearm it supplies the pronator teres, pronator quadratus, flexor carpi radialis, and palmaris longus when present. None of these muscles is actively concerned with the fingers. In addition the nerve supplies the flexor digitorum superficialis, flexor pollicis longus, and the lateral (radial) half of flexor digitorum profundus. They are concerned with the fingers.

ITEM 91-8. Trace the median nerve into the palm. Read an account of its cutaneous branches. Its motor supply in the hand is to the lateral (radial) two lumbricales and to the three muscles of the thenar eminence, namely, the opponens pollicis, flexor pollicis brevis, and abductor pollicis brevis. Occasionally, however, the opponens pollicis is supplied by the ulnar nerve.

ITEM 91-9.   Identify the radial nerve above the elbow. Read an account of its cutaneous distribution. Its motor distribution is to the brachioradialis, supinator, extensor carpi radialis longus and brevis, and extensor carpi ulnaris, none of which directly controls the digits. It also supplies the extensor digitorum and the satellite muscles to the little and index finger, as well as the abductor pollicis longus and extensor pollicis longus and brevis.

Exercise

With the aid of a textbook that deals with the applied anatomy of peripheral nerve lesions, establish the form of muscle imbalance that occurs when the median or the ulnar nerve is cut (1) at the elbow, (2) at the wrist, (3) when the radial nerve is cut above the elbow, and (4) when the posterior interosseous branch of the radial nerve is cut as it leaves the supinator.

At the same time, review the areas of sensory loss, but remember that the area of total anesthesia after a nerve lesion is much less than the area of skin actually innervated by the nerve.

Chapter 92

Joints of the Finger, Thumb, and Carpus

All joints of the upper limb are synovial joints. The typical features of a synovial joint are described on p. 270. It is recommended that the student begin the dissection of the joints of the upper limb with the joints of the hand, while the ligaments are still moist. If the student wishes to begin with the shoulder girdle he should make sure the hands are moist and well-wrapped.

The metacarpophalangeal and the interphalangeal joints of the fingers all have collateral ligaments that are significant (Fig. 92-1). Removal of the ligaments when they have become so thick and adherent that joint movement is limited is a recognized surgical procedure.

ITEM 92-1. Make a longitudinal incision into the long extensor tendon across the dorsum of the metacarpophalangeal joint of the index finger. Reflect each half of the tendon and the extensor expansion to expose the dorsal aspect of the metacarpophalangeal joint. Extending the incision throughout the length of the extensor tendon makes easier the reflection of the expansion. Examine the sides of the metacarpophalangeal joint. The obliquely-placed collateral ligaments are unmistakable. Demonstrate that each ligament is slack when the metacarpophalangeal joint is extended and taut when the joint is flexed. The interphalangeal joints have corresponding ligaments.

ITEM 92-2. The Carpometacarpal Joint of the Thumb

Identify the base of the metacarpal bone of the thumb. Make a longitudinal incision parallel to the tendon of the extensor pollicis longus from the base of the metacarpal bone proximally toward the radius. By blunt dissection, clear away the tissue released by the incision. Manipulate the thumb to show the position of the carpometacarpal joint. Then make a horizontal incision into the capsule to open the joint cavity. Open the joint wide, for it is important to see the shape of its bony surfaces. This particular articular surface of the trapezium is shaped like

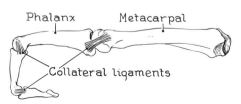

Figure 92-1. Significant collateral ligaments of the joints of the fingers.

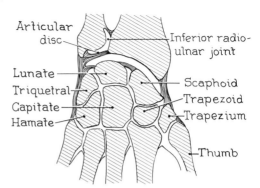

Articular
disc

Inferior radio-
ulnar joint

Lunate

Triquetral

Capitate

Hamate

Scaphoid

Trapezoid

Trapezium

Thumb

Figure 92-2. The radio-carpal joint and the carpal bones.

a saddle, and the base of the metacarpal bone is shaped to straddle the saddle. Examine the parts on a skeleton. Then demonstrate on your specimen the wide range of movement at this joint, which is such an essential part of opposition of the thumb.

It is appropriate now to study the lower (proximal) end of the meta-carpal bone of the thumb more closely and see how a force that drives the thumb in a longitudinal direction, toward the wrist, can split the lower end of the metacarpal bone. It is usually the anterior margin of the lower end of the metacarpal bone that is split off in this fashion. A metacarpal bone fractured in this way has been likened to a one legged rider astride a slippery saddle. The instability of the joint is obvious. Chronic instability of the joint is a distressing handicap.

ITEM 92-3. The Carpal Joints

The details of these joints need not be studied. The names and the general position of the various carpal bones should be studied with the aid of an atlas and a skeleton. However, several points of clinical significance should be brought out. First, the carpal joints, particularly those in the proximal row, are very mobile. Cineradiographs of the carpus during movements of the wrist demonstrate their mobility to perfection. Second, you are to be reminded that these are synovial joints and they are, therefore, subject to diseases of synovial joints. Moreover, roughening of the "tunnel" surface as a result of arthritis may affect the function of the long flexor tendons. Third, dislocations of carpal bones do occur. For example, the lunate may be dislocated anteriorly to impinge on the long flexor tendons and the median nerve. Fourth, numerous small arteries nourish the carpal bones. If a carpal bone is dislocated and these numerous small vessels are completely ruptured the bone may perish. Finally, the scaphoid bone is notable because it spans the midcarpal joint (Fig. 92-2); the waist of the scaphoid is in line with the midcarpal joint line and with the tip of the radial styloid also, when the hand is dorsiflexed and deviated to the radial side.

Chapter 93

The Wrist and Radioulnar Joints

It is more informative to call this joint the radiocarpal joint, for the lower end of the ulna is excluded from the articulation by the presence of a triangular disc (Fig. 92-2). Accordingly the proximal articular surface consists of the concave surface of the distal end of the radius and the adjoining articular disc. The distal articular surface consists of the convex proximal surface of the carpal bones, namely the scaphoid, the lunate, and the triquetrum. In the position of rest the scaphoid and lunate lie opposite specific areas of the radial articular surface, while the triquetrum adjoins the medial part of the capsule. When the hand is deviated sideways in the direction of the ulna, however, the scaphoid impinges on the lateral part of the capsule while the triquetrum meets the articular disc.

The radiocarpal joint, apparently, has a wide range of movement, for it is possible to flex the wrist so that the hand makes an angle of 90° with the forearm. In some individuals the same range of movement is possible in extension, but usually the range is considerably less. The movements, however, are not confined to the radiocarpal joint. There is considerable movement also at the midcarpal joints.

Ulnar deviation is much more extensive than radial deviation. Together the four basic movements at the wrist provide a range of circumduction almost as wide as that found in a ball and socket joint.

THE RELATIONSHIPS OF THE WRIST JOINT

Those who work in emergency departments of large or small hospitals will tell you how much of their time is devoted to the treatment of injuries of the hand and wrist. To demonstrate the challenge met in the treatment of one group of such injuries, make a mark about 2 cm. long anywhere across the front of your wrist. Now decide what nerves, arteries, and tendons you might find cut on inspecting a wound at the site of the mark. Furthermore the ends of longitudinal structures that are severed tend to retract, so they may not be immediately apparent in the wound. Sufficient, indeed, has been said to emphasize how important it is to know the relationships of all aspects of the wrist joint.

There are many structures at the wrist vital to the efficiency of the hand, but it is not difficult to learn their anatomy because all of the structures can be, and should be, identified on your own wrist. Many of the structures can be seen as well as felt. Even the median nerve can be seen when the wrist is slightly extended and the palmaris longus is absent.

The Close Relationship of Tendon to Bone

Examination of the lower end of the radius of your specimen reveals various smooth grooves, wide or narrow, in which the tendons to the hand glide. The close relationship of tendon and synovial sheath, which are relatively soft, to the underlying bone, which is hard, is of clinical importance. The tendon of the extensor pollicis longus (Fig. 80-1), for example, may wear thin with rubbing and eventually rupture; the resultant inability to extend the thumb carries the fascinating title, drummer's palsy. Furthermore, fracture of the lower end of the radius may create a rough edge that frays the tendon.

In considering how it is possible for such things to happen it must be emphasized that the tendons now being examined are embalmed and are therefore unlike their true state.

ITEM 93-1. Dissection of the Wrist

On one wrist only, identify and cut, one by one, the structures crossing the wrist until the capsule of the wrist joint is exposed.

Although anterior and posterior radiocarpal ligaments and medial and lateral ligaments are described in detail in some texts, the ligaments are merely thickenings of the capsule of the radiocarpal joint at points of maximal stress.

To demonstrate quickly the relationship of the articular disc to the joint, slice off, with an autopsy saw, the posterior third of the lower end of the ulna (Fig. 92-2). The saw will cut the triquetrum and the lunate, and perhaps more than that, but a beautiful and rapid exposure of a section of the disc is obtained.

Then cut around the capsule to open the joint cavity widely. Examine the articular surfaces and demonstrate the changing relationship of the proximal carpal bones to the disc and radius during radial and ulnar deviation.

THE INCLINATION OF THE RADIAL ARTICULAR SURFACE

On cursory examination, the articular surface of the lower end of the radius faces inferiorly when the bone is in the anatomic position. On closer inspection, however, it is seen that the surface faces slightly anteriorly as well as inferiorly. It is surprising how significant that forward inclination is in the smooth function of the radiocarpal joint, and it is imperative that it be restored after a fracture of the lower end of the radius. Furthermore, the articular surface of the radius faces slightly medially, i.e., in an ulnar direction, and that fact too must be borne in mind in reducing fractures of the lower end of the radius.

THE POSITION OF FUNCTION OF THE RADIOCARPAL JOINT

The fingers and thumb cannot grasp unless the wrist is extended (dorsiflexed is another term). No matter how tight the grasp, once the hand is forced into a position of flexion, the grasp loosens and the hand is powerless. The grip, particularly the power grip, gains strength on dorsiflexion of the wrist. The optimum position of the wrist and of the fingers in gripping is known as the position of function.

In all clinical procedures involving immobilization of the hand and wrist, the position of function is kept in mind, but just how much attention is paid to the position depends entirely on the aim of the clinician conducting the procedure.

THE JOINTS OF PRONATION AND SUPINATION

There are three joints involved in pronation and supination, two that are obvious and one that is not. The superior and inferior radioulnar joints are obvious, and they are typical synovial joints, whereas the junction of the two shafts by an interosseous membrane is not an obvious joint and is not synovial. Nevertheless, the relationship of the radial shaft to the ulnar shaft is of considerable functional significance and cannot be ignored in the restoration of function to this region. Any factor producing a limitation of movement in any one of the three radioulnar joints or in the radiohumeral joint affects the range of both pronation and supination.

Although it appears to be otherwise during the movements of pronation and supination, the ulna is virtually immobile while the radius is entirely responsible for the full range of movement. The full range of movement is determined with the elbow flexed to 90° and the shoulder fully adducted. Then, from the fully pronated position when the palm is turned down to the fully supinated position when the palm is turned up, the range of movement is nearly 180°. The axis of movement is an imaginary line drawn through the middle of the head of the radius superiorly and the center of the head of the ulna inferiorly. In the fully pronated position, the shaft of the radius crosses and lies adjacent to the ulna. In midposition, midway between pronation and supination, the radius and ulna are as far apart as possible. In full supination they lie closer together, but still are parallel. Proceed to examine the joints that make these movements possible.

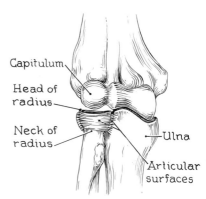

Figure 93-1.   The annular ligament fits around the head and neck of the radius to form the cuplike socket in which the head rotates.

ITEM 93-2.   In sawing through the head of the ulna to expose a cross section of the articular disc, no doubt the inferior radioulnar joint was opened. If not, cut the capsule on the anterior aspect of the joint and trim off sufficient capsule to reveal the articular surfaces. Observe the relationship of the rounded ulna head to the proximal surface of the articular disc. This disc may be perforated.

ITEM 93-3.   Opening the superior radioulnar joint involves the lateral ligament of the elbow joint. Remove the muscles attached by the common extensor tendon to the lateral epicondyle and to the lateral supracondylar ridge to expose the lateral ligament. By pronating and supinating the radius, establish the position of its head in relationship to the annular ligament that fits around the neck of the radius (Fig. 93-1). With an autopsy saw cut through the neck of the radius. Immediately superior to the margin of the head, make a horizontal incision into the lateral ligament of the elbow to open the radiohumeral joint. Remove the head of the radius. Then examine the socket from which it came. Identify the articular fossa on the lateral aspect of the ulna with which the head articulated.

THE RADIOHUMERAL JOINT

On inspection it would appear that the radiohumeral joint has built-in stability because of the shape of the head of the radius and the corresponding shape and the toughness of the annular ligament. It must be pointed out, however, that the degree of stability depends on the age group, for it is not until seven to ten years of age that the head of the radius is fully formed. Therefore, until that age it is possible for the head of the radius to slip through the annular ligament. Several names have been applied to this traumatic experience, such as nursemaid's elbow. In modern times the dislocation is known by some as supermarket elbow.

Chapter 94

The Elbow Joint

The elbow joint has two parts, namely, the humeroulnar articulation and the humeroradial articulation, which has already been examined.

The two articulations, contained in one capsule, share a common synovial cavity. The capsule is strengthened medially and laterally by the ulnar and radial collateral ligaments. There is little to be gained by cleaning those ligaments to demonstrate their fibers, which are well illustrated in anatomic texts. There is, however, much to be gained by studying the proximity of the brachial artery and the median ulnar and radial nerves to the elbow joint.

ITEM 94-1. Dissection of the Elbow Joint

To open the joint cavity wide, cut the capsule and overlying muscles. Begin laterally where the capsule and radial collateral ligament have already been cut. As you proceed, identify the major vessels and nerves to the hand. These structures are in peril in event of fractures and other injuries in this region.

ITEM 94-2. Inspect the articular surfaces of the elbow joint. The elbow is a hinge joint, but it is not like an ordinary hinge. The axis of the hinge is set at an angle to the long axis of the humerus. Accordingly, the relationship of the ulna to the humerus will vary during flexion or extension of the humeroulnar articulation.

Exercise

Stand with the upper limbs by the side palms facing forward. Observe whether or not the long axis of the humerus and the long axis of the ulna are in line. In most individuals they are not, and the angle they form is known as the carrying angle. When this angle is exaggerated, as may happen following healing of a fracture of the lower end of the humerus, the clinical term "cubitus valgus" (elbow bent outward) is applied.

What nerve crossing the elbow joint may be affected by severe cubitus valgus?

Chapter 95

The Shoulder Joint

The term shoulder refers to the rounded shape of the deltoid region; the term shoulder joint, therefore, is ambiguous because it may apply to the acromioclavicular or the scapulohumeral joint. Accordingly it is necessary to be precise and refer to each joint by its exact anatomic name. Furthermore, the acromioclavicular joint is part of the shoulder girdle, so one must distinguish between the scapulohumeral joint and the three joints of the shoulder girdle, the sternoclavicular joint, the acromioclavicular joint, and the joint involving the scapula and rib cage. To simplify description, the latter is sometimes referred to as the scapulothoracic joint. These four joints take part to a varying degree in movements of the upper limb. For ease of description, the coordinated action of these joints and their muscles is referred to as the arm-trunk mechanism. It is recommended that the student keep in mind the arm-trunk mechanism while he studies the various joints as a series of disjointed parts. Once the anatomy of the various joints has been seen, brief discussion of the arm-trunk mechanism can proceed.

ITEM 95-1. Dissection of the Sternoclavicular Joint

To examine this joint, move the clavicle and manubrium in opposite directions in order to establish the joint cavity. In life the range of movement of this joint is considerable; its importance becomes more vivid when one realizes that the joint is the only connection between the skeleton of the trunk and the skeleton of the upper limb.

The joint is surrounded by a capsule that may be cleaned and cut into to open the joint cavity, but one of the quickest and easiest ways to open the joint is to slice off the anterior aspect of the joint with an autopsy saw. Explore the cavities of the joint created by the intervening articular disc. Observe that superiorly the capsule of the joint is quite thin, but observe also that the articular disc is attached superiorly to the clavicle and inferiorly to the sternum. It may well be that the disc is the principle structure preventing dislocation superiorly of this joint.

Next clear away tissues from the inferior aspect of the joint to demonstrate (1) how the manubrial articular surface extends on to the first costal cartilage and (2) the costoclavicular ligament. Finally, it is important to recall the close proximity posteriorly of the major vessels of the neck and head.

499

Exercise

At some convenient time palpate the medial end of your clavicle while you put the upper limb through a wide range of movement. In life the sternoclavicular joint provides for a much greater range of circumduction of the clavicle than one can glean from an examination of a cadaver.

ITEM 95-2.   The Acromioclavicular Joint

In an embalmed cadaver this joint is always so firmly fixed that it is difficult to appreciate its mobility in life. Furthermore, it is not easy to establish quickly the position of the joint unless the following procedure is adopted. Move the clavicle and scapula in opposite directions to establish roughly the location of the acromioclavicualr joint. Then skim off the superior aspect of the joint with an autopsy saw.

Observe that an oval articular facet on the posterolateral and inferior aspect of the lateral end of the clavicle articulates with a corresponding facet on the medial aspect of the acromion. Probe into the joint cavity and establish the strength of the capsule. The strongest links, however, between clavicle and scapula extend between the superior aspect of the coracoid and the lateral part of the clavicle. To see the coracoclavicular ligaments clear away fatty areolar tissue between the coracoid and the clavicle. The coracoclavicular ligaments are so powerful that they are unmistakable, provided you proceed far enough posteriorly along the coracoid process.

Once some mobility has been created in the acromioclavicular articulation as a result of your dissection, test the various directions of movement. The acromion can glide anteriorly and posteriorly upon the clavicle as well as rotate.

ITEM 95-3.   The Scapulohumeral Joint

Although movement of the shoulder girdle contributes a great deal to the range of movement of the upper limb, most of the movement occurs in the scapulohumeral joint. It has been calculated that the contribution of the scapulohumeral joint is twice that of the joints of the shoulder girdle. Thus the scapulohumeral joint assumes considerable importance and the factors accounting for its great mobility should now be examined.

Identify the following muscles and their attachments to the humerus: the subscapularis, the supraspinatus, the infraspinatus, and the teres minor. Those muscles form the rotator cuff, which blends with the capsule of the scapulohumeral joint anteriorly, superiorly, and posteriorly. Slip an index finger in behind the subscapularis, press superiorly, and establish that the inferior part of the capsule of the scapulohumeral joint is devoid of immediate support inferiorly. The inferior capsule is slack and, in error, is described as redundant. The slack is taken up when the limb is raised above the head; presumably in that position the superior capsule is slack.

The Subscapularis

This muscle is of importance in the treatment of anteromedial dislocations of the scapulohumeral joint. As a result of the dislocation, the attachments of the muscle come to lie close together and the muscle fibers shorten accordingly. Retraction is the term commonly applied to muscle-shortening of this kind. The manipulation to reduce an anteromedial dislocation of the glenohumeral joint takes into account retraction of the subscapularis muscle.

ITEM 95-4. Examine the subscapularis and observe its extensive attachment to the anterior aspect of the scapula and how the muscle narrows to its humeral attachment.

ITEM 95-5. To open the scapulohumeral joint, cut the subscapularis and reflect it medially. A bursa deep to the tendon of the subscapularis communicates with the synovial cavity. Slit the capsule open and expose the head of the humerus and the glenoid cavity. Look for thinning or an actual deficiency of the anterior capsule, where the synovial cavity of the joint communicates with the subscapularis bursa. It is through this part of the capsule that the head of the humerus is pushed in anteromedial dislocation of the glenohumeral joint. The margin of the glenoid cavity is elevated by the labrum glenoidale, which is triangular on cross section. How much the labrum glenoidale contributes to the stability of the joint is debatable. Compare the area of the articular surface of the glenoid with that of the head of the humerus. That the glenoid faces anteriorly and superiorly as well as laterally may not be obvious at this late stage in the dissection; the orientation is of some consequence in the arm-trunk mechanism.

ITEM 95-6. To expose the tendon of the biceps, slit the ligament that holds the tendon into the bicipital groove. Demonstrate that the tendon passes deep to the joint capsule to reach the superior end of the glenoid cavity. By injecting latex into the synovial cavity it is possible to demonstrate that the tendon does not actually enter the synovial cavity but remains extrasynovial.

The Rotator Cuff

For reasons that are not clearly understood, the rotator cuff degenerates at or near its humeral attachment and, as a consequence, the cuff may either rupture or become the site of calcified deposits. The diagnosis and treatment of these clinical problems cannot be dealt with here, but you can consider carefully the anatomy of the cuff.

The tendinous fibers of the supraspinatus, infraspinatus, teres minor, and subscapularis all contribute to the cuff. In this manner they strengthen the capsule of the shoulder joint before they are attached to the humerus. Superiorly the rotator cuff is related to the subacromial bursa and at a slightly higher level to the coracoacromial arch. The distance between the greater tuberosity of the humerus and the arch is very small, so that the "free" space for the rotator cuff is negligible. Indeed the proximity of the tuberosity to the arch with a bursa interposed between them has led to the concept that they form a functional, but not truly anatomic, joint.

When the shoulder is abducted and the greater tuberosity moves toward and under the arch, sufficient space between them is maintained in two ways: First, the head of the humerus slides a few millimeters inferiorly, on the glenoid cavity; second, the humerus rotates externally. These two adjustments are controlled by the rotator cuff muscles. Once the rotator cuff has degenerated to a certain degree, the adjustments are imperfect. Limitation of abduction is one consequence.

In order to give the student a straightforward introduction to the anatomy of the cuff a very simple outline has been given. It is as well, therefore, to add that each time a clinician is called on to diagnose a lesion in the vicinity of the cuff he meets a fresh challenge, for there are numerous causes of limitation of movement and pain in the shoulder.

The Arm-Trunk Mechanism

The arm-trunk mechanism is a comprehensive term for the movements of the upper limb in relation to the trunk. The mechanism is subordinate to the needs of the hand, yet effective movement of the hand into an optimal position—in short, the reach—depends in large measure on the arm-trunk mechanism. When the arm-trunk mechanism is defective the reach is limited and the function of the hand is impaired.

The outstanding feature of the arm-trunk mechanism is the imperceptible adjustment of both the shoulder girdle and the scapulohumeral joint while the upper limb sweeps through a wide range of movement. It is not necessary to sweep the limb through a wide range of movement to test the efficiency of the arm-trunk mechanism of the ordinary person. Certainly such a thorough test would be necessary for a boxer, for example, whose success depends on a perfect physique. But for the ordinary person, placing the hand on top of the head or on the back of the neck and then putting the hand in the hip pocket is an adequate simple test.

The test just described combines abduction and rotation of the humerus (the scapulohumeral joint), rotation of the scapula (the scapulothoracic and acromioclavicular joints), and elevation and rotation of the lateral end of the clavicle (the sternoclavicular joint). Some textbooks give measurements of the range of movement at each joint, but to give precise measurements is misleading for two reasons: first, the range varies from person to person; second, loss of mobility in one of the joints concerned with the arm-trunk mechanism can be compensated for, often to a considerable degree, by increased mobility in the other joints. However, it serves a useful purpose to bear in mind that two-thirds of the movement apparent when the limb is raised above the head occurs at the scapulohumeral joint.

In raising the limb above the head there are two movements, external rotation and abduction, occurring in the scapulohumeral joint. Of those two movements, external rotation is more basic to the mobility of the joint. Clinically, in the treatment of patients with stiff scapulohumeral joints, external rotation must be restored before any actual increase in abduction can occur. If external rotation cannot be fully restored, perhaps because of a surgical procedure, actual abduction in the scapulohumeral joint remains limited.

The muscles responsible for external rotation are the rotator cuff muscles. They also control gliding of the humeral head on the glenoid fossa. The muscle responsible for abduction is the deltoid. The supraspinatus, too, is classed as an abductor of the scapulohumeral joint. However, the respective parts played by the deltoid and the supraspinatus are not as clear-cut as is sometimes stated. A clear summary of evidence concerning their respective parts is given by Gardner, Gray, and O'Rahilly (1963) with the conclusion that the muscles should be investigated further.

The basic movements of the scapula are four in number, forward movement (also called protraction) backward movement (also called retraction), and upward and downward rotation. Rotation changes the direction in which the glenoid faces. In upward rotation the glenoid fossa faces superolaterally; in downward rotation inferolaterally. In all four movements the scapula slides on the chest wall. The basic movements of the lateral end of the clavicle are elevation, depression, protraction, retraction, and rotation; all these basic movements combine in circumduction of the clavicle when the upper limb is swung in a wide circle. It is apparent that movements of the clavicle cannot be divorced from movements of the scapula.

All the muscles attached to the scapula and clavicle play some part in powerful movements of the upper limb against resistance. In simple daily activities however, the trapezius and serratus anterior are the muscles with most control. Figure 95-1 illustrates how the segments of the trapezius swivel the scapula. Much of the serratus anterior is at-

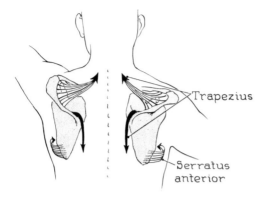

Figure 95-1. Rotation of the scapula is controlled in large measure by the trapezius and serratus anterior.

tached to the inferior angle of the scapula; those muscle fibers, too, play a large part in swiveling the scapula so that the glenoid fossa looks superiorly and laterally. Paralysis of either the trapezius or serratus anterior limits the apparent range of abduction of the upper limb. Under those circumstances, the imperceptible adjustment of both the shoulder girdle and the scapulohumeral joint during movement of the upper limb comes to light.

Winged Scapula

The concentration of muscle fibers of the serratus anterior upon the inferior angle of the scapula (Fig. 95-1), seemingly keeping the angle against the chest wall, is probably why the inferior angle becomes extraordinarily prominent when the serratus anterior is paralyzed. A prominent scapula is referred to as a "winged scapula." Winging of the scapula is commonly associated with paralysis of the nerve to the serratus anterior, but bilateral winged scapula does occur as a physical abnormality unconnected with any form of paralysis.

REFERENCES

Basmajian, J. V., and Latif, A.: Integrated actions and functions of the chief flexors of the elbow. Journal of Bone and Joint Surgery, *39A*:1106, 1957.
Bunnell, S.: Surgery of the Hand. Philadelphia, J. B. Lippincott Co., 1948.
Gardner, E., Gray, D. J., and O'Rahilly, R.: Anatomy. Philadelphia, W. B. Saunders Co., 1963.
Hall, M. C.: Luschka's Joint. Springfield, Ill., Charles C Thomas, 1965.
Jones, F. W.: The Principles of Anatomy as Seen in the Hand. London, Bailliere, Tindall & Cox, 1944.
Mitchell, G. A. G.: The Essentials of Neuroanatomy. Edinburgh, E. & S. Livingstone Ltd., 1966.
Turek, S. L.: Orthopaedics. Philadelphia, J. B. Lippincott Co., 1959.

PART 8

ANATOMY AND
CLINICAL DIAGNOSIS

Function, not structure, is the manifestation of life. Surely no anatomist was more aware of this than John Hunter, an eighteenth century surgeon and anatomist who gained lasting renown because of his remarkable capacity for investigation. His interests were wide. His experiments, including those on tissue transplantation and hypothermia, were crude by present day standards, but from them he developed a profound appreciation of function, as his writings reveal:

> Mere composition of matter does not give life because the dead body has all the composition it ever had.

That death reduces all to a common denominator, structure, is very obvious in a dissecting laboratory, where one cadaver bears a striking resemblance to another but no two students look alike. Patients, too, are different. True, sleeping, eating, and so on are functions common to all, yet each patient is just that little bit different in the performance of these functions. Individual differences in function are recognized by the diagnostician. Examining his patient he soon faces the decision, "is this variation in function normal or abnormal."

The normal function of the human body is hard to understand because it lacks concrete form. Accordingly, for scientific purposes, function is reduced to certain specific phenomena easily recognized, readily measured, and attributed, often too rigidly, to definite structures. Once function is reduced in this way, very artificial boundaries are created and the ubiquitous nature of function can easily be overlooked. The worst that can happen is that function will be overlooked entirely while the attention centers upon structure alone. This can happen both in the basic science laboratories and in the hospital. Therefore, the student looking at the electron micrograph of a cell, the photomicrograph of an organ, or the obvious features of an anatomic dissection, must recognize that he is looking at structure devoid of function, and, what is more, during only a moment of time.

In the previous paragraph the student was warned not to overlook the ubiquitous nature of function. A similar warning is necessary now in the introduction to three classes of patient's complaints. The lines of division between these classes are muted and indistinct. Nevertheless classification of subject matter is a useful point of departure for the beginner. Thus it may be said that patients' complaints fall broadly into two main groups, namely disorders of function and disorders of structure. An example of the first group is as follows: "Doctor, I get breathless very easily these days." An example of the second group is thus: "Doctor, there is a lump here and it is getting bigger." There is, however, a large intermediate group, in which a disorder of function is the manifestation of a disorder of structure. For example, one cause of breathlessness is narrowing of the bronchi, as in asthma.

As the student's experience of this intermediate group grows he will learn that he must establish the true nature of the disorder of function before he establishes the presence or absence of a disorder of structure. A disorder of function is usually established by means of a careful medical history, but it is also true that a disorder of function is frequently observed during the medical interview or in the course of the physical examination; rapid breathing and rapid pulse are common examples, and there are many others. A disorder of structure, on the other hand, is established by means of a complete physical examination. In this chapter the medical history is not referred to again because it is a subject in its own right. The student, nevertheless, will remember the priority of the medical history in the practice of medicine.

Tissues and Systems

An abnormality found on physical examination is commonly termed a physical sign. In his first few weeks as a clinical student, even the best student has difficulty in applying his anatomic knowledge when he is confronted for the first time with a physical sign that is unfamiliar. On enquiry it is found that the difficulty stems not from his lack of anatomic knowledge so much as from his ignorance of the gross pathologic changes that can occur in the tissues of the body. The beginner is not aware how much disease can alter the size, shape and substance of an organ or a structure. To understand these changes a knowledge of pathology is essential.

Having established that disease can produce profound changes in structure, we can now consider two simple methods of applying anatomy in the evaluation of physical signs. The student has a choice of action. He may recall the tissues of the body, skin, fat, muscle, bone, nerve, vessel, and so forth; thus he may succeed in linking the abnormality with a tissue. If he is unsuccessful, his second choice is to review the systems of the body, including the hemopoetic system and the endocrine and lymphatic systems, and in this way he may establish the system in which the abnormality is located. These two simple approaches, arbitrarily termed the tissue and the system approach, are extremely useful to the beginner, who will be quick to observe that there is a minimum of anatomic detail required in their application. The beginner will recognize also that the two approaches take time. However, as his clinical experience grows, he will soon be able to recognize quickly any one of the common range of physical signs.

Negative and Positive Observations

For success in a physical examination, the ability to observe is an essential prerequisite. Frederick Wood-Jones (1879-1954), one of the greats in anatomy, wrote ". . . the man who seeks success in medicine does so in vain if he remains unobservant." It has been said that the powers of observation increase rapidly up to the age of seven years and then decrease steadily. The student can judge for himself how acute are his own powers of observation. Accordingly, he should extend his powers of observation, and, in doing so, he must recognize that successful observation is more than a hasty look. It is a deliberate study, the eyes methodically scanning the field.

> Horatio: Before my God, I might not this believe,
> Without the sensible and true avouch
> Of mine own eyes . . .
>
> Hamlet.

So much stress is laid upon the positive identification of structures in gross anatomy that it is necessary to point out that negative observations are equally important, if not more, in the practice of medicine and in other walks of life. At sea, for instance, it is of supreme importance to record that during a watch, no land, no ship, and no iceberg was seen on the radar screen. Then if an iceberg does appear during the next watch the captain will know precisely when and where. In medicine this is equally true. The lower limb, for instance, is normal because certain pathologic features are not present. The record may state "no skin blemishes, no muscle wasting, no joint displacement, and no bone deformity." Such observations, dated on a medical record, are especially valuable when, sometime later, all four abnormal features are present.

Systemic Anatomy

In the process of dissection the student moves from region to region, and he may easily complete his dissection with an understanding of regional anatomy, yet without any appreciation of systemic anatomy. In each region each structure belongs to a body system and is in fact just a small part of that system. A concept of the systems of the body is fundamental in the practice of medicine, for disease apparent in a structure in one region of the body may be a local manifestation of similar disease in other regions of the body. For example, if the student finds that the arteries of the upper limb are diseased, he may discover that the arteries to the head, heart, gut, and lower limbs are also diseased. Systemic disease can occur in other systems of the body too. Accordingly, in the physical examination of a region the separate part must be set into an image of the total system to which it belongs.

The Lymphatic System

For a particular reason this system warrants special mention. The clinical student is asked time and again, "what is the lymphatic drainage of this organ, tissue or region?" It is unfortunate, therefore, that the lymphatic system, playing such a fundamental part in diseases of the body, cannot be adequately studied in the cadaver because it is largely unseen except for one or two congregations of lymph nodes, the occasional vessel, and possibly certain trunks or ducts if they were distended with lymph at death. The lymphatic system can only be studied either experimentally on live animals or in the course of a clinical radiologic investigation, when radiopaque fluid injected into the system is conspicuous on a radiograph. At present, therefore, much of our knowledge of the anatomy of the normal lymphatic system is based on pathologic and clinical experience.

In clinical practice, when a group of lymph nodes is found to be enlarged then the doctor must examine all the organs and regions from which lymph drains to this particular group of nodes. On the other hand, when an organ is found to be diseased the doctor must examine one or more groups of lymph nodes, each of which receives some lymph from the organ. In the first instance the investigation moves from one group of lymph nodes to several organs. In the second instance the investigation moves from one organ to several groups of nodes. In keeping with these procedures, the student will find listed in major anatomy texts not only the lymphatic field of individual groups of nodes, but also the lymph drainage of each organ, structure or region.

To test your understanding of these different approaches to the lymphatic system here are two examples. First, on examination of a patient the right axillary lymph nodes are found to be abnormally large. Second, on the examination of a woman's right breast there is found a cancer known to spread through the lymphatic system. Using the principles outlined above, how would you continue the physical examination of these two patients?

Total Body Concept

In a previous paragraph the need for a concept of body systems was stressed. A further and related need is a concept, a vision if you like, of the total body, because medical care is concerned with the total body, including the mind. The need for this concept is urgent in the care of a victim of a violent highway accident; he is unconscious, and has suffered fractured bones in his limbs, fractured ribs and a punctured lung, bruising of the abdominal wall, a damaged kidney, a ruptured spleen, and a split of the wall of the duodenum. His whole body requires immediate care and the nervous, locomotor, respiratory and cardiovascular, alimentary, urinary, and hemopoietic systems demand simultaneous attention while the effect of the accident upon his endocrine system cannot be ignored. In addition the possibility of a psychologic effect from the trauma must be anticipated. The patient's life and future well-being depend without question upon a total body concept.

> Only those who know man both in his parts and in his entirety, simultaneously under his anatomical, physiological and mental aspects, are capable of understanding him when he is sick.
>
> Alexis Carrel.

All the Ages of Man

The practice of medicine is concerned with all age groups and both sexes, although ultimately a doctor can specialize in the health of a specific sex or age group. Such specialization, however, comes later. Presently the undergraduate clinical student is concerned with all age groups, and he must learn how the anatomy of the unborn, newborn, infant, child, adolescent, and adult differs from the anatomy of old age, to which he is over-exposed in the dissecting laboratory. The student is advised, therefore, to read, and reread, an excellent chapter, "Anatomical Changes through the Ages" in *Anatomy of the Human Body* (Lockhart, Hamilton, and Fyfe, 1959), a lively and easily-assimilated account of the changes occurring in Man as his years advance.

CONCLUSION

Sir William Osler, writing in 1903 on the need of radical reform in the method of teaching senior students, said this:

> We expect too much of the student and we try to teach him too much. Give him good methods and a proper point of view, and all other things will be added, as his experience grows.

Greatly influenced by those words in the writing of this book, I have presented to the student methods I judge to be good and a point of view I believe to be sound. I know that all else will be added as his experience grows.

Index

Note: Numbers in *italics* indicate pages on which illustrations appear; t after number indicates table on page.